Healthy Aging in Asia

HEALTHY AGING IN ASIA

Edited by Karen Eggleston

Stanford | Walter H. Shorenstein Asia-Pacific Research Center
Freeman Spogli Institute

THE WALTER H. SHORENSTEIN ASIA-PACIFIC RESEARCH CENTER
(Shorenstein APARC) addresses critical issues affecting the countries of Asia, their regional and global affairs, and U.S.-Asia relations. As Stanford University's hub for the interdisciplinary study of contemporary Asia, we produce policy-relevant research, provide education and training to students, scholars, and practitioners, and strengthen dialogue and cooperation between counterparts in the Asia-Pacific and the United States.

The Walter H. Shorenstein Asia-Pacific Research Center
Freeman Spogli Institute for International Studies
Stanford University
Encina Hall
Stanford, CA 94305-6055
http://aparc.fsi.stanford.edu

Healthy Aging in Asia
may be ordered from:
Brookings Institution Press
https://www.brookings.edu/bipress/
books@brookings.edu

Walter H. Shorenstein Asia-Pacific Research Center, 2020.
Copyright © 2020 by the Board of Trustees of the Leland Stanford Junior University.

Library of Congress Control Number: 2020934262

First printing, 2020

ISBN 978-1-931368-54-4

Contents

Tables and Figures

Tables

Abbreviations

ACSC	ambulatory care-sensitive condition
AMED	Agency for Medical Research and Development
AMI	acute myocardial infarction
AOD	age-of-death
ASIRC	age-standardized incidence rate
BKPAI	Building Knowledge Base on Population Ageing in India
CCSV	Community Care Service Voucher
CDC	center for disease control
CDM	chronic disease management
CDR	cancer detection rate
CGAT	Community Geriatric Assessment Teams
CHARLS	China Health and Retirement Longitudinal Study
CHC	community health center
CHCC	Community Health Call Centre (Hong Kong)
CI	confidence interval
CIR	cancer incidence rate
COPD	chronic obstructive pulmonary disease
CSIRO	Commonwealth Scientific and Industrial Research Organization
CSSA	Comprehensive Social Security Assistance (Hong Kong)
CVD	cardiovascular disease
DALYS	disability-adjusted life-years

DM	diabetes mellitus
DRAH	diabetes-related avoidable hospitalization
EHCV	Elderly Health Care Voucher (Hong Kong)
EHI	Employees' Health Insurance (Japan)
GDHP	Global Digital Health Partnership
GP	general practitioner
HAQ	Healthcare Access and Quality (Index)
HBV	hepatitis B virus
HCV	hepatitis C virus
HIRA	Health Insurance Review & Assessment Service (Korea)
HMD	Human Mortality Database
HPV	human papilloma virus
HRS	Health and Retirement Study
HTA	Health Technology Assessment
JDS	Japan Diabetes Society
JMA	Japan Medical Association
JMPT	joint management by three professionals
KAM	Korean Academy of Medical Sciences
KCDC	Korea Centers for Disease Control and Prevention
KDA	Korea Diabetes Association
KDB	Kokuho Database
KNHANES	Korea National Health and Nutrition Examination Survey
KPI	key performance indicator
LDP	Liberal Democratic Party (Japan)
LMIC	low- and middle-income country
LYG	life-years gained
MCI	mild cognitive impairment
METI	Ministry of Economy, Trade and Industry (Japan)
MEXT	Ministry of Education, Culture, Sports, Science, and Technology (Japan)
MHLW	Ministry of Health, Labour and Welfare (Japan)
NATCM	National Administration of Traditional Chinese Medicine (China)
NCD	noncommunicable (chronic) disease

NCMS	New Rural Cooperative Medical System (China)
NCSP	National Cancer Screening Program (Korea)
NDB	National Insurance Claim and Health Checkup Database (Japan)
NGO	non-governmental organization
NHC	National Health Commission (China)
NHI	National Health Insurance (Taiwan and Japan)
NHIS	National Health Insurance Services (Korea)
NHS	National Health Service
NICE	National Institute for Health and Care Excellence
OECD	Organisation for Economic Cooperation and Development
OOP-PD	out-of-pocket expenditure for prescription drugs
OWPH	One-way Permit Holders
P4P	pay-for-performance
PC-CDM	Primary Care-Chronic Disease Management
PEP	Patient Empowerment Programme (Hong Kong)
PMDA	Pharmaceutical and Medical Device Agency (Japan)
PPM	personalized and precision medicine
PPP	public-private partnerships
QALY	quality-adjusted life-years
RAMP	Risk Factor Assessment and Management Programme (Hong Kong)
RCHE	residential care home for the elderly
RCSV	Residential Care Service Voucher (Hong Kong)
SD	standard deviation
SES	socioeconomic status
SHC	specific health checkup
SHG	specific health guidance
SHCSHG	specific health checkups and specific health guidance
UEBMI	Urban Employee Basic Medical Insurance (China)
URBMI	Urban Resident Basic Medical Insurance (China)
WHO	World Health Organization

Contributors

Chapter 1

KAREN EGGLESTON is a senior fellow at the Freeman Spogli Institute for International Studies (FSI) at Stanford University, director of the Stanford Asia Health Policy Program, and deputy director of the Shorenstein Asia-Pacific Research Center at FSI. She is also an affiliate of the National Bureau of Economic Research. Eggleston earned her PhD in public policy from Harvard University, after completing MA degrees in economics and Asian studies from the University of Hawaii and a BA in Asian studies summa cum laude (valedictorian) from Dartmouth College. She studied in China for two years and was a Fulbright scholar in Korea. Her research focuses on government and market roles in the health sector; Asia health policy; healthcare productivity; and the economics of the demographic transition. She served as an adviser to the Asia Pacific Observatory on Health Systems and Policies and as a consultant to the World Bank, Asian Development Bank, and WHO regarding health system reforms in the PRC.

Chapter 2

VICTOR FUCHS is the Henry J. Kaiser, Jr., Professor of Economics and of Health Research and Policy, emeritus at Stanford University. He received a BS in business administration from New York University, and an MA and PhD in economics from Columbia University. Fuchs is a member of the Institute of Medicine and was president (1995) and distinguished fellow (1990) of the American Economic Association. He received the Distinguished Investigator Award (1988) and the Distinguished Fellow Award (1996) from the Association for Health Services Research, and was awarded the Baxter Foundation's Health Services Research Prize (1991). Fuchs uses economic theory to provide a framework for the collection and analysis of healthcare data. He has been particularly interested in the role of physician behavior and financial incentives in determining healthcare expenditures, as well as the role of attitudes and beliefs in public support for national health insurance.

DAEJUNG KIM is a research fellow at the Korea Institute for Health and Social Affairs. He received a PhD in economics from Toulouse School of Economics, Toulouse University. Kim is an executive fellow at the Korean Association of Health Economics and Policy. He is interested in health industry regulation and health expenditure.

ZHI PING TEO graduated from Stanford University in 2019 with a master's degree in East Asian studies and a bachelor's degree in political science. She is passionate about the intersections between public policy and addressing societal challenges such as health inequities. Her thesis studied China's Belt and Road Initiative, particularly the political and economic logic of partner countries' decision-making processes. Her interests include international relations and institutions, and she has worked at the United Nations Mechanism for International Criminal Tribunals and with UN Women/ASEAN. She works at the Ministry of Defense in Singapore.

Chapter 3

CHIYO HASHIMOTO is a research assistant at APARC at Stanford University, working on a wide variety of topics related to healthcare policy in Japan. She has worked as a health economics researcher at a private institute in Japan. She received a BA in Occidental history from the University of Tokyo, and a master of public policy from Hitotsubashi University, focusing on health economics. She published a paper based on her master's thesis, "Installation and Utilization of MRI scanners in Japan" (in Japanese), and co-authored a working paper, "The Welfare Consequences of Free Entry in Vertical Relationships: The Case of the MRI Market."

Chapter 4

MINORI ITO earned an MA from Stanford University in international policy and economics. Her current research focuses on the economics of technology and econometric methods for analyzing technology's impact on industrial structure and efficiency. Her capstone project was on the global economic impacts of artificial intelligence and value chain analysis, and another project focused on the impacts of technology and robots on healthcare in Japan. Prior to Stanford, she worked at the Ministry of Foreign Affairs of Japan, focusing on multilateral negotiations. She received the bachelor of laws from Keio University, while also studying abroad at Georgetown University.

Chapter 5

HOKUTO ASANO is an official of the Government of Japan. Since joining the government, he has worked for the Railway Division, Real Estate Division, and Cabinet Secretariat. Currently, he is a deputy director in charge of the G20 Tourism Ministerial Meeting. He is interested in the financial sustainability of Japan's healthcare system. He has written a paper on "Equivalence Scales, the Cost of Children, and the Cost of Living in Japan's Public Assistance System." He received bachelor's and master's degrees in economics from the University of Tokyo, and the master of arts in international policy studies from Stanford University.

Chapter 6

HONGSOO KIM is a professor at the Graduate School of Public Health at Seoul National University (SNU), South Korea. Her research areas include aging and health policy, long-term care systems, and health system performance assessment. She was formerly the scientific committee chair of the Korean Academy of Long-term Care, the Korean Gerontological Society, and the Korean Society of Health Policy and Administration, as well as a 2016–17 Fulbright Visiting Scholar and Takemi Fellow in International Health at the Harvard School of Public Health. She received her PhD from New York University, where she worked as assistant professor before she joined SNU.

Chapter 7

JANET TIN KEI LAM is a doctor in training; she expects to receive her medical degree and master of public health (specializing in health economics, policy and management) from the University of Hong Kong in 2020. She previously worked as a research assistant at the School of Public Health, University of Hong Kong; has received a presentation prize at the WONCA conference; and has published in the *European Journal of Health Economics*.

SABRINA CHING TUNG WONG is a doctor in training; she expects to receive her medical degree from the University of Hong Kong in 2020. She previously worked as a research assistant at the School of Public Health, University of Hong Kong, and has been a reviewer for the *International Journal of Rheumatic Diseases*. She is especially interested in health inequity and the chronic care model.

JIANCHAO QUAN joined the School of Public Health in 2013, and was appointed clinical assistant professor in 2017 at the University of Hong Kong. He graduated with a degree in medicine from the University of Oxford. After his clinical training in London, he specialized in public health and subsequently obtained an MPH with Distinction. He received his BA and MA in medical sciences (infection and immunity) from the University of Oxford, and his postgraduate degree in economics from the University of Hong Kong. His research interest lies in the economic analysis of healthcare services and health policy.

Chapter 8

JIANQUN DONG is a professor at the National Center for Chronic and Non-communicable Disease Control and Prevention, Chinese Center for Disease Control and Prevention. Dr. Dong graduated from Peking Union Medical College/Chinese Academy of Medical Sciences with a doctoral degree in epidemiology and biostatistics. He graduated from Heidelberg University in the 1990s with a master of science. Dr. Dong has dedicated himself to noncommunicable disease epidemiology, community health, and health promotion for many years. He has had a number of enriching experiences in international academic exchanges and cooperation.

FAN MAO is an MS and MD candidate and assistant researcher working in the Department of Chronic Disease Prevention and Evaluation, National Center for Chronic and Noncommunicable Disease Control and Prevention, Chinese Center for Disease Control and Prevention. He is devoted to chronic disease prevention and health promotion, as well as the evaluation and scaling up of public health programs.

WENLAN DONG is a chief physician at the National Center for Chronic and Noncommunicable Disease Control and Prevention, Chinese Center for Disease Control and Prevention. Dr. Dong has for years been greatly involved in noncommunicable disease risk factor control, health promotion, disease burden, and health resource studies, and she has published many scientific papers and monographs.

YINGYING JIANG is an associate researcher at the Department of Comprehensive Prevention and Evaluation, National Center for Chronic and Noncommunicable Disease Control and Prevention, Chinese Center for Disease Control and Prevention. She has an MS in public health and has long been engaged in the field of chronic disease prevention and control, community-based intervention, and health promotion.

SHIWEI LIU is a professor of epidemiology and director of the Division of Comprehensive Intervention of Noncommunicable Disease and Evaluation, National Center for Chronic and Noncommunicable Disease Control and Prevention, Chinese Center for Disease Control and Prevention. He received his PhD in epidemiology and biostatistics from Peking Union Medical College in 2009. His current work and research interests focus on the epidemiology of noncommunicable diseases (NCDs), comprehensive strategies of NCD control and prevention, NCD intervention using mobile health technology, the evaluation of public health policy or intervention, and burden of disease study.

MAIGENG ZHOU is an MD, professor/senior researcher, and deputy director of the National Center for Chronic and Noncommunicable Disease Control and Prevention, Chinese Center for Disease Control and Prevention. Dr. Zhou is a core member on the expert panel for the Global Burden of Disease. He has presided over numerous research studies, such as a study of environment pollution and health in the Huai River, the effects on health of climate change, the relationship between air pollution and health, a study of the sub-national burden of disease in China, and has published many papers in journals including *Lancet*, the *New England Journal of Medicine*, *JAMA*, and *BMJ*.

Chapter 9

MIN YU is deputy director of the Zhejiang Provincial Center for Disease Control and Prevention. He was awarded as one of the New-Century 151 Talents of Zhejiang Province, China. He is a committee member of the epidemiology branch of the Chinese Preventive Medicine Association. He is a leader in the key discipline of noncommunicable diseases (NCD) epidemiology and led the establishment of the NCDs and behavioral risk factor surveillance system in Zhejiang Province. Yu earned his medical degree at Zhejiang University and the master of public health at Peking Medical University. Currently, his research focuses on the epidemiology of NCDs, strategy for NCD control and prevention, and disease burden.

YIWEI CHEN earned his PhD in economics from Stanford University. His research focuses on identifying and addressing important policy questions in healthcare systems across the United States and China. His work has won the "Rising Star" prize in health economics, which is awarded to the top health economics papers from the 2018–19 academic job market by the

Becker Friedman Institute at the University of Chicago. Prior to his doctoral study, he obtained his bachelor's degree in economics from the University of Chicago and was a management consultant at TGG Group, LLC.

HUI DING is a PhD candidate in economics at Stanford University. She received the bachelor's degree in economics and psychology from Peking University. Her current work mainly focuses on health economics in both the United States and China. In particular, she is interested in the supply side of the healthcare market, as well as in the role of insurance in containing costs, promoting new technology, adjusting patients' and providers' behavior, and affecting health outcomes.

JIEMING ZHONG graduated from the school of public health of Zhejiang University and received the master of public health from the Chinese Center for Disease Control and Prevention. He is the director of the Department of Noncommunicable Disease Control and Prevention in the Zhejiang Center for Disease Control (CDC). He served as deputy director of the Department of Tuberculosis Control and Prevention in the Zhejiang CDC during 2008–14. Zhong is a member of the Zhejiang Preventive Medicine Association and has engaged in and chaired several international cooperation and local research projects. He has conducted in-depth research on the control and prevention of NCDs and tuberculosis.

RUYING HU graduated with a BA from Tongji Medical College of Huazhong University of Science and Technology. She is the deputy director of the Department of Noncommunicable Disease (NCD) Control and Prevention in the Zhejiang Center for Disease Control and has been leading the work on NCD surveillance in Zhejiang Province. She is a member of the Disability Prevention and Control Committee of the Chinese Preventive Medicine Association and has led several national and local research projects. She has conducted in-depth research on disease burden and diabetes control and prevention.

CHUNMEI WANG graduated with a BA from Wenzhou Medical University. She is the deputy director of Tongxiang County Center for Disease Control and Prevention and the deputy section chief of Tongxiang Health Bureau. She is a deputy chief technician and skilled in noncommunicable disease control and prevention.

KAIXU XIE graduated with a BA from Wenzhou Medical University. He is a researcher at the Noncommunicable Disease Control and Prevention Department in Tongxiang County Center for Disease Control and Prevention. He is a deputy chief physician of public health and skilled in noncommunicable disease control and prevention.

XIANGYU CHEN is a public health physician and working staff member at the Noncommunicable Disease Control and Prevention Department in the Zhejiang Provincial Center for Disease Control and Prevention. Chen's ongoing areas of research include the development of risk prediction models using health check-up data, and the cost-effectiveness evaluation for flu shots among individuals with diabetes. He completed his MS in epidemiology and BA in preventive medicine at Soochow University.

PEDRO GALLARDO recently graduated from Stanford University with a BA in East Asian studies, with a concentration of coursework focused on the Chinese healthcare system. Gallardo is interested in the interplay of culture, language, and health, especially as it relates to noncommunicable chronic diseases. He has explored this interest through work in Chinese public health initiatives, serving as a Spanish interpreter through multiple channels, and managing a free health clinic. He hopes to continue his work in health advocacy through a career in medicine.

Chapter 10

RIZE JING is currently a PhD candidate in the School of Public Health at Peking University. He received the master of public health degree from Peking University in 2018. Mr. Jing's research areas include health economics, health policy, and health system research, and focus on analyses of primary health care, hospital efficiency, health insurance, and health economics evaluation in China. His PhD thesis studies family physician behaviors and impacts on clinical outcomes in China. He has published more than 10 peer-reviewed Chinese and English research articles.

HAI FANG is a professor of health economics at Peking University. He received the master of public health and the PhD in economics from the State University of New York at Stony Brook in 2006. Prior to teaching at Peking University, he taught at the University of California, Davis; the University of Miami; and the University of Colorado, Denver. Dr. Fang's research areas include health economics, vaccine economics, and health policy. He has published 80 peer-reviewed articles in English and has been the principle investigator for 20 research grants from the National Natural Science Foundation of China, Gates Foundation, and British Medical Research Council, among others.

Chapter 11

JASON LI is a medical student at Harvard Medical School interested in population health and health equity. He holds a BS in human biology with honors from Stanford and was a U.S. Fulbright Fellow at Shaanxi Normal University in China, where he conducted research on healthcare quality, access, and reform in rural China. During his time at Stanford, Li worked on public health projects at Peking University, Xinan University, and at the White House Initiative on Asian Americans and Pacific Islanders.

Chapter 12

JOHN D. DONAHUE is the Raymond Vernon Senior Lecturer in Public Policy, Kennedy School, Harvard University. He is also faculty chair of the Master in Public Policy (MPP) Program and the SLATE Curriculum Initiative Co-Chair for Cases and Curriculum. His teaching, writing, and research mostly deal with public sector reform and with the distribution of public responsibilities across levels of government and sectors of the economy, including extensive work with the HKS-HBS joint degree program. Donahue has consulted for business and governmental organizations, including the National Economic Council, the World Bank, and the RAND Corporation, and serves as a trustee or advisor to several nonprofits. A native of Indiana, he holds a BA from Indiana University and an MPP and PhD from Harvard.

YIJIA JING is a professor in public administration and associate director of foreign affairs at Fudan University. He is the editor-in-chief of *Fudan Public Administration Review*, and serves as the vice president of the International Research Society for Public Management. He is associate editor of *Public Administration Review* and co-editor of the *International Public Management Journal*. He is also the founding co-editor of the Palgrave book series, *Governing China in the 21st Century*.

RICHARD ZECKHAUSER is the Frank P. Ramsey Professor of Political Economy, Kennedy School, Harvard University. He graduated from Harvard College (summa cum laude) and received his PhD there. He is an elected fellow of the Econometric Society, the Institute of Medicine (National Academy of Sciences), and the American Academy of Arts and Sciences. In 2014, he was named a Distinguished Fellow of the American Economic Association.

His contributions to decision theory and behavioral economics include the concepts of quality-adjusted life years (QALYs), status quo bias, betrayal aversion, and ignorance (states of the world unknown) as a complement to the categories of risk and uncertainty. Many of his policy investigations explore ways to promote the health of human beings, to help markets work more effectively, and to foster informed and appropriate choices by individuals and government agencies.

Chapter 13

JUI-FEN RACHEL LU is a professor in the Department of Health Care Management and dean of the College of Management at Chang Gung University in Taiwan, where she teaches comparative health systems, health economics, and healthcare financing. Her research focuses on equity issues in Taiwan's healthcare system; the impact of the National Health Insurance program on the healthcare market and household consumption patterns; and comparative health systems in the Asia-Pacific region. She earned her BS from National Taiwan University, and her MS and ScD from Harvard University. Lu has served as a member of various government committees dealing with healthcare issues in Taiwan and is the recipient of various awards. She is the author of *Health Economics.* and has published papers in journals including *Health Affairs*, *Medical Care*, and *Journal of Health Economics.*

CHRISTINA PING is an undergraduate student in biology at Stanford University. Her interests lie in oncology and also in global health policy and economics, specifically regarding the accessibility and scalability of current cancer treatment technology, as well as insurance coverage for cancer treatment among different countries. Previously, Ping conducted clinical trials research at Memorial Sloan Kettering Cancer Center on tumor surveillance using blood biomarkers, and mechanisms of drug resistance in metastatic breast cancer patients. Upon graduation in June 2020, she will be working as a healthcare consultant as part of IQVIA's consulting services team.

NANCY HANZHUO ZHANG is a graduate student in international policy at Stanford University. Her work and interests revolve around development economics, more specifically health, education, and trade in the emerging markets. Holding a BA in economics from UC Berkeley, Zhang has gained research and policy analysis experiences from the World Bank, the Bill & Melinda Gates Foundation, and the Economist Group. She has lived extensively in Belgium, China, and the United States, acquiring native fluency in French, English, and Chinese. In August 2020, she will start a position at an economic litigation consulting firm to further enhance her quantitative and analytical skills in practice.

Chapter 14

KAVITA SINGH is an epidemiologist by training and works as a research scientist at the Public Health Foundation of India. Her research work has primarily focused on evaluating the long-term effectiveness and cost-effectiveness of a multicomponent quality improvement intervention in 1,146 patients with type 2 diabetes attending 10 tertiary care clinics in India and Pakistan, as part of the National Heart Lung Blood Institute–funded CARRS Trial. Recently, she has been awarded the Emerging Global Leader Award (K43 grant, 2019–24), funded by the National Institutes of Health, Fogarty International Centre, to conduct a research project that aims to develop and test the feasibility of a multicomponent cardiovascular quality improvement strategy for patients with established cardiovascular diseases in India.

DORAIRAJ PRABHAKARAN is professor of chronic disease epidemiology at the Public Health Foundation of India, and executive director of the Center for Chronic Disease Control. Dr. Prabhakaran has participated in and led several major international and national research studies, and heads one of only 11 funded global centers of excellence funded by the National Heart, Lung and Blood Institute and the UnitedHealth Group, the Center of Excellence – Center for Cardio-metabolic Risk Reduction in South Asia. Dr. Prabhakaran's research has produced major insights into the epidemiology, developmental origin, and biomarkers of cardiovascular diseases (CVDs) and diabetes in India, practice patterns on acute coronary syndrome; translation research in CVDs, and development of low-cost combination drugs for primary and secondary prevention of CVDs in South Asia. Currently, he is working to establish a model surveillance system for CVD, evaluating the role of community health workers and mobile technology health programs to prevent and manage chronic diseases, undertaking two CVD cohorts, and involved in several clinical trials evaluating low-cost strategies.

Preface

As this book goes to press in April 2020, the world is in the midst of pandemic COVID-19 (coronavirus disease caused by SARS-CoV-2, a new coronavirus identified in 2019 with similarities to the SARS virus). First identified in Wuhan, People's Republic of China, other parts of Asia and the rest of the world have been dealing with the pandemic, along with the social and economic costs of the measures needed to control its spread. While such a crisis may overshadow any of the more mundane and humdrum topics of healthy aging, it actually accentuates many of the themes highlighted in the chapters of this book: the importance of strengthening health systems, especially primary care; the need for policies across multiple sectors (e.g., public health, urban planning, transportation, education) that support healthy aging; the imperative of supporting the vulnerable and addressing disparities so that the blessings of longevity can be equitably enjoyed. Since those with chronic conditions and the frail elderly are most susceptible to severe disease or death from COVID-19 or other pathogens, including the seasonal influenza, societies need to focus on healthy aging to build resilience to the periodic threat of epidemics and pandemics, as well as to the day-to-day killers such as cardiovascular disease, stroke, and cancer. Moreover, measures to ensure social connectedness and civil society support for the vulnerable, whether during mandatory social distancing or not, can support mental health and healthy aging.

Only in the coming years will the health impacts of current crisis become evident, from the lives saved by proactive responses, to the numbers who suffered acute myocardial infarction, stroke, and other events from not keeping up with routine anti-hypertensive and anti-diabetic medications during "lockdown"; from the lessons learned in governance and public-private partnerships for future crises, to the festering weaknesses in health financing and delivery never addressed; from the reduced traffic accidents from less commuting and reduced ill health from air pollution, to those who suffered catastrophic social and economic consequences from loss of livelihood or mental strain; from the many lives improved from better handwashing (perhaps fewer influenza deaths in future flu seasons?), to those lost from reversion to poorer hygiene when everyday life resumes its rush and complacency. May the suffering from this pandemic in Asia and beyond reinforce the interconnections between effective health systems and resilient civil society; the importance of transparent, scientific leadership that embraces Li Wenliang's message that "there should be more than one voice in a healthy society";[1] and the prudence and humanity of equitable investments in healthy aging, based on scientific analysis of the "value for money" spent on alternative policies or interventions. Perhaps from this crisis will emerge new ways of using telemedicine and leveraging other technologies to support the health of the rural, poor, and vulnerable; innovative protocols for bringing together resources in a public health emergency; and a renewed conviction that investment in strong health systems undergirds the very social and economic fiber of our societies.

We dedicate the research in this volume to all those suffering from COVID-19, especially those who have been denied the possibility of healthy aging.

I thank all the authors who contributed their research and policy expertise to the chapters of this book. I acknowledge and thank the numerous Stanford research assistants who assisted with various stages of the research included in this volume, including Pedro Gallardo, Rebecca Spencer, Karissa Dong, Helen Chen, Janice Zhang, Renata Starbird, Yanghe Iven Sha, Jillayne Ren, and others noted in the respective chapters. I extend special thanks to George Krompacky for his professionalism and patience during the editing and production work for this volume.

Finally, many thanks to my loving family for all your support. I dedicate my work on this volume to Adrian and Alanna: may you continue to thrive and cultivate healthy habits to enjoy long, full lives; and with love to Chris 可思, looking forward to healthy aging together.

Karen Eggleston
Stanford, California

---

1 Gao Yu, Ding Gang, Dave Yin, Qin Jianhang, and Timmy Shen, "Chinese Coronavirus Whistleblower Li Wenliang Dies of the Disease," *Caixin*, February 7, 2020, accessed 20 March 2020, https://www.caixinglobal.com/2020-02-07/chinese-coronavirus-whistleblower-dies-101512456.html.

Healthy Aging in Asia

1 Healthy Aging in Asia

Introduction

Karen Eggleston

Population aging and the economic (re)emergence of Asia—two of the most important phenomena of the twenty-first century—converge in the challenges Asian economies face in promoting healthy aging. The demographic transition from high to low fertility and mortality has been more rapid in much of Asia than in Europe and North America, and high-income East Asia leads the world in life expectancy and proportion of elderly, with middle-income China rapidly catching up at lower per capita income. Will most of the population benefit from longevity? And will these longer lives be healthy ones?

Much research reinforces the conclusion that investing in health brings economic benefits, when focused on priority health investments (Jamison et al. 2016). The probability that newborns will survive to age 90 has increased dramatically—in high-income countries from 4.8% in 1950 to 26.7% today and 50% by 2060, according to United Nations (UN) data (Eggleston and Mukherjee 2019). This triumph of longevity, along with low (frequently below-replacement) fertility, has important social and economic implications. Families, communities, and policies must adjust in ways that support healthy aging throughout the life course. For example, gains in longevity are increasingly accumulating at the end of life in conventional retirement years, rather than by reducing infant mortality (Eggleston and Fuchs 2012); therefore, working to older ages will be necessary. But extending work-lives is feasible only if the added years are healthy ones, and equitable only if the least advantaged also benefit from healthy aging. The great blessing of longer lives dims when later years are clouded by pain, disability, and loss of dignity.

How are health systems in Asia promoting evidence-based policies for healthy aging? What strategies have been tried to prevent noncommunicable chronic diseases (NCDs), screen for early detection, raise quality of care, improve medication adherence, reduce unnecessary hospitalizations, and increase "value for money" in health spending? The chapters of this book contribute to the literature on how diverse economies of Asia are preparing for older population age structures and transforming health systems to support patients who will live with chronic disease for decades. Fourteen concise chapters are arranged by country and topic. Authors are social scientists and policymakers (e.g., Daejung Kim from Korea, and Maigeng Zhou, Min Yu, and colleagues from the central and provincial centers for disease control [CDCs] in China) sharing their empirical evidence and policy insights from recent and ongoing programs in each country or jurisdiction covered. They include experts in multiple disciplines and from multiple generations— from Professor Victor R. Fuchs, the "Dean of Health Economics," now in his ninth decade, to students and recent graduates with fresh perspectives (Pedro Gallardo, Jason Li, Christina Ping, Zhi Ping Teo). Topics include precision health and personalized medicine in Japan; China's evolving family doctor system and its national demonstration areas for chronic disease control; cancer disparities and public-private roles in Taiwan; and policies for healthy aging in Korea and India. Several chapters draw on research led by the Stanford Asia Health Policy Program on the net value of chronic disease management programs throughout Asia, starting with analysis of detailed longitudinal, patient-level data on diabetes management as a lens for understanding the net value of medical spending for patients with complicated chronic diseases across diverse health systems.

In this brief introduction to the book, I discuss patterns of demographic and epidemiologic change in the region and the contributions of each chapter, while highlighting the importance of addressing disparities in healthy aging.

Aging Asia

Regions vary in their historical experience of demographic transition. Some areas, such as the former Soviet Union or Eastern Europe, experienced a prolonged stagnation or even dramatic decline in life expectancy during the transformational recession accompanying the demise of socialism, followed in some cases by rapid improvement and greater variation in life span (Kornai and Eggleston 2001; Aburto and van Raalte 2018). In contrast, the Asian economies undergoing systemic transformation from central planning to market-based economies, China and Vietnam, have seen steady increases in life expectancy. Among high-income countries, Case and Deaton (2015) highlight "deaths of despair" (such as opioid overdoses) among the middle class and middle-aged in the United States and their relationship to the recent U.S. decline in life expectancy. Japan, meanwhile, has achieved world-leading longevity, and South Korea also exceeds the average for high-income countries, as shown in figure 1.1.

FIGURE 1.1 Life expectancy at birth, 2013 (in years)

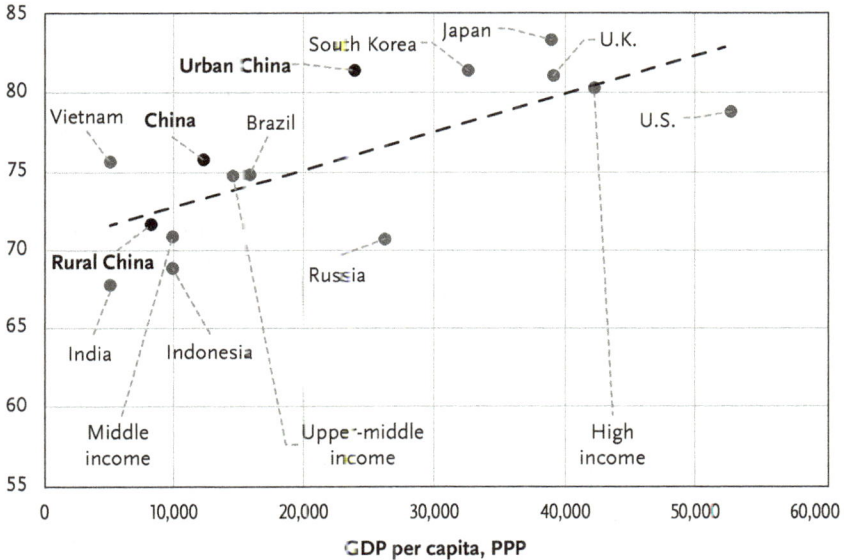

SOURCES: World Development Indicators, World Bank, and Global Burden of Disease estimates in Zhou et al. (2016).
NOTE: Horizontal axis shows per capita gross domestic product (GDP) in purchasing power parity (PPP).

Chapter 2 explores inequality in these longevity trends. Victor Fuchs and co-authors describe the distributions in age of death and their changes over time in three high-income countries of East Asia—Japan, South Korea, and Singapore—and the United States, compared with other high-income countries. The authors show that differences in life span between advantaged and disadvantaged groups generally decrease over time and with economic development, but remain large, especially among men. This greater survival gap among men echoes findings from many other studies. In Europe, for example, Permanyer et al. (2018) find that in Spain between 1960 and 2015 life expectancy increased for all, but with differences between the low and highly educated, especially among men. Chapter 2 concludes with a discussion of how policy might address inequalities by focusing on the causes of death among youth and the middle-aged. Clearly, to support healthy aging, policymakers must pay attention to the entire life course.

Research can help to inform policy, not only by understanding patterns of change, but also by helping to monitor how societies adapt to aging along multiple dimensions. Some studies propose individual-based measures of healthy aging, while others focus on societal adaptation. For example, Chen et al. (2018) develop an "Aging Society" index that assesses the status of older populations across five specific domains, including productivity and engagement, well-being, equity, economic and physical security, and intergenerational cohesion, using data from the Organisation for Economic Cooperation and Development (OECD). They find that Japan lags behind Norway and Sweden, according to their index.

In this book, chapters 3, 4, and 5 explore dimensions of Japan's policies for healthy aging, followed by expert accounts of South Korea and Hong Kong, all high-income economies with rapidly aging populations. The next five chapters provide different perspectives on China's demographic change and health system reforms. As evident in figure 1.1, China truly embodies "multiple countries within one," at least in terms of health. In figure 1.1, I disaggregate urban and rural China as if they are two separate countries. I illustrate internal disparities by showing the average life expectancy (with data from Zhou et al. [2016]) for the top four provinces (Shanghai, Beijing, Tianjin, and Zhejiang)—labeled "urban China"—compared to the average for the lowest four provinces (Tibet, Xinjiang, Qinghai, and Guizhou), which are labeled "rural China." A few conclusions are inescapable. The 2013 gap in life expectancy between these proxies for urban and rural China—almost 10 life years—is equivalent to the gap between high- and middle-income countries. Residents of the top four provinces enjoy first-world health outcomes, virtually a different country from that of their compatriots in the lowest four provinces.

The Social Determinants of Health
and Disparities in Healthy Aging

These wide regional and urban-rural disparities in health outcomes stem from a plethora of factors; access to healthcare is one, but much previous research (e.g., Fuchs 2004; Marmot 2015) highlights the importance of many (often highly correlated) non-medical factors, termed "social determinants of health," including poverty, low educational attainment, and lack of local public goods (such as clean water, modern toilets, protection from harmful toxins, and community-wide control of vectors for infectious disease). Income, education, occupation, age, sex, marital status, and ethnicity are all correlated with health (Fuchs 2004). Moreover, the direction of causation is two-way: poor health can interfere with schooling and earning income, while poor education and low income can contribute to ill health and premature mortality. The virtuous cycle between better health and socioeconomic status has as its counterpart the vicious cycle of "illness-induced poverty" from causes ranging from childhood malnutrition to catastrophic medical spending.

To lay the foundation for healthy aging, societies must address these social determinants of health. Chapter 13, for example, discusses the many infection-caused cancers prevalent in China that contribute to urban-rural health disparities. Screening, as discussed in multiple chapters, can be effective in catching cancer at stages early enough to treat, as well as detecting other chronic diseases and avoiding disabling complications. But screening can also lead to false positives and over-treatment, as is potentially the case with the rapid increase in the incidence of thyroid cancer and its treatment (Vaccarella et al. 2016).[1] Chapter 3 speaks to this theme by discussing Japan's screening program for metabolic syndrome and other policies within the Healthy Japan 21 (2013–22) plan, as well as the importance of tobacco control.

Several chapters in this book describe policies aimed at promoting healthy behaviors and addressing the non-medical determinants of health. For example, chapter 4 discusses the political economy of "precision health" and its prospects in Japan. Chapter 8 discusses how China seeks to promote local innovations for control of risk factors leading to chronic disease. Here, Jianqun Dong and colleagues from the China National Center for Disease Control and Prevention describe China's efforts to motivate local government

---

[1]   Du et al. (2018, 291) discuss the experience of Zhejiang Province, showing rapid increase in diagnosis of thyroid cancer with low and stable mortality, concluding "this increase in incidence might be due to increased diagnosis with advanced technology." These trade-offs, as well as public and private roles, feature in chapter 13.

responsibility in the prevention and control of NCDs with inter-sectoral coordination and by promoting multi-department cooperation in the construction of national demonstration areas and National Health Cities.

Managing Chronic Disease

In additional to the social determinants of healthy aging, the role of appropriate healthcare remains quite important, especially in managing patients with chronic disease. Several chapters discuss economic research on diabetes and hypertension, two increasingly prevalent conditions in aging Asia.

In chapter 9, Min Yu of the Zhejiang provincial CDC and co-authors note that diabetes poses a critical public health issue in many countries, especially for health systems ill-prepared to manage chronic disease within primary care. China's efforts to strengthen population health and primary care management for diabetes, especially in rural areas, deserve careful study and benchmarking to international experience to inform further progress. Improved prevention and control may not only improve patients' quality of life, but also potentially save resources by reducing avoidable hospital admissions. The authors propose age- and sex-standardized medical expenditures on avoidable admissions, alongside the more standard metric of number of admissions, as a new way of measuring primary care management of diabetes and comparing progress over time and across regions.

Chapter 11 provides empirical evidence about hypertension control in China and its relationship with the country's expansion of health insurance. Here, Jason Li argues that, given China's growing elderly population and chronic disease burden, controlling hypertension has been called the most urgent and cost-effective public health strategy the country could pursue, and shows through his analysis of the "care cascade" that China still struggles with poor hypertension management: 59.7% of all hypertensives were diagnosed, 51.4% were treated, and only 22.3% achieved effective control. Insurance coverage depth remains shallow for many citizens; increased insurance generosity was associated with a higher likelihood of treatment but not of diagnosis and control. Thus, Li suggests that factors beyond insurance may be limiting the positive effect of insurance generosity on hypertension management, an area for evidence-based policy to contribute to better chronic disease control.

Confronting the challenges of aging societies will require thinking carefully about the value of investments in methods for managing chronic conditions. Several chapters in this book showcase careful empirical research on this theme. For example, chapter 3 summarizes research on the net value of diabetes management in Japan; and the appendix provides detailed methods for others to consult in providing research evidence for other patient populations. This net value approach seeks to measure the productivity of resources devoted to chronic disease management, with detailed patient-level data to include the monetary value of improved health outcomes. As Dunn and Fernando (2019) argue, "a complete understanding of the growth trends in the medical care sector, as well as our overall economy, hinges on properly accounting for quality alongside costs." Eggleston, Grossman, and Cutler (2004) suggest that productivity research could be considered the "genome" of healthcare delivery innovation, given its foundational role in guiding reforms of healthcare delivery systems to achieve quality and efficiency.

Indeed, careful research can help society to avoid across-the-board cost control measures that stifle healthcare innovations that would deliver health improvement at a reasonable cost, or even cut cost. Chapter 7 provides another valuable perspective in this line of research.

Healthcare Access and Quality: Raising Averages, Addressing Disparities

The contributors to this volume also point to health system innovation beyond specific chronic disease control measures—innovation aimed to to improve healthcare more generally and to reduce inequality. Disparities in healthcare access and quality remain vital policy priorities, especially for large, diverse countries such as India and China.

Ethical challenges are the focus of several studies of health sector reforms. For example, Kornai and Eggleston (2001) argue that reforms of health sectors in transition economies should promote individual sovereignty and choice, on the one hand, while assuring social solidarity—i.e., helping the suffering, the troubled, and the disadvantaged—on the other. These two ethical principles have their counterparts in the phenomena of innovation and shortage (or access): can a health system sustain both choice (i.e., allowing the wealthy to purchase health improvements) *and* solidarity to provide access to those same health improvements for those less fortunate?

Science, population health, and economic development, although uneven, have expanded the possibilities for all; social policies determine how soon and how completely those same possibilities for healthy longevity are made available to those less fortunate. Angus Deaton (2013) emphasizes a similar point: innovations, first in population health and later in medical care, increased inequality but also brought progress with "trickle down" access for the poor. Indeed, this idea that innovations first accessed by the rich eventually diffuse to the poor has been called the "inverse equity hypothesis," and seems to apply to multiple cases (e.g., Lee et al. [2015] on cancer screening). Vaccines are one of the most cost-effective technologies for health over the life course (Bloom 2018), yet the net benefit of their use for specific populations remains a critical policy question.

Policies to assist countries in responding effectively to population aging should give disproportionate weight and financial support to speeding up the inverse equity diffusion process to narrow health and healthcare inequalities, such as between rural and urban areas or between the poor and the non-poor. This lesson is highlighted in multiple chapters of this book, with detailed experiences and policies in various Asian economies illustrating progress and the challenges of equitable access to technologies for healthy aging, especially acute for low- and middle-income countries.

For measuring disparities, new metrics have also been developed that could be refined and extended over time. For example, a recent study develops the "Healthcare Access and Quality" (HAQ) index, which measures premature mortality from causes preventable by access to high-quality healthcare (Fullman et al. 2018). According to this metric (figure 1.2), India improved significantly between 1990 and 2016, but is still working to catch up with Indonesia, Vietnam, and Brazil. China's rapid improvement in access and quality is evident from the fact that even China's *lowest* region in 2016 was above the 1990 national median. Among 195 countries and territories, China shows the highest absolute change in the HAQ Index during 2000–16, overtaking Brazil and approximating South Korea in 2000. China's HAQ index in 2016 was the highest among all countries with the same or lower medical spending per capita.

Despite this progress, sizable disparities remain in both health and healthcare within large low- and middle-income countries such as China and India. For example, although China achieved universal health coverage and improved healthcare utilization in both rural and urban areas over the past two decades, there are still substantial inter-regional gaps in service coverage, availability, and affordability. To illustrate, the 43-point regional disparity in HAQ within China (i.e., between Beijing and Tibet) is the equivalent of the difference between Iceland (ranked highest in the world) and North Korea. India also exhibited huge disparities—between Goa and Assam is a 30.8-point difference—whereas Japan recorded the smallest range in subnational HAQ performance in 2016 (a 4.8-point difference). Fullman et al. (2018) also note fast improvements in healthcare access and quality in southeast Asia.

FIGURE 1.2 Changes in the Healthcare Access and Quality (HAQ) Index, 1990–2016

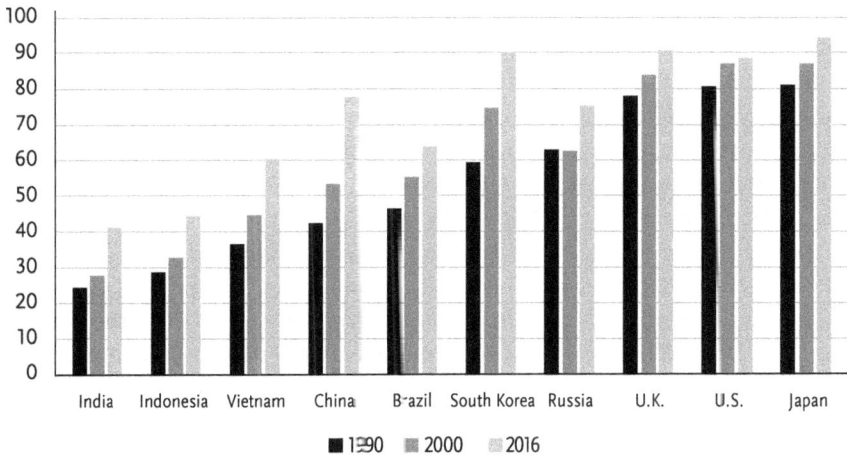

SOURCE: Data extracted from Fullman et al. (2018).

To improve healthcare access and quality, health system innovations play an important role. Several chapters discuss such efforts in aging Asia. For example, chapter 10 on the family doctor system in China describes the many efforts to re-orient China's health service delivery system away from crowding at tertiary hospitals and establish reliable systems for community-based care.

Another aspect of health system adjustment to aging involves the role of the public and private sectors in delivering health services and providing long-term care to the frail elderly. Public needs far outstrip the abilities of the government alone to deliver, including the broad array of social services that support healthy aging. These are the topics of two chapters. In chapter 12, Donahue and co-authors report results from a survey of 17 medium-sized cities in China on how local governments are seeking ways to create public value through contracting with the private sector and collaborative arrangements with some shared discretion, what the authors label "collaborative governance." The chapters on Hong Kong, Korea, and India all touch upon different roles of public and private actors in each system. And in chapter 13 Eggleston, Lu, Ping, and Zhang discuss how government and private actors take on complementary roles in addressing cancer as a leading cause of death, from drug discovery and development, to negotiating drug prices on insurance formularies, to delivering innovative target therapies.

Demographic changes interact with new technologies, such as personalized medicine therapies, to challenge the sustainable financing of medical care. Hokuto Asano, in chapter 5, focuses on this issue. He explains Japan's policies regarding personalized and precision medicine, including data collection, policy support, and how insurance coverage for new therapies works in Japan, comparing four drugs and companion diagnostic tests to their coverage and pricing in the United Kingdom. He also notes the importance of cost-effectiveness analyses in this process. Cautious optimism could be warranted regarding the power of innovation to produce both "miracle drugs" and the new approaches to financing and payment that will spread their benefits more widely (Eggleston 2018).

In sum, the contributors to this volume provide detailed empirical evidence and rich policy experience, covering multiple aspects of policy initiatives for healthy aging in health systems as diverse as those of the cities Singapore and Hong Kong to large economies such as Japan, India, and China. I thank the authors for their contributions and hope you, the reader, will find our work useful.

References

Aburto, José Manuel, and Alyson van Raalte. 2018. "Lifespan Dispersion in Times of Life Expectancy Fluctuation: The Case of Central and Eastern Europe." *Demography* 55 (6): 2071–96.

Bloom, David E. 2018. "Valuing Vaccines: Deficiencies and Remedies." *Vaccine* 33 (Suppl. 2): B29–33.

Case, Anne, and Angus Deaton. 2015. "Rising Morbidity and Mortality in Midlife among White Non-Hispanic Americans in the 21st Century." *Proceedings of the National Academy of Sciences* 112 (49): 15078–83.

Chen, Cynthia, Dana P. Goldman, Julie Zissimopoulos, and John W. Rowe. 2018. "Multidimensional Comparison of Countries' Adaptation to Societal Aging." *Proceedings of the National Academy of Sciences* 115 (37): 9169–74.

Deaton, Angus. 2013. *The Great Escape: Health, Wealth, and the Origins of Inequality*. Princeton University Press.

Du, Lingbin, Youqing Wang, Xiaohui Sun, Huizhang Li, Xinwei Geng, Minghua Ge, and Yimin Zhu. 2018. "Thyroid Cancer: Trends in Incidence, Mortality and Clinical-Pathological Patterns in Zhejiang Province, Southeast China." *BMC Cancer* 18 (1): 291.

Dunn, Abe, and Lasanthi Fernando. 2019. "Medical Expenditures Are Likely 'Worth it.' But Can We Measure How Much They Are Worth?" *Health Affairs Blog, Health Affairs*. February 20, 2019. http://www.healthaffairs.org/do/10.1377/hblog20190215.71093/full/.

Eggleston, Karen. 2018. "Innovation and Shortage: The Yin and Yang of the Health Sector." *Acta Oeconomica* 68 (supplement): 99–114.

Eggleston, Karen, and Victor R. Fuchs. 2012. "The New Demographic Transition: Most Gains in Life Expectancy Now Realized Late in Life." *Journal of Economic Perspectives* 26 (3): 137–56.

Eggleston, Karen, Jerome Grossman, and David Cutler. 2004. "Productivity Research and Healthcare Delivery Innovation." *Applied Health Economics and Health Policy* 3 (3): 133–41.

Eggleston, Karen, and Anita Mukherjee. 2019. "Financing Longevity: The Economics of Pensions, Health, and Long-Term Care—Introduction to the Special Issue." *Journal of the Economics of Ageing* 13 (special issue guest editor with Anita Mukherjee): 1–6.

Fuchs, Victor R. 2004. "Reflections on the Socio-Economic Correlates of Health." *Journal of Health Economics* 23 (4): 653–61.

Fullman, Nancy, et al. (GBD 2016 Healthcare Access and Quality Collaborators). 2018. "Measuring Performance on the Healthcare Access and Quality Index for 195 Countries and Territories and Selected Subnational Locations: A Systematic Analysis from the Global Burden of Disease Study 2016." *The Lancet* 391 (10136): 2236–71.

Jamison Dean, Gavin Yamey, Naomi Beyeler, and Hester Wadge. 2016. "Investing in Health: The Economic Case." In *Doha: WISH Investing in Health Forum*. http://www.wish.org.qa/wp-content/uploads/2018/01/IMPJ4495_WISH_Investing_in_Health_WEB.pdf.

Kaslow, David C., Steve Black, David E. Bloom, Mahima Datla, David Salisbury, and Rino Rappuoli. 2018. "Vaccine Candidates for Poor Nations Are Going to Waste." *Nature* 564 (7736): 337–39.

Kornai, János, and Karen Eggleston. 2001. *Welfare, Choice and Solidarity in Transition: Reforming the Health Sector in Eastern Europe*. Cambridge University Press.

Lee, John Tayu, Zhilian Huang, Sanjay Basu, and Christopher Millett. 2015. "The Inverse Equity Hypothesis: Does It Apply to Coverage of Cancer Screening in Middle-Income Countries?" *Journal of Epidemiology and Community Health* 69 (2): 149–55.

Marmot, Michael. 2015. "The Health Gap: The Challenge of an Unequal World." *The Lancet* 386 (10011): 2442–44.

Permanyer, Iñaki, Jeroen Spijker, Amand Blanes, and Elisenda Renteria. 2018. "Longevity and Lifespan Variation by Educational Attainment in Spain: 1960–2015." *Demography* 55 (6): 2045–70.

Vaccarella, Salvatore, Silvia Franceschi, Freddie Bray, Christopher P. Wild, Martyn Plummer, and Luigino Dal Maso. 2016. "Worldwide Thyroid-Cancer Epidemic? The Increasing Impact of Overdiagnosis." *New England Journal of Medicine* 375 (7): 614–17.

Zhou, Maigeng, Haidong Wang, Jun Zhu, Wanqing Chen, Linhong Wang, Shiwei Liu, Yichong Li, et al. 2016. "Cause-Specific Mortality for 240 Causes in China During 1990–2013: A Systematic Subnational Analysis for the Global Burden of Disease Study 2013." *The Lancet* 387 (10015): 251–72.

2 Healthy Aging, and Inequality in Age-of-Death

Comparing Trends in Japan, Korea, Singapore, and the United States

Karen Eggleston, Victor R. Fuchs, Daejung Kim, and Zhi Ping Teo

In recent years, income inequality has become a subject of major interest, not only to economists, sociologists, and other social scientists but also to public policy analysts and politicians around the globe (e.g., Piketty 2014; Piketty and Saez 2014; World Economic Forum 2015; Jones and Kim 2018). Less attention has been paid to another significant contributor to disparities in people's overall well-being: inequality in age-of-death (AOD).

Although the subject of much research by demographers (see, e.g., Lee 2003; Edwards and Tuljapurkar 2005; Edwards 2011; Gillespie, Trotter, and Tuljapurkar 2014; Seligman, Greenberg, and Tuljapurkar 2016; Zuo et al. 2018), the dramatic reduction in AOD inequality at the beginning of the demographic and epidemiologic transitions (e.g., in the first half of the twentieth century in most now-high-income economies) and the rather limited decline in recent decades has not been widely discussed despite its importance. Globally, valuing health and survival greatly adds to measures of human welfare improvement, despite the challenges of financing longevity (Eggleston and Mukherjee 2009). For example, Jones and Klenow (2016) estimate that a consumption-equivalent measure of economic welfare that takes account of life expectancy and leisure shows a 20-fold increase over a century rather than a seven-fold increase for per capita incomes alone.

A few studies of how health and survival gaps by socioeconomic status (SES) have evolved over time—across birth cohorts and generations—suggest a widening gradient (Cutler, Deaton, and Lleras-Muney 2006; Meara, Richards, and Cutler 2008; Costa 2015); others have focused on changes in inequality

The authors thank Rui Du, Shannon Xue, Emily Nguyen, and Pedro Gallardo for excellent research assistance, and a Shorenstein APARC faculty research award for financial support.

of income and health over time, and whether they are causally related (e.g., Pickett and Wilkinson 2015). Recent contributions within economics highlight the importance of inequality in components of well-being beyond income and wealth (Becker, Philipson, and Soares 2005; Fleurbaey 2009; Jones and Klenow 2016) and their implications for public policy (National Academies of Sciences, Engineering, and Medicine 2015).[1] For the United States, Chetty et al. (2016) focus on inequality in average life expectancy according to income and geography, while Currie and Schwandt (2016) highlight the decreasing inequality in mortality among younger cohorts of Americans by race and county-level measures of poverty. Case and Deaton (2015) highlight the recent U.S. decline in life expectancy and its relationship to "deaths of despair" (such as opioid overdoses) among the middle class and middle-aged.

We contribute to this developing area of research by describing AOD distributions and their changes over time in three high-income countries of East Asia—Japan, South Korea (hereafter Korea), and Singapore—and the United States, compared with other member countries of the Organisation for Economic Co-operation and Development (OECD).

Taking the U.S. case as illustrative (Fuchs and Eggleston 2018), figure 2.1 shows the well-known increase in survival, illustrated by the upward/rightward shift of the AOD distribution over time. In the first half of the twentieth century the large shift from death at younger ages to older ages has been attributed primarily to rising living standards and population health measures such as clean water and sanitation (e.g., Alsan and Goldin 2019). Advances in medical care began to be important after the discovery and diffusion of antibiotics mid-century and with improvements in cardiovascular care, among other factors (Cutler and Miller 2005; Cutler, Deaton, and Lleras-Muney 2006; Costa 2015). As Catillon, Cutler, and Getzen (2018, 2) argue, "there is a stronger case that personal medicine affected health in the second half of the twentieth century than in the preceding 150 years." As striking as the increase in average AOD is the decline in inequality of AOD in the first half of the twentieth century, although data limitations mean that the estimates for 1900–02 should be interpreted with caution. Figure 2.1 shows that the AOD distribution becomes much more concentrated between 1900–02 and 1949–51—in other words, inequality in AOD sharply declined over the period. After 1949–51 there is a further decline.

---

1   For example, the spring 2016 issue of the *Journal of Economic Perspectives* features five papers on the theme "Inequality Beyond Income" that discuss inequalities in consumption, crime, family and fertility, and mortality. Currie and Schwandt (2016) highlight that survival inequality among children and youth has declined substantially in the United States since 1990, suggesting that "today's children are likely to face considerably less inequality in mortality as they age than current adults" (Currie and Schwandt 2016, 30).

FIGURE 2.1 Distribution of age-of-death in the United States, total population (1900–02, 1949–51, and 2010)

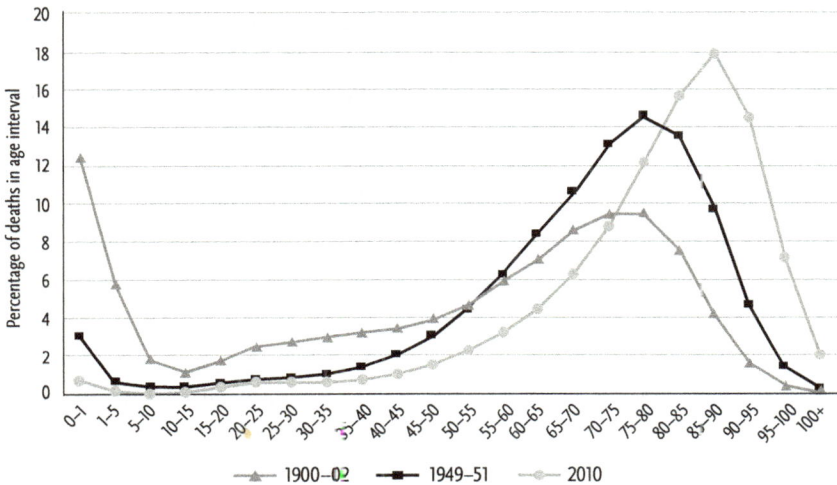

SOURCE: *National Vital Statistics Reports* 63, no. 7 (November 6, 2014), table 20, "Survivorship by age, race, and sex: Death registration States, 1900–1902 to 1919–21, and United States, 1929–31 to 2010," all races (men and women combined), p. 47.

In this chapter, we focus on how inequality in AOD in three countries of East Asia declined much faster than in the United States between the 1950s and 2010 (table 2.1). Japan, Korea, and Singapore changed dramatically as they developed and passed through the demographic transition toward low mortality and low fertility. After World War II their average per capita income and life span quickly converged with that of the OECD countries. Japan, notably, achieved world-leading life expectancy. Healthy aging, and inequality in healthy aging, is of particular policy importance for these economies in the coming decades, since (like most of East Asia) they have experienced more rapid population aging than have Europe and North America. Consider a commonly used metric, the number of years a society takes to increase its population's share of people aged 65 or more from 7 percent to 14 percent. This process took 115 years in France (1864–1979) and 73 years in the United States (1942–2015), but only 24 years in Japan (1970–94) and only 18 years in Korea (2000–18) (Kim 2018). Unsurprisingly, the proportion of medical expenditures on the elderly has increased rapidly, too—in Korea, from 24 percent in 2005 to over 35 percent by 2014 (Kim 2018). As policymakers confront the challenges of longer lives, they need to keep in mind the inequality in gains in life span and address the causes of death among youth and the middle-aged as well as the elderly.

In addition to illustrating trends in AOD inequality, we also discuss how it may be related to income, income inequality, and other factors, across countries and across regions within countries (i.e., Korean provinces, Japanese prefectures). We conclude with a brief discussion of whether any of these associations can be interpreted as causal pathways, and what the resulting implications might be for public policy to reduce inequality in a central component of well-being: years of life lived. For example, logical policies—such as promoting longer work-lives and higher ages of pension eligibility—may have unequal impact on the less fortunate (such as those at the low end of the survivorship distribution).

The remainder of the chapter is organized as follows. The next section provides a description of data sources and our methods for assessing inequality in AOD. The following sections present our results regarding AOD inequality in Japan, Korea, Singapore, the United States, and other OECD countries, followed by the univariate and multivariate correlates of AOD inequality across Korean provinces and Japanese prefectures. The final section discusses our findings in the context of related literature and suggests how policy should focus on causes of death among youth and middle-aged populations to raise overall survival while reducing disparities.

Data, Methods, and Measures

The national AOD distributions presented here come from period life tables based on national vital statistics data. For the United States, they are derived from the period life tables published by the Center for Disease Control and Prevention, National Center for Health Statistics, National Vital Statistics System. These life tables are useful for their historical breadth (going back to the beginning of the twentieth century, albeit only for a sub-sample of the population, in states with a death registry) and for their disaggregation by race and ethnicity. The results are broadly consistent with those derived from U.S. life tables within the Human Mortality Database (HMD, a project created by the University of California, Berkeley, and the Max Planck Institute), a high-quality demographic data source that is the basis for our analysis of Japan and of all other OECD countries it covers. Data for Singapore come from the Singapore Department of Statistics and the HMD, and for Korea from the National Vital Statistics System and associated official life tables.

The survivorship tables and the life expectancy tables provide all necessary data for calculating the AOD distributions and other summary measures. AOD distribution for a given year, taken from the period life tables for that year, differs from the age distribution of actual deaths in that year; the latter is influenced by past mortality, fertility, and immigration, as well as current age-sex-specific mortality. It also differs from a distribution describing the actual AOD that a birth cohort experiences as it lives out its life span. Cohort distributions can only be estimated many decades after the year of birth of the cohort. The period distributions described in this chapter are analogous to estimates of life expectancy at birth; that is, they describe outcomes conditional on the cohort experiencing the age-sex-specific mortality prevailing in the given year.

For income, income inequality, and other correlates of national and sub-national inequality, we also draw from standard national statistics as listed in the reference list as well as the World Development Indicators database of the World Bank.

Methods

The distributions of AOD depart significantly from a normal distribution. The modal age of death is typically 10 years higher than the mean age of death; the median is typically about halfway between the mean and the mode. Thus, following Fuchs and Eggleston (2018), we emphasize non-parametric measures of inequality such as comparison of age at the 20th percentile (A20) and at the 80th percentile (A80) of the AOD distribution.[2]

To examine correlates of AOD inequality across OECD countries, U.S. states, Japanese prefectures, and Korean provinces, we first report population-weighted univariate Pearson correlations between area characteristics and a measure of AOD inequality. For Japan, we also estimate multivariate ordinary least squares regressions with population-weighted A20 and A80/A20 by sex as dependent variables to explore whether statistically significant correlations remain after simultaneously controlling for other predictor variables. Since these are descriptive regressions or ecologic models of AOD inequality, the associations we report are not causal relationships between the predictor variables and AOD inequality. The relationships do, however, provide input to compare with other studies with designs that pinpoint specific causal mechanisms and to inform study of how public policy can mitigate AOD inequality.

---

2   We look at both the absolute difference and the ratio of A80 to A20, which is highly correlated (>0.90) with the inter-quartile ratio in cross-section (U.S. states) and in time series. Results are similar when we measure inequality in AOD by dividing a survival distribution at the median AOD (A50) into a bottom and a top half of survivors, and calculating life expectancy at birth (the mean AOD) for each half.

Results

Table 2.1 provides specific measures of inequality in AOD in the four countries, calculated as the differences between AOD at the 80th and 20th percentiles of the AOD distributions. Results show a dramatic improvement in A20, and steady improvement in A80 across for the four. Only for the United States do we have data back to the dawn of the previous century, and those numbers should be interpreted with caution. Nevertheless, looking back, it is shocking to see how much inequality there was at the beginning of the twentieth century. In 1900–02 approximately one out of five Americans died before reaching 10 years of age, while another only one-fifth lived past the age of 75. By 1949–51, AOD at the 20th percentile had increased to 55 years; AOD at the 80th percentile underwent a more modest increase to 85 years. Thus, as infant mortality fell substantially, the absolute difference between the 80th and 20th percentiles decreased by 35.0 years, but between 1949–51 and 2010, it decreased by only 7.6 years.

Conclusions are similar when instead we summarize the major changes in inequality in AOD by dividing the survivorship table into two halves: the bottom half includes all in the cohort who die before the median age of death; the top half includes all who die after the median age of death. Most of the decline in AOD inequality was achieved by large gains in survival by the bottom half of the AOD distribution. For example, for the United States between 1900–02 and 2010, life expectancy at birth for the bottom half of the distribution increased from 24.4 years to 67.1 years, while the increase for the top half was from 74.1 to 90.2.

For the East Asian countries, we focus on the period after 1950, when their demographic and economic development converged rapidly with the levels of other high-income countries. All three countries saw a decline in AOD inequality, with a more rapid rise in AOD at the 20th percentile than at the 80th percentile as the primary reason. This pattern resembles the overall trend in the United States from 1900 to 2010.

The bottom set of rows in table 2.1 show AOD inequality as measured by the ratio A80/A20. Japan and Singapore at first had higher AOD inequality than did the United States, but had lower inequality by 2010. Over this period Japan caught up with and surpassed U.S. longevity. To illustrate the large welfare improvements in that country, Japan's A20 in 2010 (75 years old) equaled U.S. A80 in 1900.

TABLE 2.1 Inequality in age-of-death in Japan, Korea, Singapore, and the United States as measured at the 20th and 80th percentiles of the distribution, 1950 and 2010

	1900–02	1950	2010
A20*			
Japan	—	39	75
Korea	—	47†	71
Singapore	—	52‡	73
United States	10	55	69
A80*			
Japan	—	80	94
Korea	—	79†	89
Singapore	—	80‡	92
United States	75	85	91
A80/A20			
Japan	—	2.02	1.26
Korea	—	1.68†	1.25
Singapore	—	1.55‡	1.27
United States	7.49	1.53	1.34

SOURCES: See text; National Vital Statistics for each country, except Human Mortality Database for Japan. For United States, *National Vital Statistics Reports* 63, no. 7 (2010).
NOTE: *A20 and A80 values are in years of age; †Korea values are for 1970; ‡Singapore values are for 1957.

The patterns are similar for Singapore—described in more detail in the next section—and for sub-populations, with lower survival and wider disparities among males. Figures 2.2a and 2.2b show the decreasing inequality in AOD for Japan and Korea among males and females separately, as well as for the total population. Female A20 in Japan by 2016 had caught up to female A80 in 1950; while male A20 had not similarly caught up with 1950's A80, it exhibited a larger absolute increase. AOD inequality is higher among males (table 2.2).

For all cases studied, increasing average life expectancy is associated with a faster increase in A20 than A80 (figures 2.2a, 2.2b).[3] This differen-

3   For example, for the United States since 1950 (the more reliable data), the standard deviation of the A20 series exceeds that of A80, at 3.72 vs. 2.54, but part of this difference can be explained by a greater long-term trend for A20, at 0.192 vs. 0.132. The most appropriate comparison is the average (absolute) year-to-year change net of long-term trends. The difference between A20 and A80, 0.222 vs. 0.185, is statistically significant, p<.01. More generally, A20, A80, and life expectancy are all positively correlated and increasing across all countries and sub-national populations studied. It would be only in extraordinary circumstances that one or two of the three measures changed in one direction while the other(s) changed in the opposite direction.

FIGURE 2.2A Decreasing inequality in age-of-death in Japan at the 20th and 80th percentiles of the distribution, by sex, 1947–2016

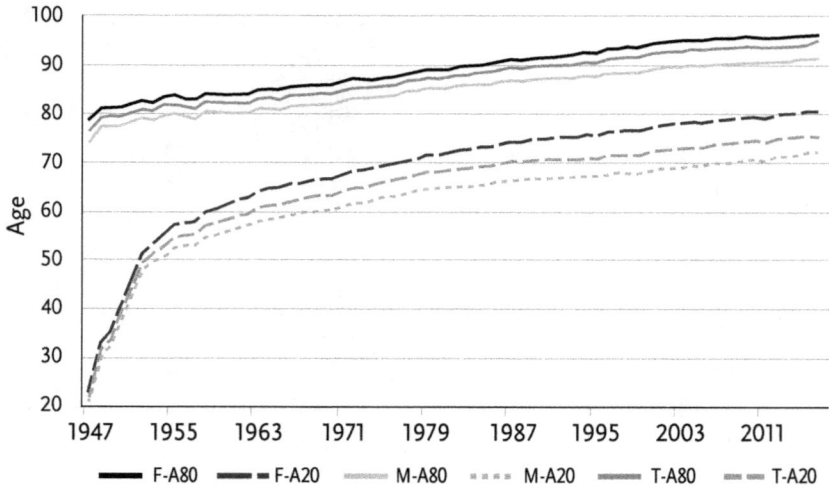

SOURCE: Human Mortality Database.
NOTE: F = female; M = male; T = total.

FIGURE 2.2B Decreasing inequality in age of death in Korea at the 20th and 80th percentiles of the distribution, by sex, 1970–2016

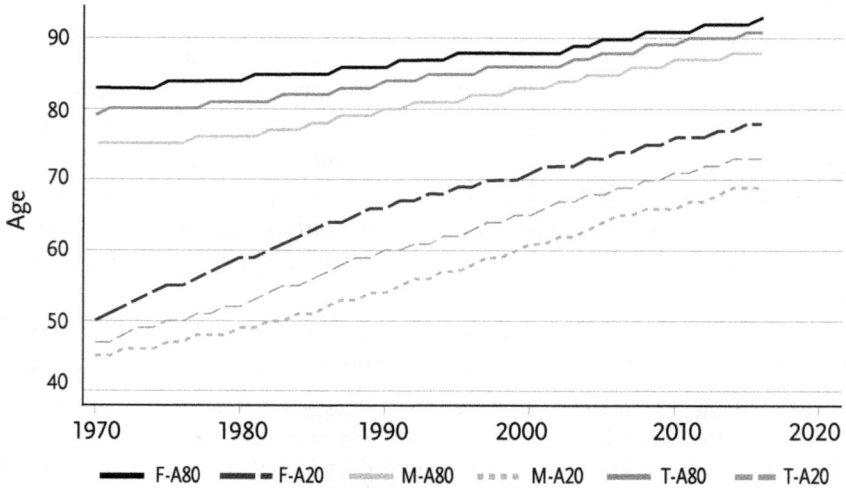

SOURCE: Statistics Korea, "Life Tables."
NOTE: F = female; M = male; T = total.

TABLE 2.2 Mean age-of-death at the 20th and 80th percentiles of the distribution, by sex, across OECD countries and within Japan and the United States

	Year	Males		Females	
		A80	A20	A80	A20
U.S. total population	2010	89.5	65.6	92.7	72.6
Other OECD countries, excluding United States	2010	89.3 (2.12)	68.7 (93.96)	92.5 (1.33)	75.4 (2.17)
Other OECD countries, excluding former socialist countries	2010	89.6 (0.98)	69.8 (2.10)	93.0 (0.88)	76.2 (1.43)
U.S. states	2000	88.2 (1.37)	64.4 (1.85)	91.7 (0.90)	70.6 (1.74)
Japanese prefectures	2010	90.5 (0.43)	70.6 (1.07)	95.8 (0.44)	79.6 (0.37)
Japanese prefectures	2000	89.1 (0.52)	68.2 (0.89)	94.4 (0.41)	77.5 (0.54)

SOURCES: OECD Statistics (OECD.stat, https://stats.oecd.org); for Japan, Human Mortality Database; for United States, *National Vital Statistics Reports* 63, no. 7 (2010).
NOTE: Unweighted means with standard deviations in parentheses.

tial improvement in the survival of the least advantaged drives decreasing inequality in AOD, although substantial inequality remains. Further decrease in inequality depends on addressing the causes of death among youth and middle-aged populations, which differ from those among the elderly (who suffer to a much greater degree from the leading causes of overall mortality such as cardiovascular disease and cancer). As shown in figures 2.3a and 2.3b, the proportion of deaths caused by accidents and suicides is much greater at younger ages. Thus, relatively high inequality in AOD generally indicates that early causes such as accidents and suicides have declined relatively slowly.

Inequality in AOD across OECD countries

Figures 2.4a–2.4c illustrate inequality in AOD across the relatively high-income countries, the OECD. The United States has relatively high inequality in AOD, compared not only to East Asia but also to other high-income economies. Figure 2.4a shows the A20 and A80 for the total population in year 2010 or latest available year. Countries are arrayed in order of the gap, A80–A20, from smallest (Iceland) to the largest (Hungary). The United States has higher inequality in AOD than all but three other OECD countries, all formerly socialist countries with low A20.[4]

---

4   Indeed, the United States is the only country with high inequality in AOD that also has a high A80 (around 90 years); all other countries where the difference between A80 and A20 is greater than 23 have much lower A20 and A80.

FIGURE 2.3A Korean causes of death by age, 2014 (percent share)

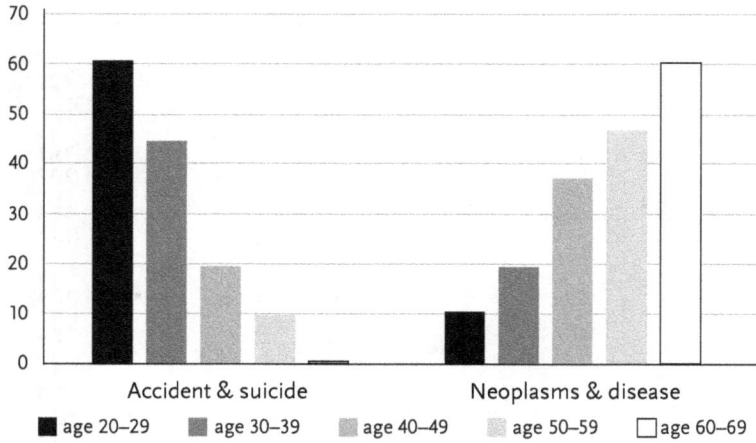

■ age 20–29   ■ age 30–39   ▨ age 40–49   ▨ age 50–59   ☐ age 60–69

SOURCE: *Journal of the Korean Medical Association* 59 (3): 221.

FIGURE 2.3B U.S. causes of death by age and sex, 2014 (percent share)

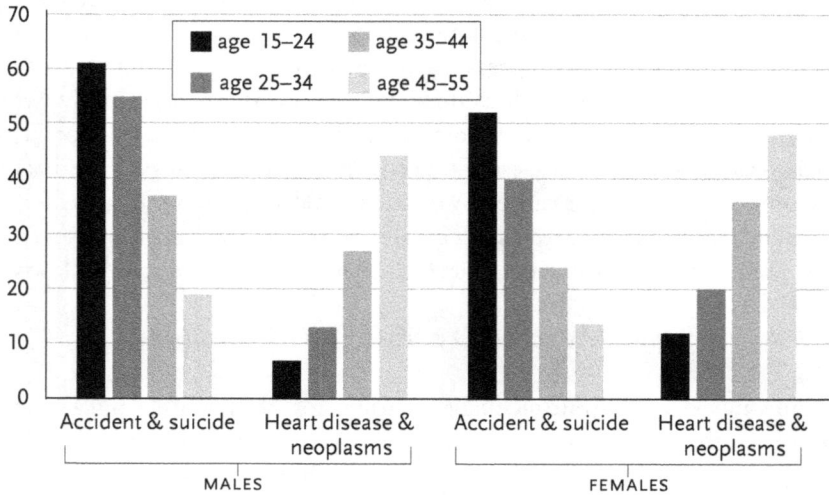

SOURCES: *National Vital Statistics Report* 65, no. 5; Fuchs and Eggleston (2018), figure 3.

Heterogeneity in AOD inequality:
Male-female, black-white, other race/ethnicity differences

Figures 2.4b and 2.4c show inequality in AOD among males and females separately for the OECD countries. As noted, AOD inequality in general is higher, and more heterogeneous, among males (figure 2.4b) than among females (figure 2.4c). The United States ranks highest among these OECD countries in terms of female AOD inequality.

Looking across the 26 high-income countries with reliable life tables compiled in the HMD, we also see that variation in AOD is far higher among males than females. The United States compares quite unfavorably to other high-income countries in terms of gender inequality in AOD; indeed, for both men and women in the HMD sample, the U.S. inequality is exceeded only by countries of the former Soviet Union. For men, the United States is slightly worse than the Czech Republic and slightly better than Bulgaria; for women, the U.S. inequality in AOD is about the same as those of Lithuania and Scotland.

The countries achieving the lowest gender inequality in AOD overlap considerably with the countries with the highest life expectancy (since, mechanically, bringing up the survival of the shortest-lived segments of the population yields the greatest boost to average life expectancy). Thus it is not surprising that Japan and Switzerland are among the top five countries for both men and women in terms of lowest inequality in AOD.

Within the United States, substantial differences also exist between different racial and ethnic groups. Tables 2.3a and 2.3b show that race differences and sex differences in age of death at the 80th and 20th percentiles are substantial, but small relative to the 80th–20th differences within each race-sex group.[5]

Inequality in age of death in Singapore

Inequality in the AOD in Singapore has changed significantly since the mid-twentieth century. In 1957, approximately one out of five Singaporeans died before reaching 52 years of age, while the top one-fifth of the survivor population lived past 80 years of age. From 1957 to 2017, AOD at the 20th percentile increased by 23 years to 75 years of age. In contrast, AOD at the 80th percentile increased by 13 years to 93 years of age. The more rapid rise

---

5   When describing differences in life expectancy and AOD inequality distributions by race and ethnicity, it is important to remember that data can be confounded by changes in reporting of these underlying characteristics and the prevalence of multiple-race individuals, especially over time and by birth cohort. Currie and Schwandt (2016) emphasize that trends in survival and its inequality by race and ethnicity over time are complicated by changes in the ways that race and ethnicity are measured in the numerator and denominator over time. For example, there has been a large increase among younger cohorts in the self-report of multiple races, such that "if the observed exponential growth of multiple-race reporting continues into the future, the last single-race African-American and single-race white persons will be born in 2050 and 2080, respectively!" (Currie and Schwandt 2016, 42).

FIGURE 2.4A Age-of-death at the 20th and 80th percentiles of the distribution for the total population of 31 OECD countries, 2010

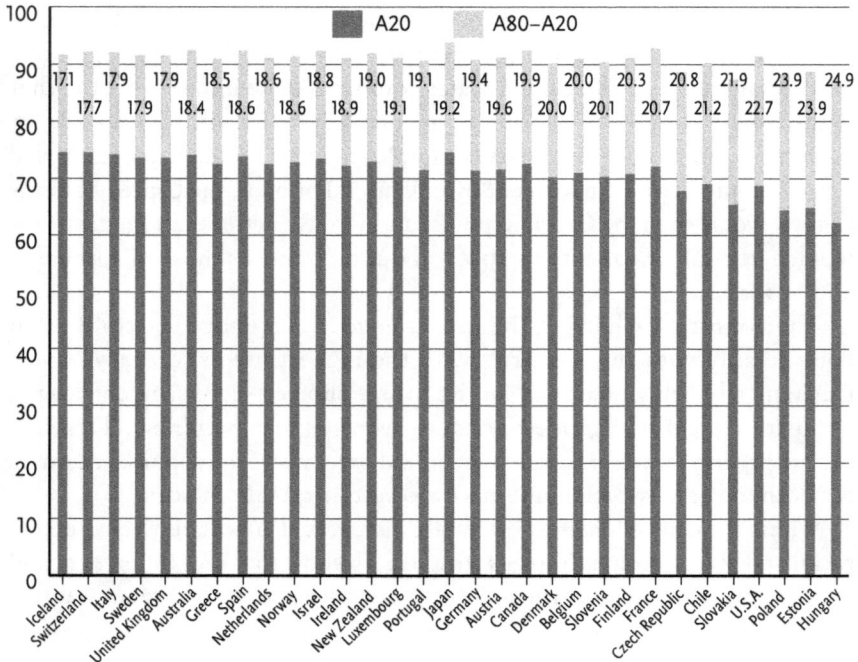

SOURCE: Authors' analysis of data from OECD.stat and Human Mortality Database.
NOTE: Chile, Hungary, and Poland are based on 2009 data.

in AOD at the 20th percentile contributed to the decline in inequality.

In terms of inequality in AOD, the absolute difference between the 80th and 20th percentiles decreased by five years from 28 years in 1957 to 23 years in 1962, three years before Singapore's independence in 1965. For the 60-year period from 1957 to 2017, absolute inequality in AOD decreased by 10 years.

The gains for the total population in life expectancy at birth (mean AOD) over the period from 1957 to 2017 were significant: 19.9 years over 60 years or approximately 3.3 years per decade.[6] In terms of inequality in AOD across the relatively high-income countries (figures 2.4a–2.4c), Singapore is close to the median of the distribution with an A80–A20 of 19.5 in 2010. Singapore has a relatively low male A80–A20 of 19.8, in the lower half of the OECD distribution. For females, Singapore's absolute inequality in AOD is 17.9, above that of Japan but considerably lower than that of the United

6   This is comparable to the gains for the United States in the first half of the century, at 3.8 years per decade, but substantially higher than the gains in the United States for the time period of 1949–51 to 2010, at 1.8 years per decade.

FIGURE 2.4B Age-of-death at the 20th and 80th percentiles of the distribution for males in OECD countries, 2010

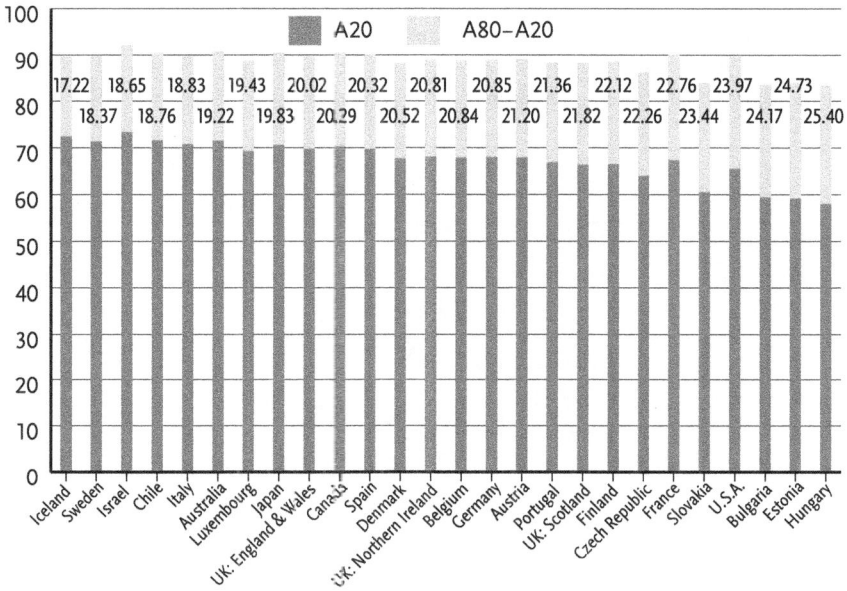

SOURCE: Authors' analysis of data from OECD.stat and Human Mortality Database.
NOTE: Slovakia, Luxembourg, Israel, Italy, and Hungary are based on 2009 data.

FIGURE 2.4C Age-of-death at the 20th and 80th percentiles of the distribution for females in 32 OECD countries, 2010

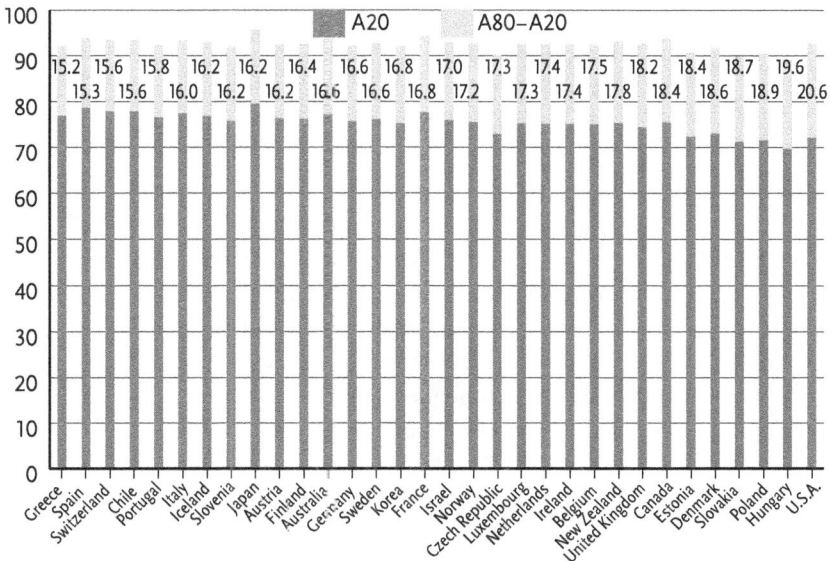

SOURCE: Authors' analysis of data from OECD.stat and Human Mortality Database.
NOTE: Chile is based on 2005 data; Poland and Hungary are based on 2009 data.

States. Singapore's relatively moderate inequality in AOD is paired with high life expectancy at birth: 81.7 in 2010. By 2017, inequality in AOD decreased to 18.5 and life expectancy at birth increased to 83.1.

TABLE 2.3A U.S. life expectancy at birth for four race-sex groups, 1970 and 2010 (years)

Race-Sex Group	1970	2010	Change 1970 to 2010	
			Absolute	Percent
White males	67.94	76.54	8.60	12.6
White females	75.49	81.29	5.80	7.7
Black males	60.00	71.85	11.85	19.8
Black females	68.32	78.00	9.68	14.2

SOURCE: Authors' analysis of life table data from National Center for Health Statistics, National Vital Statistics System, Fuchs 2016 and sources cited therein.

TABLE 2.3B Percent of each race–sex group with life expectancy at birth below the median of the total U.S. population, 1970 and 2010

Race-Sex Group	1970	2010	Change 1970 to 2010
White males	59	57	−2
White females	36	43	+7
Black males	74	69	−5
Black females	57	52	−5

SOURCE: Authors' analysis of life table data from National Center for Health Statistics, National Vital Statistics System, Fuchs 2016 and sources cited therein.

Exploring the correlates of AOD inequality

Cross-sectional studies of the relation between income and AOD show a significant positive relation, albeit diminishing at higher income levels (Preston 1975). Figures 2.5a and 2.5b show that poverty is correlated with inequality in AOD across Japanese prefectures and Korean provinces.

Given the association between income and AOD, and the increase in income *inequality* in many countries, including the United States, in recent years, we might expect increasing income inequality to be associated with greater inequality in AOD. Data shown in Fuchs and Eggleston (2018), however, do not support that hypothesis. Further research using detailed micro data on income and its distribution, and study designs able to identify causal pathways, would be useful to explore this association between income inequality and AOD inequality over time (see, e.g., Chetty et al. 2016; Currie

FIGURE 2.5A Inequality in male age-of-death and poverty rate by Japanese prefecture, 2010

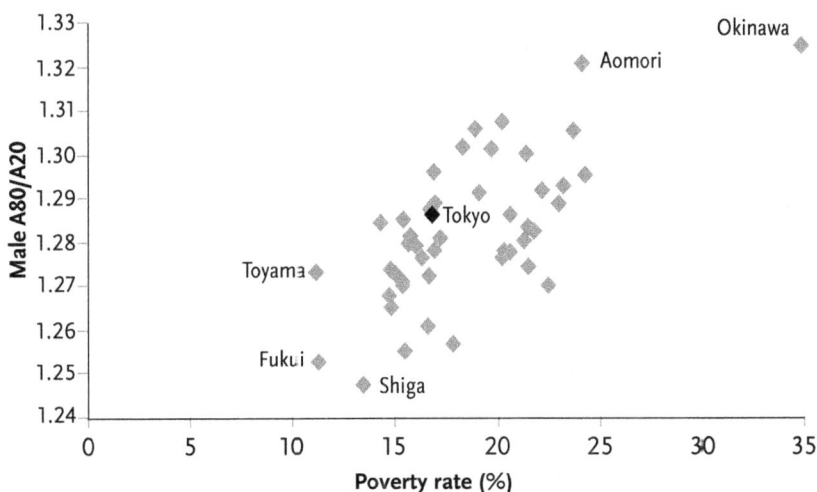

SOURCE: Authors' analysis of data from Japanese Vital Statistics, Human Mortality Database, and Tomuro (2016).

FIGURE 2.5B Regional income in Korean provinces and inequality in age-of-death, 2008, 2011, 2014, and 2017

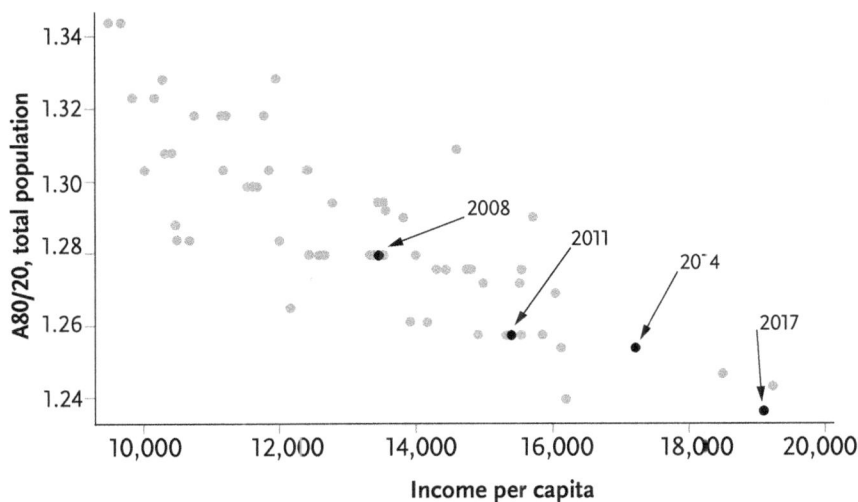

SOURCE: Statistics Korea, "Life Tables by Province of 2008, 2011, 2014, 2017."
NOTE: Seoul is represented by the four dark dots.

and Schwandt 2016).[7]

Correlates of AOD inequality
across regions within Korea and Japan

In this section, we describe the association between various potential predictor variables and inequality in AOD across regions within Asia's two OECD countries, Korea and Japan. Table 2.4a shows the results for Korea. Higher income, and lower male smoking, are correlates of higher A20 and lower A80/A20 across provinces. The Pearson correlation coefficient between male smoking and male A20 is -0.6, almost twice the value Chetty et al. (2016) report for the U.S. correlation between smoking and life expectancy in the top income quartile. Other patterns are less easy to interpret, given the strong correlations among SES markers; for example, obesity (which is correlated with higher female A20) is higher among high-SES women in Korea.

Table 2.4b explores what area characteristics are correlates of AOD inequality for Japan's 47 prefectures in 2010. Among Japanese men, those in the bottom 20 percent of the survival distribution survive to a higher age (A20), and inequality in AOD (A80/A20) is lower, in prefectures with fewer smokers, fewer overweight people, more college graduates, a lower percentage of people in poverty or relying on government assistance, and lower unemployment. The Gini index of income inequality in a prefecture is not a statistically significant univariate correlate of prefecture-level AOD inequality (as measured by A80/A20). Similar patterns are observed for women, but with fewer significant correlates of AOD inequality than for men; interestingly, AOD inequality among women is lower in prefectures with a larger share of rural residents, suggesting that rural residence may be protective of survival (higher female A20, lower A80/A20), or that selective migration/urbanization is more pronounced in shaping the survival distribution among women than men in Japan. These results are consistent with those of Nomura et al. (2017); the two leading behavioral risk factors in Japan in 2015 were unhealthy diets and tobacco smoking.

---

7   Other potentially important correlates of AOD inequality include other SES markers, such as education, and details about communities and geography, such as urban/rural residence, population density, percentage of immigrants, regional or local unemployment rates, and local policies that may mediate pathways between AOD and individual or household characteristics (such as policies regarding income support, nutrition, health care and insurance, and other social spending). We provide exploratory analyses with a few of these variables across Japanese prefectures and Korean provinces.

TABLE 2.4A Correlation between province characteristics and measures of inequality in age-of-death in Korea, 2008, 2011, 2014, and 2017

	Total A20	Total A80/A20	Male A20	Male A80/A20	Female A20	Female A80/A20
Income per capita	0.8713*	−0.8351*	0.8699*	−0.8080*	0.7551*	−0.8123*
GRDP per capita	0.2880*	−0.3404*	0.3038*	−0.3937*	0.2786*	−0.4445*
Unemployment rate‡	0.3206*	−0.4959*	0.3613*	−0.4447*	0.0733	−0.1975
Male smokers†	−0.5587*	0.5316*	−0.6180*	0.5438*	—	—
Obesity	0.3753*	−0.0573	0.2899	−0.0452	0.6019*	−0.2071
Population density	0.3836*	−0.4298*	0.3988*	−0.3421*	0.205	−0.2561

SOURCES: Statistics Korea, "Life Tables by Province of 2008, 2011, 2014, 2017."
NOTE: GRDP = gross regional domestic product; *Pearson correlation, 5 percent significance; †current smoking rate available only for males; ‡unemployment rate available for both males and females.

In a multivariate framework, several of the same correlates remain statistically significant, including the association of population density with greater AOD inequality (now for men as well as women; results not shown).[8]

Discussion

The challenge of healthy aging involves not only increasing average survival, but also addressing inequality in survival and quality of life. In this chapter, we have focused on inequality in AOD to measure disparities in three high-income East Asian countries and the United States compared with other OECD countries.

Many previous studies have focused on the increase over time in average AOD, not its distribution. Some economists have estimated a high value of such improvements in survival for a representative consumer. See, for example, the estimates put forward by Murphy and Topel (2006) of the present value of a longer life for a representative American, based on expected lifetime utility, with the value of non-market time included. Such studies make no

8   Rather counterintuitively, the Gini index is statistically significant in the multivariate framework but negatively correlated with AOD inequality (i.e., controlling for poverty, education, unemployment, etc., a wider income distribution is associated with less AOD inequality). In other words, attributes of some prefectures such as Tokyo are such that survival is more equal than other prefectures even though income inequality is higher, similar to the finding highlighted by Chetty et al. (2016) that life expectancy among males in the lowest quartile of income varies across localities and is often higher in localities with substantial income inequality.

TABLE 2.4B Correlation between Japanese prefecture characteristics and measures of inequality in age-of-death, 2010

	Male A20		Female A20		Male A80/A20		Female A80/A20	
	Coeff.	95% CI	Coeff.	95% CI	Coeff.	95% CI	Coeff.	95% CI
% smokers[*]	-0.413	-0.626 -0.143	-0.152	-0.421 0.141	0.355	0.076 0.583	0.091	-0.202 0.368
% overweight[†]	-0.679	-0.809 -0.487	-0.477	-0.672 -0.22	0.67	0.474 0.803	0.529	0.285 0.708
% college graduates	0.374	0.097 0.597	-0.034	-0.318 0.256	-0.329	-0.563 -0.047	-0.022	-0.307 0.267
% rural pop	-0.012	-0.299 0.276	0.296	0.009 0.537	-0.016	-0.301 0.273	-0.288	-0.531 -0.001
pop density	-0.069	-0.349 0.223	-0.28	-0.525 0.008	0.089	-0.203 0.367	0.279	-0.009 0.524
GPP per capita[‡]	-0.017	-0.303 0.271	-0.123	-0.396 0.17	0.043	-0.247 0.326	0.092	-0.201 0.369
% poverty rate[§]	-0.597	-0.755 -0.374	-0.179	-0.443 0.114	0.671	0.475 0.803	0.468	0.209 0.666
% on assistance	-0.572	-0.738 -0.341	-0.394	-0.612 -0.12	0.629	0.417 0.776	0.609	0.39 0.763
Gini index	-0.32	-0.556 -0.036	-0.241	-0.494 0.049	0.265	-0.024 0.513	0.222	-0.069 0.479
Unemployment rate	-0.677	-0.807 -0.484	-0.349	-0.578 -0.069	0.697	0.513 0.82	0.506	0.256 0.693
Unemployment rate (by gender)	-0.665	-0.799 -0.466	-0.437	-0.644 -0.172	0.682	0.491 0.81	0.57	0.338 0.736

SOURCES: Japanese government statistics (http://www.stat.go.jp, http://www.mhlw.go.jp); Tomuro 2016; see text and chapter by Hashimoto and Eggleston for additional sources.

NOTE: [*]Male smoking rate only available for those ages 20 and over; [†]male overweight rate available only for ages 20–69; [‡]gross prefectural product; [§]Tomuro 2016; Coeff. = coefficient; CI = confidence interval.

attempt to measure the utility gain from a decrease in the *variation* in AOD, or reduced uncertainty regarding length of life, although they do suggest that the value of such a change would be substantial for any reasonable monetary value assumed for a quality-adjusted life-year.[9] Murphy and Topel (2006) estimate that cumulative gains in life expectancy after 1900 were worth over US$1.2 million to the representative American in 2000. If that estimate were applied to the gains in survival at the bottom of the distribution (e.g., A20), and to all the other countries with similar or greater gains in survival over the past century, such as Korea, Japan, and Singapore, the monetary value would be orders of magnitude more impressive. The remaining inequality in AOD across and within countries points to the large welfare improvements possible from policies focused on helping those most disadvantaged.

Previous literature on differences in AOD has often focused on average AOD within specific groups classified according to SES. Numerous empirical studies document that individuals with higher income generally enjoy better health and survival—a relationship known as the SES gradient—across a wide range of health status indicators, as measured in different countries and at different points of time (Marmot et al. 1991; Hurt, Ronsmans, and Saha 2004; Khang, Lynch, and Kaplan 2004; Lleras-Muney 2005; Cutler, Deaton, and Lleras-Muney 2006; Cutler and Lleras-Muney 2008; Marmot et al. 2008; Kim and Ruger 2010; Stringhini et al. 2010; Heckman et al. 2014; Chen et al. 2016 for China). Both theory (e.g., Becker 1962, 2009) and empirical research confirm that the SES-survival relationship reflects causality both from income to health and vice versa (Fuchs 2004). For example, in multiple studies of the educational gradient in mortality, causality runs both from health to schooling and vice versa, with part of the correlation explained by income (Grossman 1972; Preston 1975; Fuchs 1992, 2004; Deaton 2006; Cutler, Deaton, and Lleras-Muney 2006; Lleras-Muney 2005; Mazumder 2008; Clark and Royer 2013).

Studies of inequality of AOD have become more numerous in recent years, focusing primarily on widening disparities in AOD across income and

---

9   Despite accusations that economists unfairly "price the priceless"—with the value of survival gains depending directly on lifetime earnings and the associated value of leisure—it should be noted that Murphy and Topel's estimations impute to the poor and to the rich the income of the average. Similarly, Murphy and Topel (2006) use the same value of a life-year for men and women when valuing gains across the twentieth century, although clearly the lifetime earnings of women were much smaller than for men during most of that century. Thus, the technique can be used to value survival gains for the poor or those without a market wage, assuming the same lifetime earnings as a comparator, and need not make the assumption that lives of the poor are worth less than those of the better off because the latter have greater ability to pay for survival.

education classes and their implications for policy (e.g., National Academy of Sciences 2015; Chetty et al. 2016). We focus on inequality in AOD in three Asian countries, illustrating their rapid demographic and epidemiologic transitions that compress many socioeconomic processes into only two or three generations. Their rapid declines in AOD inequality represent an achievement of healthy aging meriting study and emulation.

Salient preventable causes of premature mortality remain, of course. Heavy smoking among men contributes to the socioeconomic disparity in health in all three East Asian countries. There also are large health disparities within the population of older adults, suggesting the need to focus on effective policies for healthy aging. For example, in Korea, there is a significant gradient in the prevalence of hypertension by SES. A socioeconomic gradient in health is also evident for diabetes prevalence (Kim 2018). As noted, Korean men still smoke heavily despite a recent decline, and disparities widen with age because higher SES men are more likely to quit smoking as they age.

Our study complements several within demography that highlight differences between average AOD and dispersion in AOD across countries. For example, Gillespie, Trotter, and Tuljapurkar (2014), measuring life-span inequality by the variance in AOD (and for main analyses, focusing on AOD among adults, 15 and older), find that differences among countries in life-span inequality appear to be linked to stagnation in mortality decline among young and middle-aged men.[10] Seligman, Greenberg, and Tuljapurkar (2016) further show that the causes of death that contributed most to declines in the variance in AOD (e.g., causes most prominent for children and young adults) are different from those that contributed most to increases in average life expectancy.

A question naturally arises as to whether any future additional years of life gained will be healthy years or instead be marred by increasing disability and morbidity. Fries (1980, 1996) developed the "compression of morbidity" hypothesis, envisioning a compression of morbidity between an increasing age of onset of disability and the age of death. Many scholars have studied the compression of morbidity in high-income countries (e.g., Crimmins and Beltran-Sanchez 2010) including in Asia (e.g., Lee, Lee, and Mason 2016; Jeon and Kwon 2017), often finding evidence of compression. However, a countervailing factor might arise from medical interventions that reduce mortality among those in the worst health (Zeckhauser, Sato, and Rizzo 1985),

---

10   Moreover, analysis of the young-old threshold age, below and above which mortality decline respectively decreases and increases life-span inequality, suggests that mortality change among working-aged adults, especially men, will determine whether life-span inequality will decrease or increase as life expectancy continues to increase. Gillespie et al. (2014) argue that we may be entering an era of rising life-span inequality.

which suggests the possibility that the longer-lived elderly could be sicker for a longer period. The net effect of rising longevity on age-specific morbidity is an empirical question that deserves study (Eggleston and Fuchs 2012).

Among the many research questions that should be of high priority for the future, rigorous work on trends in the "compression of morbidity" across countries and socioeconomic contexts ranks highly. Such research would contribute to a better understanding of this important component of well-being across diverse societies and populations. Using years before death rather than before birth could be one retrospective measure used to highlight the importance of quality of life at the end of life (Fuchs 2018). Evidence, and policies supported by that evidence, should address healthy aging by focusing on reducing causes of premature mortality and improving quality of life (Fuchs 2018). As Fuchs and Eggleston (2018) note, "preventing a death at age 25 or 35 will have more effect on life expectancy and inequality than preventing a death at 65 or 75." Policies should emphasize further enhancing maternal and child health, reducing smoking, preventing accidents, including on the road, and fostering life-long habits of resiliency and social connectedness for longer work-lives and healthy aging.

References

Alsan, Marcella, and Claudia Goldin. 2019. "Watersheds in Child Mortality: The Role of Effective Water and Sewerage Infrastructure, 1880–1920." *Journal of Political Economy* 127 (2): 586–638.

Becker, Gary S. 1962. "Investment in Human Capital: A Theoretical Analysis." *Journal of Political Economy* 70 (5, Part 2): 9–49.

Becker, Gary S. 2009. *Human Capital: A Theoretical and Empirical Analysis, with Special Reference to Education.* Chicago: University of Chicago Press.

Becker, Gary S., Tomas J. Philipson, and Rodrigo R. Soares. 2005. "The Quantity and Quality of Life and the Evolution of World Inequality." *American Economic Review* 95 (1): 277–91.

Case, Anne, and Angus Deaton. 2015. "Rising Morbidity and Mortality in Midlife among White Non-Hispanic Americans in the 21st Century." *Proceedings of the National Academy of Sciences* 112 (49): 15078–83.

Catillon, Maryaline, David Cutler, and Thomas Getzen. 2018. "Two Hundred Years of Health and Medical Care: The Importance of Medical Care for Life Expectancy Gains." NBER Working Paper No. 25330, National Bureau of Economic Research, Cambridge, MA.

Chen, Brian K., Hawre Jalal, Hideki Hashimoto, Sze-chuan Suen, Karen Eggleston, Michael Hurley, Lena Schoemaker, and Jay Bhattacharya. 2016. "Forecasting Trends in Disability in a Super-Aging Society: Adapting the Future Elderly Model to Japan." *The Journal of the Economics of Ageing* 8: 42–51.

Chen, Qiulin, Karen Eggleston, Wei Zhang, Jiaying Zhao, and Sen Zhou. 2017. "The Educational Gradient in Health in China." *China Quarterly* 230: 289–322.

Chetty, Raj, Michael Stepner, Sarah Abraham, Shelby Lin, Benjamin Scuderi, Nicholas Turner, Augustin Bergeron, and David Cutler. 2016. "The Association Between Income and Life Expectancy in the United States, 2001-2014." *Jama* 315 (16): 1750–66.

Clark, Damon, and Heather Royer. 2013. "The Effect of Education on Adult Mortality and Health: Evidence from Britain." *American Economic Review* 103 (6): 2087–120.

Costa, Dora L. 2015. "Health and the Economy in the United States from 1750 to the Present." *Journal of Economic Literature* 53 (3): 503–70.

Crimmins, Eileen M., and Hiram Beltrán-Sánchez. 2010. "Mortality and Morbidity Trends: Is There Compression of Morbidity?" *Journals of*

Gerontology Series B: Psychological Sciences and Social Sciences 66
(1): 75–86.

Currie, Janet, and Hannes Schwandt. 2016. "Mortality Inequality: The
Good News from a County-Level Approach." *Journal of Economic
Perspectives* 30 (2): 29–52.

Cutler, David, and Grant Miller. 2005. "The Role of Public Health
Improvements in Health Advances: The Twentieth-Century United
States." *Demography* 42 (1): 1–22.

Cutler, David, and Adriana Lleras-Muney. 2008. "Education and Health:
Evaluating Theories and Evidence." In *Making Americans Health-
ier: Social and Economic Policy as Health Policy*, edited by Robert F.
Schoeni, James S. House, George A. Kaplan, and Harold Pollack. New
York: Russell Sage Foundation.

Cutler, David, Angus Deaton, and Adriana Lleras-Muney. 2006. "The
Determinants of Mortality." *Journal of Economic Perspectives* 20 (3):
97–120.

Deaton, Angus. 2006. "The Great Escape: A Review of Robert Fogel's
The Escape from Hunger and Premature Death, 1700-2100." *Journal
of Economic Literature* 44 (1): 106–14.

Edwards, Ryan D. 2011. "Changes in World Inequality in Length of Life:
1970–2000." *Population and Development Review* 37 (3): 499–528.

Edwards, Ryan D., and Shripad Tuljapurkar. 2005. "Inequality in Life
Spans and a New Perspective on Mortality Convergence Across
Industrialized Countries." *Population and Development Review* 31 (4):
645–74.

Eggleston, Karen N., and Anita Mukherjee. 2019. "Financing Longevity:
The Economics of Pensions, Health, and Long-Term Care—Introduction to the Special Issue." *The Journal of the Economics of Ageing* 13:
1–6.

Eggleston, Karen N., and Victor R. Fuchs. 2012. "The New Demographic
Transition: Most Gains in Life Expectancy Now Realized Late in Life."
Journal of Economic Perspectives 26 (3): 137–56.

Fleurbaey, Marc. 2009. "Beyond GDP: The Quest for a Measure of Social
Welfare." *Journal of Economic Literature* 47 (4): 1029–75.

Fries, James F. 1980. "Aging, Natural Death, and the Compression of
Morbidity." *New England Journal of Medicine* 303 (3): 130–35.

Fries, James F. 1996. "Physical Activity, the Compression of Morbidity,
and the Health of the Elderly." *Journal of the Royal Society of Medicine* 89 (2): 64–68.

Fuchs, Victor R. 1992. "Poverty and Health: Asking the Right Questions." *The American Economist* 36 (2): 12–18.

Fuchs, Victor R. 2004. "Reflections on the Socio-Economic Correlates of Health." *Journal of Health Economics* 23 (4): 653–61.

Fuchs, Victor R. 2006. *The Rise of Income Inequality in the United States, 1978-2001*. Stanford Institute for Economic Policy Research Policy Brief, Stanford.

Fuchs, Victor R. 2011. *Who Shall Live?: Health, Economics and Social Choice Second Edition Expanded*. World Scientific Publishing Company.

Fuchs, Victor R. 2016. "Black Gains in Life Expectancy." *Jama* 316 (18): 1869–70.

Fuchs, Victor R. 2018. *Health Economics and Policy: Selected Writings by Victor Fuchs*. World Scientific Publishing Co. Pte. Ltd.

Fuchs, Victor R., and Karen Eggleston. 2018. *Life Expectancy and Inequality in Life Expectancy in the United States*. Stanford Institute for Economic Policy Research Policy Brief, Stanford.

Gillespie, Duncan OS, Meredith V. Trotter, and Shripad D. Tuljapurkar. 2014. "Divergence in Age Patterns of Mortality Change Drives International Divergence in Lifespan Inequality." *Demography* 51 (3): 1003–17.

Grossman, Michael. 1972. "On the Concept of Health Capital and the Demand for Health." *Journal of Political Economy* 80 (2): 223–55.

Heckman, James J., John Eric Humphries, Greg Veramendi, and Sergio S. Urzua. 2014. "Education, Health and Wages." NBER Working Paper No. w19971, National Bureau of Economic Research, Cambridge, MA.

Hurt, Lisa, Carine Ronsmans, and Sajal Saha. 2004. "Effects of Education and Other Socioeconomic Factors on Middle Age Mortality in Rural Bangladesh." *Journal of Epidemiology and Community Health* 58 (4): 315–20.

Jeon, Boyoung, and Soonman Kwon. 2017. "Health and Long-Term Care Systems for Older People in the Republic of Korea: Policy Challenges and Lessons." *Health Systems & Reform* 3 (3): 214–23.

Jones, Charles I., and Jihee Kim. 2018. "A Schumpeterian Model of Top Income Inequality." *Journal of Political Economy* 126 (5): 1785–826.

Jones, Charles I., and Peter J. Klenow. 2016. "Beyond GDP? Welfare Across Countries and Time." *American Economic Review* 106 (9): 2426–57.

Khang, Young-Ho, John Lynch, and George Kaplan. 2004. "Health Inequalities in Korea: Age- and Sex-Specific Educational Differences in the 10 Leading Causes of Death." *International Journal of Epidemiology* 33 (2): 299–308.

Kim, Daejung, Jay Bhattacharya, Karen Eggleston, Bryan Tysinger, and M. Zhao. 2018. "Impacts of Smoking Interventions on the Chronic Disease Burden of South Korea's Future Elderly: Adapting the Future Elderly Model to South Korea." Forthcoming.

Kim, Daejung. 2018. "Impact of Inequality on the Future Elderly in South Korea." Presentation at the OECD conference in Inequality of Ageing, April 5, 2018, Paris.

Kim, Hak-Ju, and Jennifer Prah Ruger. 2010. "Socioeconomic Disparities in Behavioral Risk Factors and Health Outcomes by Gender in the Republic of Korea." *BMC Public Health* 10 (1): 195.

Lee, Ronald, Sang-Hyop Lee, and Andrew Mason. 2016. " 'Introduction' for Special Issue of Journal of the Economics of Aging Titled 'The Demographic Dividend and Population Aging in Asia and the Pacific.'" *Journal of the Economics of Ageing*: 1–4.

Lee, Ronald. 2003. "The Demographic Transition: Three Centuries of Fundamental Change." *Journal of Economic Perspectives* 17 (4): 167–90.

Lleras-Muney, Adriana. 2005. "The Relationship Between Education and Adult Mortality in the United States." *Review of Economic Studies* 72 (1): 189–221.

Marmot, Michael G., Stephen Stansfeld, Chandra Patel, Fiona North, Jenny Head, Ian White, Eric Brunner, Amanda Feeney, and G. Davey Smith. 1991. "Health Inequalities among British Civil Servants: The Whitehall II Study." *The Lancet* 337 (8754): 1387–93.

Marmot, Michael, Sharon Friel, Ruth Bell, Tanja AJ Houweling, Sebastian Taylor, and Commission on Social Determinants of Health. 2008. "Closing the Gap in a Generation: Health Equity through Action on the Social Determinants of Health." *The Lancet* 372 (9650): 1661–69.

Mazumder, Bhashkar. 2008. "Does Education Improve Health? A Reexamination of the Evidence from Compulsory Schooling Laws. *Economic Perspectives* 32 (2): 2–17.

Meara, Ellen R., Seth Richards, and David M. Cutler. 2008. "The Gap Gets Bigger: Changes in Mortality and Life Expectancy, by Education, 1981–2000." *Health Affairs* 27 (2): 350–60.

Murphy, Kevin M., and Robert H. Topel. 2006. "The Value of Health and Longevity." *Journal of Political Economy* 114 (5): 871–904.

National Academies of Sciences, Engineering, and Medicine. 2015. *The Growing Gap in Life Expectancy by Income: Implications for Federal*

Programs and Policy Responses. Washington, DC: The National Academies Press.

Nomura, Shuhei, Haruka Sakamoto, Scott Glenn, Yusuke Tsugawa, Sarah K Abe, Md M. Rahman, Jonathan C. Brown, et al. 2017. "Population Health and Regional Variations of Disease Burden in Japan, 1990–2015: A Systematic Subnational Analysis for the Global Burden of Disease Study." 2015. *The Lancet* 390 (10101): 1521–38.

Pickett, Kate E., and Richard G. Wilkinson. 2015. "Income Inequality and Health: A Causal Review." *Social Science & Medicine* 128: 316–26.

Piketty, Thomas, and Emmanuel Saez. 2014. "Inequality in the Long Run." *Science* 344 (6186): 838–43.

Piketty, Thomas. 2014. *Capital in the 21st Century.* Harvard University Press.

Preston, Samuel H. 1975. "The Changing Relation between Mortality and Level of Economic Development." *Population Studies* 29 (2): 231–48.

Seligman, Benjamin, Gabi Greenberg, and Shripad Tuljapurkar. 2016. "Equity and Length of Lifespan Are Not the Same." *Proceedings of the National Academy of Sciences* 113 (30): 8420–23.

Statistics Korea. "Life Tables." Accessed December 1, 2019. http://kosis.kr/statHtml/statHtml.do?orgId=101&tblId=DT_1B42&vw_cd=MT_ZTITLE&list_id=A5&seqNo=&lang_mode=ko&language=kor&obj_var_id=&itm_id=&conn_path=MT_ZTITLE.

Statistics Korea. "Life Tables By Province." Accessed December 1, 2019. http://kosis.kr/statHtml/statHtml.do?orgId=101&tblId=DT_1B44&vw_cd=MT_ZTITLE&list_id=A5&seqNo=&lang_mode=ko&language=kor&obj_var_id=&itm_id=&conn_path=MT_ZTITLE.

Stringhini, Silvia, Séverine Sabia, Martin Shipley, Eric Brunner, Hermann Nabi, Mika Kivimaki, and Archana Singh-Manoux. 2010. "Association of Socioeconomic Position with Health Behaviors and Mortality." *Jama* 303 (12): 1159–66.

Tomuro, Kensaku 戸室健作. 2016. "都道府県別の貧困率, ワーキングプア率, 子どもの貧困率, 捕捉率の検討" [Trends observed in poverty rates, working poor rates, child poverty rates and take-up rates of public assistance across 47 prefectures in Japan.] 山形大学人文学部年報 [Yamagata University Faculty of Humanities annual report] no.13. https://www-hs.yamagata-u.ac.jp/wp-content/uploads/2017/10/nen-pou13_03.pdf.

World Economic Forum. 2015. *Outlook on the Global Agenda 2015.* http://reports.weforum.org/outlook-global-agenda-2015.

Zeckhauser, Richard J., Ryuzo Sato, and John Rizzo. 1985. "Hidden Heterogeneity in Risk: Evidence from Japanese Mortality." *Health Intervention and Population Heterogeneity: Evidence from Japan and the United States* 26 (3): 137–56.

Zuo, Wenyun, Sha Jiang, Zhen Guo, Marcus W. Feldman, and Shripad Tuljapurkar. 2018. "Advancing Front of Old-Age Human Survival." *Proceedings of the National Academy of Sciences* 115 (44): 11209–14.

3 Healthy Aging and Economic Research on the Net Value of Noncommunicable Disease Management in Japan

Chiyo Hashimoto and Karen Eggleston

Japan's population has the oldest age structure of any country in the history of the world, and population aging and decline will continue for at least the next few decades. Accordingly, Japan epitomizes the challenges societies face in adjusting social institutions to a much older age structure.

While Japan has achieved strong health outcomes, its disease and disability burden will continue to increase in the foreseeable future due to aging. Both medical and long-term care spending are projected to increase continuously into the future. With a rapidly aging and declining overall population, and specifically a shrinking working-age population, ensuring financial sustainability of the health insurance and long-term care systems requires careful economic analysis and adjustment. The growth of regional health disparities also spurs concern.

To address this formidable challenge of financing and providing services to an aging population, multiple arenas of research can provide vital inputs for decision-making. For example, economic analysis can help assess financing options and the cost-effectiveness of different approaches to promoting healthy aging. Demography and epidemiology contribute important methods for assessing trends and projecting future scenarios. Chapters 4 and 5 provide examples of different and complementary approaches to Japan's policies for healthy aging, from precision health to personalized medicine.

In this chapter, we first briefly describe Japan's policies for prevention and control of noncommunicable diseases (NCDs), which account for 82 percent of deaths in Japan. The burden of NCDs is expected to increase with aging. Aiming to reduce the NCD burden, the Japanese government implemented policies for healthy aging starting in 2001 under the rubric of "Healthy Japan 21" (referred to as "Health Japan 21" in official policy documents).

This plan, now in its second iteration (2013–22), focuses on primary and secondary prevention through lifestyle improvements and changes to social environments (Terahara 2015). To provide illustrative policy detail, we focus on a few specific programs for addressing prominent risk factors: tobacco control, and screening for metabolic syndrome, diabetes, and cancer.

Second, we provide an overview of recent empirical research on policies and programs to promote healthy aging, the cost of NCDs, and the "value for money" in chronic disease management, especially for the most prevalent and costly chronic diseases such as hypertension and diabetes. We end with a brief discussion.

Population Aging and Chronic Disease in Japan

Japan is aging rapidly and its population is shrinking.[1] The share of its population aged 65 and over is expected to increase from 26.6 % in 2015 to 31.2% in 2030 and 38.1% in 2060, while the share of its working-age population aged 15–64 is projected to decrease from 60.8% in 2015 to 57.7% in 2030 and 51.6% in 2060[2] (National Institute of Population and Social Security Research 2017).

Japan has consistently achieved top-ranked health outcomes as measured by many health indicators such as life expectancy and age-adjusted mortality rate. Table 3.1 shows Japan fares better than the average in member countries of the Organisation for Economic Co-operation and Development (OECD) across all indicators related to health outcomes (OECD 2017a). The average life expectancy is projected to further increase to 82.39 years for men and 88.72 years for women by 2030 (Cabinet Office 2018).[3] Meanwhile, due to population aging, Japan's burden of disease and disability is also expected to increase.[4] Chen et al. (2016) project a large increase in the disability burden among elderly people, showing the simulation result that over 27 percent of Japan's elderly will face some limitations in the activities of daily living by 2040. The government thus set a goal of extending *healthy* life expectancy more than the increase in life expectancy by 2022, in Healthy Japan 21.

---

1   Japan's population is expected to shrink from 127,095,000 in 2015 to 119,125,000 in 2030 and 92,840,000 in 2060.

2   Medium-fertility and medium-mortality is assumed.

3   Japan's healthy life expectancy is 71.19 years for men and 74.21 years for women in 2013.

4   Kasajima et al. (2019) project the population health distribution for Japan using a pseudo-panel method.

TABLE 3.1 Health outcomes, Japan vs. OECD average, 2015

	Japan	OECD average
Life expectancy at birth, total	83.9	80.6
Male	80.8	77.9
Female	87.1	83.1
Life expectancy at 65, total	21.9	19.5
Ischemic heart disease mortality*	34.0	112.0
Cancer mortality*	176.6	203.7
All cancers incidence*	217.1	270.5
Share of adults with diabetes[†]	5.7	7.0
Adult population smoking daily[‡]	18.2	18.4
Recorded alcohol consumption among adults[§]	7.2	9.0
Obesity (measured, BMI>30)[‡]	3.7	19.4
Overweight (measured, BMI≥25)[‡]	20.1	34.5

SOURCE: OECD 2017a.
NOTE: *Age-standardized rate per 100 000 population; [†] those aged between 20 and 79 years with Type 1 or Type 2 diagnosed diabetes; [‡] percent of population aged 15 years and over; [§] in liters per capita (15 years and older). BMI = body mass index.

In addition to the extension of healthy life expectancy, a reduction in health disparities among prefectures is one of the main goals of Healthy Japan 21. Despite achieving strong health outcomes, Japan faces the growth of health disparities in several forms, including regional variation in the disease burden among prefectures (Nomura et al. 2017).[5] For example, life expectancy at birth increased by 4.2 years between 1990 and 2015, but the gaps between prefectures with the lowest and highest life expectancies widened from 2.5 to 3.1 years (Nomura et al. 2017). Many of the indicators related to cancer, such as the age-adjusted mortality rate and incidence rate, also vary widely between prefectures (Foundation for Promotion of Cancer Research 2018). The government promotes developing health policies at the prefecture level, which can address region-specific health issues and meet the health needs of local residents.

Also, rising healthcare expenditure has been a major policy concern. Japan's healthcare expenditure as a share of gross domestic product (GDP) has been above the OECD average since 2009 (figure 3.1), as its pace of spending growth has been quicker than that of other OECD countries, partly due to rapid growth in pharmaceutical spending amid rapid aging and the increasing prevalence of NCDs (OECD 2015, 2017b). In 2017, Japan's health spending

5 Fullman et al. (2018) show that the regional variation of personal healthcare access and quality has narrowed in Japan.

per person was estimated at US$4,717, above the OECD average of $4,069, and spending as a share of GDP was estimated at 10.7 percent, higher than the OECD average of 8.9 percent (OECD 2018).

FIGURE 3.1 Healthcare expenditure in Japan and OECD 35, 2003–16

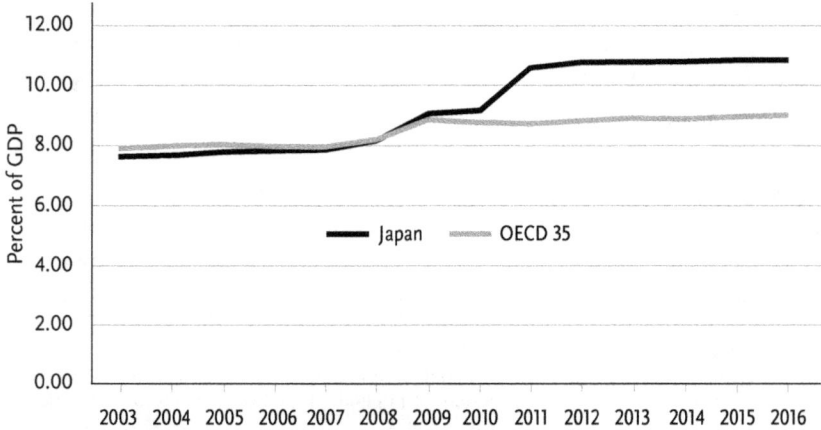

SOURCE: OECD 2017a.

With this increasing health spending and rapid aging, ensuring the financial sustainability of Japan's health system requires urgent policy action. Unami (2018) points out that the large increase in population aged 75 and over in the next 10 years will further increase the heavy financial burden on the social security system in Japan, because the per-capita cost of medical and long-term care increases significantly with age after the mid-70s. The Japanese government has updated a projection of social security costs and their financing (MHLW 2018b). Figure 3.2a shows the projection result, assuming business as usual (i.e., without reform). Both medical and long-term care benefit expenses[6] are expected to increase continuously into the future. Figure 3.2b shows the projection of financing. Both government subsidies and insurance contributions would need to be raised to finance increasing medical and long-term care benefit expenses.[7]

---

6   Benefit expenses do not include patient copayment.

7   In Japan, medical care and long-term care costs are financed by government subsidies, premium contributions, and patient copayments. For national medical spending in FY2016, around half of the expenditure was paid through premium contributions (49.1%), with the remainder financed by government subsidies (38.6%) and patient copayments (11.5%). Long-term care spending has a statutory rule for splitting its financing: 45% by government subsidies, 45% by premium contributions, and 10% by patient copayments.

FIGURE 3.2A Japan's FY2018 medical and long-term care benefit expenses, projected to FY2025 and FY2040

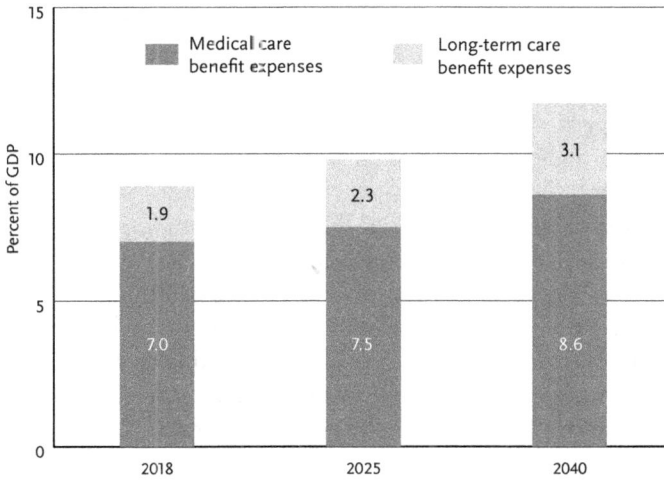

SOURCE: MHLW 2018b.
NOTE: Medical care benefit expenses in 2040 are projected to be 8.6–8.9 percent of GDP, depending on the assumption of the growth rate of per-capita cost by service.

FIGURE 3.2B Japan's FY2018 financing of medical and long-term care benefit expenses, projected to FY2025 and FY2040

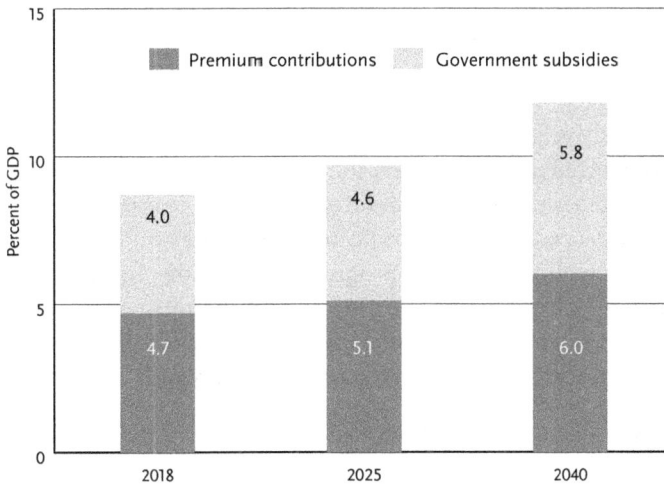

SOURCE: MHLW 2018b.
NOTE: Premium contributions and government subsidies in 2040 are projected to be 6.0–6.1 percent and 5.8–5.9 percent of GDP respectively, depending on the assumption of the growth rate of per-capita cost by service.

However, such increases would be difficult because Japan has already borne large increases in the financing burden of social security cost increases. For example, the social security expenditure within the national budget tripled between FY1990 and FY2015, whereas the total amount of other policy expenditures stayed almost the same (Unami 2018). Also, the Japanese government spent 23.2 percent of its total expenditures on health in 2015, which was the highest among OECD countries (OECD 2017a). Not only the government but also many non-governmental health insurance societies in Japan have fallen into financial difficulties, spurring mergers, reorganization, and other consolidation. For example, *Asia Insurance Review* (2018) reported that over 40 percent of the 1,394 health insurance societies for employees of large firms and their family members have already been disbanded or started moving toward dissolution due to premium increases and other financial strains. Numerous economic projections reinforce the urgency of Japan's financing challenge. To illustrate, Nozaki, Kashiwase, and Saito (2014) project that the increase in government subsidies for medical and long-term care spending in the period 2010–30 would be equivalent to raising the consumption tax rate by 7 percent.[8] Also, several studies project a large and growing inter-generational inequity in the burden of social security spending, with heavier burdens on the younger generations (Tajika and Kikuchi 2004; Fukui and Iwamoto 2007; Suzuki et al. 2012).

Despite some decline in the age- and sex-specific disease burden from NCDs during the past decades (Ikeda et al. 2011; Sakamoto et al. 2018), the number of deaths attributable to NCDs still accounts for 82 percent (an estimated 1,072,000 people) in Japan. Also, the pace of reduction in the mortality rate from NCDs has leveled off since 2005 (Nomura et al. 2017).[9] As the incidence of NCDs is expected to increase with continued aging, the government urgently needs to implement health policies to prevent and control NCDs.

Consider, for example, the case of one complex and costly chronic disease, diabetes mellitus. Given its progression to serious complications, some projections consider diabetes will be one of the most costly diseases for Japan among the prevalent chronic diseases, such as cardiovascular diseases (CVDs), cancer, respiratory diseases, and mental health conditions (Bloom

---

8   Nozaki, Kashiwase, and Saito (2014) and Ueda, Horiuchi, and Tsutui (2011) project that the share of government subsidies would be higher than that of premium contributions for financing Japan's health spending in the future. Ueda, Horiuchi, and Tsutui (2011) obtain the result that the ratio of government subsidies will increase and exceed premium contributions in the 2020s.

9   Gilmour et al. (2014) and Iso (2011) point out that the large decline in high blood pressure and smoking would contribute to better controlling NCDs.

et al. 2017). In spite of good control of diabetes in recent years (Charvat et al. 2015; Ikeda et al. 2017), Japan's healthcare expenditure (US$28 million) on its 7.2 million people with diabetes aged 20–79 ranked fifth highest worldwide (International Diabetes Federation 2017). Despite a reduction in age-specific incidence, the disease's overall prevalence may continue to rise as the proportion of oldest-old increases, since incidence increases with age. Therefore, it is not surprising that the prevalence of diabetes is expected to increase in Japan, mainly due to aging (Charvat et al. 2015). The International Diabetes Federation (2017) predicts diabetes prevalence in Japan will be 8.3 percent in 2045, an increase of 0.6 percentage points from 2017. Those with the highest risk of diabetes in Japan are older men, reflecting men's less favorable profiles of risk factors and lifestyle habits such as body mass index, blood pressure, tobacco smoking, and alcohol drinking (Charvat et al. 2015; Ikeda et al. 2017; Goto et al. 2015).

Cancer has been the leading cause of death in Japan since 1981. The age-adjusted mortality rate for cancer has been constantly decreasing in recent years, recording a rate of 161.7 for men and 87.3 for women per 100,000 population in 2016. The total number of cancer deaths was approximately 370,000, which accounts for 28.5 percent of total deaths in 2016 (Foundation for Promotion of Cancer Research 2018). On the other hand, the age-adjusted cancer incidence rate has been increasing for both males and females in all age groups since 1985. The incidence rate, which is the annual number of newly diagnosed cases per 100,000 population, was 805.6 for men and 556.3 for women, and the total number of cancer incidence was approximately 862,000 in 2013 (Foundation for Promotion of Cancer Research 2018). The medical care cost of cancer accounted for 14.1 percent of total national medical expenditure in FY2016.

The mortality from CVDs in Japan is among the lowest in OECD countries (OECD 2017c). However, FY2016 medical spending for CVDs accounted for 19.7 percent of total medical spending—the highest by disease category (MHLW 2018d). Compared with other OECD countries, Japan spends more on circulatory disease per hospital discharge, which could be due to the very long hospital stays the disease requires (OECD 2016).

Chronic obstructive pulmonary disease (COPD) was the tenth leading cause of death in both 1995 and 2015 (Sakamoto et al. 2018). Japan ranks lowest for admissions for asthma and COPD among OECD countries, which suggests primary care is generally of high quality for these diseases (OECD 2017b).

Policies to Promote Healthy Aging and Chronic Disease Control in Japan

Aiming to make its social security system sustainable into the future, the Japanese government is implementing progressive policies to reduce the NCD burden through Healthy Japan 21 (2013–22). Table 3.2 shows examples of numerical goals set by the government to tackle NCD prevalence. The midterm evaluation report of the program points out that although approximately 60 percent of the indicators among prefectures—including extension of healthy life expectancy and reduction of health disparities—improved, the number of people who definitely had or were at risk for metabolic syndrome increased by 120,000 between FY2008 and FY2015, contrary to the goal of reducing that number (MHLW 2018a).

The Japanese government has been developing NCD prevention and control policies.[10] Tobacco control and a screening program for metabolic syndrome would play a primary role. Diabetes management and cancer control programs would be representative examples of secondary prevention.

Tobacco control

Tobacco smoking is one of the main contributors to deaths from NCDs. Tobacco smoking causes an estimated 130,000 deaths in Japan annually, while another 15,000 deaths are associated with secondhand smoke (MHLW 2016). Smoking is strongly associated with the development of diabetes. Akter, Goto, and Mizoue (2017) estimate 18.8 percent of type 2 diabetes cases in men and 5.4 percent of type 2 diabetes cases in women were attributable to smoking. The socioeconomic loss of smoking was estimated at more than ¥2.05 trillion in FY2015 (Kyodo News 2018).

Japan has been reluctant to implement strong tobacco smoking controls[11] despite its relatively high rate of male smoking among developed countries. Notably, in 2017 the adult smoking rate for men fell below 30 percent for the first time since 1986, and the combined share of male and female smokers was 17.7 percent, a reduction partly due to a growing health consciousness

---

10   Ezoe et al. (2017) review the history of health promotion policies to prevent and control NCDs in Japan.

11   The reason that the Japanese government cannot strengthen the tobacco control policy could be related to the fact that the tobacco tax has been one of the most important sources of revenue for the government, which still retains about 33 percent of the stocks of Japan Tobacco (Ikeda et al. 2011; Tsugawa et al. 2017).

TABLE 3.2 Example goals of Healthy Japan 21

Indicators		2010		2022 Goal
Healthy life expectancy	Male	70.42 years		To extend healthy life expectancy more than the increase of life expectancy
	Female	73.62 years		
Healthly life expectancy disparities among prefectures*	Male	2.79 years		To reduce gaps among prefectures
	Female	2.95 years		
Age-adjusted mortality rate of cancer under age 75 (per 100,000)	84.3			73.9*
Participation in cancer screenings	Gastric:	Male	36.6%	50% (40% for gastric, lung, and colorectal cancer)†
		Female	28.3%	
	Lung :	Male	26.4%	
		Female	23.0%	
	Colorectal :	Male	28.1%	
		Female	23.9%	
	Cervical :	Female	37.7%	
	Breast :	Female	39.1%	
Average systolic blood pressure	Male	138 mmHg		Male 134 mmHg
	Female	133 mmHg		Female 129 mmHg
Number of definite and at-risk people with metabolic syndrome	14,000,000‡			25% less than 2008*
Participation rates of specified health checkups and specified health guidance	Checkups: 41.3% Guidance: 12.3%§			Checkups: ≥70% Guidance: ≥45%‖
Number of patients newly introduced to dialysis due to diabetic nephropathy	16,247			15,000
Percent of individuals with elevated blood glucose levels (HbA1c (NGSP) ≥8.4%)	1.2%§			1.0%
Increase in number of diabetic persons	8,900,000#			10,000,000
Recognition of COPD	25%**			80%
Mean salt intake	10.6g			8g
Percent of individuals who consume alcohol over recommended limits††	Male	15.3%		Male 13.0%
	Female	7.5%		Female 6.4%
Adult smoking rate	19.5%			12%

SOURCE: Health Japan 21 (the second term), National Institute of Health and Nutrition, http://www.nibiohn.go.jp/eiken/kenkounippon21/en/kenkounippon21/mokuhyou.html.
NOTE: *Goal is for 2015; †goal is for 2016; ‡2008 data; §2009 data; ‖goal is for 2017; #2007 data; **2011 data; ††recommended daily limits of alcohol consumption: male 40g, female 20g.
COPD = chronic obstructive pulmonary disease.

among people (Japan Times 2018). The World Health Organization (WHO) also projects Japan's adult smoking rate will decrease to 15.6 percent (male 24.3 percent, female 7.5 percent) by 2025 (WHO 2015).

The Japanese government has raised the tobacco tax several times in order to discourage smoking, with notable effects (Yuda 2013; Tabuchi, Fujiwara, and Shinozaki 2016). The Healthy Japan 21 goal for adult smoking prevalence was set at 12 percent by 2022. Also, in July 2018, an amendment was passed that for the first time bans smoking in public facilities (Osaki 2018a). However, smoking is still permitted in smaller restaurants and bars capitalized at ¥50 million or lower and with a floor space of no more than 100 square meters, which would exempt an estimated 55 percent of all eateries. The Tokyo Metropolitan government also passed an anti-smoking ordinance that is stricter than the national version, aiming for a smoke-free 2020 Tokyo Olympics (Osaki 2018b), now postponed to 2021.

Screening program for metabolic syndrome

High blood pressure and obesity are also major NCD risk factors. A mandatory annual checkup[12] for all citizens has played an important role in mitigating these risk factors in Japan. In addition to this basic checkup, in 2008 a screening program for metabolic syndrome, making use of specific health checkups (SHCs) and specific health guidance (SHG), was initiated. All health insurers are required to provide SHCs for their beneficiaries aged 40–74 for the screening of metabolic syndrome risk factors. Based on the results of exams, including such factors as waist size and body mass index (BMI), people who are diagnosed with metabolic syndrome will be urged to receive a series of SHGs (Inui et al. 2017). Health insurers have access to both the health checkup data and the healthcare expenditure data of each insured individual. Each health insurer is expected to use these data to plan effective health interventions in order to maintain their financial stability (Kohro et al. 2008).

However, participation in these screening programs has been limited: 51.4 percent of the target individuals received checkups and 18.8 percent received counseling sessions in 2016, far from the goal set by the government of 70 and 45 percent, respectively. Also, there are huge gaps in participation among insurers and/or insurances. In FY2017, the highest SHC participation rate was 77.9 percent (Mutual Aid Association Insurance) and the lowest was

12   In Japan, all insurers must provide this annual checkup for their insured. The checkup includes a basic examination, with measurement of height and weight, blood pressure, and some other tests.

35.8 percent (seamen's insurance), while the highest SHG participation rate was 25.6 percent (municipality controlled national health insurance) and the lowest was 6.8 percent (seamen's insurance) (MHLW 2018e). To increase participation in these screening programs, the government introduced financial incentives and decided to disclose the participation rate by insurer (MHLW 2018c). Another problem of SHCs and SHGs is a lack of evaluation (Ikeda et al. 2011; Inui et al. 2017). Inui et al. (2017) doubt the efficiency of these checkups, pointing to great regional disparity in their prevalence and its meager improvement during the period 1995–2013. Also, the authors find that SHCs/SHGs have little effect on health status, smoking behavior, and medical expenses. Iizuka et al. (2017) find people respond to health signals by increasing medical care utilization, but no evidence is found that additional care, such as diabetes mellitus–related physician visits for individuals surpassing the checkup thresholds, is cost-effective. Hirakawa and Uemura (2013) show that SHCs/SHGs did not help to improve the health status of rural people with newly diagnosed metabolic conditions. By contrast, Tsushita et al. (2018) conclude that SHC has made a great contribution to preventing metabolic syndrome and its complications.

Diabetes management

While Japan has successfully controlled diabetes for the past decade, there is still room for further improvement. For example, in 2017 Japan ranked seventh highest in the world for the number of people aged 20–79 with impaired glucose tolerance—12 million people, or 12.8 percent prevalence (International Diabetes Federation 2017). Also, a large number of people with diabetes are still left untreated (Ikeda et al. 2017), and an estimated 3.4 million people are undiagnosed (International Diabetes Federation 2017). Regarding the quality of primary care for diabetes, a key factor in diabetes management, OECD (2017c) points out weaknesses in Japan based on the fact that hospital admissions for diabetes are higher than the OECD average. On the other hand, Quan et al. (2017) find Japan had a low proportion of people with diabetes who required inpatient admission and a high rate of outpatient visits, which implies a higher quality of primary care for diabetes in Japan, compared with Singapore, Hong Kong, and communities in rural and peri-urban Beijing.

The Japan Diabetes Society (JDS) provides guidelines for the diagnosis and treatment of diabetes in Japan. It recommends that the initial test measuring hemoglobin A1c (HbA1c) and plasma glucose should be performed for the diagnosis of diabetes. The targets for glycemic control are an HbA1c ≥ 6.5

percent and fasting plasma glucose ≥ 126 mg/dL, or an oral glucose tolerance test 2 hours ≥ 200 mg/dL or random (casual) plasma glucose ≥ 200 mg/dL. The guideline emphasizes the measurement of plasma glucose level for the diagnosis of diabetes, and not solely relying on HbA1c tests. The JDS treatment guide stresses the importance of glycemic control to prevent complications, such as an HbA1c level below 7 percent (below 6 percent when aiming for normal glycemia). In patients with type 2 diabetes, the guide recommends diet therapy and exercise therapy first. If the target value for glycemic control is not achieved despite continuation of these treatments for 2–3 months, then oral hypoglycemic agents or insulin preparations are recommended to be administered initially in small doses, depending on the type, disease condition, age, metabolic abnormality, and status of diabetic complications.

Cancer control

While the mortality from cancer has been decreasing, the incidence rate has been increasing in recent years. One reason for this increase could be the low participation rate in cancer screening programs: at 30–40 percent in Japan, it is lower than in other developed countries. The screening rate for breast cancer is especially low: only 41 percent of women aged 50–69 receive mammography, which is much lower than the 59 percent average for OECD countries (OECD 2017c). These lower screening rates might be related to the Japanese health insurance system's historic focus on tertiary prevention and disease treatment (Sauvaget et al. 2016). Sano, Goto, and Hamashima (2014) find that sending personal invitation letters would be particularly effective in improving cancer screening rates in all municipalities, which are responsible for conducting gastric, lung, colorectal, cervical, and breast cancer screenings. The government aims to increase the participation rate of cancer screening to 50 percent by 2022 in Healthy Japan 21.

With wide regional variations in screening rates, cancer mortality rates, and incidence rates, developing localized cancer control policies will be an important step (Foundation for Promotion of Cancer Research 2018; Matsuda and Saika 2018). The government expects all prefectures to have a system for monitoring cancer incidence (Matsuda and Saika 2018) and to use those data for setting appropriate control policies.

The third-term Basic Plan to Promote Cancer Control Programs, which was approved in October 2017, clearly mentions that Japan will further step up its efforts to develop personalized and precision medicine (PPM) for cancer patients (MHLW 2017). The government selected core hospitals for genome cancer treatment and is now preparing for insurance coverage for genetic testing. Multiplex gene panel testing was approved as "advanced medical care"[13] on April 1, 2018, so that the test can be conducted in combination with other healthcare services covered by public health insurance, though the test itself is not covered by public health insurance yet. This test can examine the 114 kinds of gene mutations and helps in the search for the most effective medication or treatment for particular kinds of cancer. The government has established a study group for a consortium of genomic medical care for cancer and has been making efforts to further develop PPM for cancer, as Hokuto Asano discusses in chapter 5 on personalized medicine in Japan (Asano 2017).

Research on the Economics of Chronic Disease Control in Japan

Numerous studies estimate the economic costs associated with NCDs in Japan. Bloom et al. (2017) estimate the economic burden of chronic conditions in five domains (CVDs, cancer, respiratory diseases, diabetes, and mental health conditions) for Japan, China, and South Korea. The total losses associated with these diseases in the period 2010–30 is estimated to be US$16 trillion for China, $5.7 trillion for Japan, and $1.5 trillion for South Korea.

Though Japan has the lowest admissions for COPD among OECD countries, several studies point out that COPD presents a significant socioeconomic burden in Japan due to a high use of healthcare resources and a higher impact on work impairment and productivity loss for patients of working age (Foo et al. 2016; Igarashi et al. 2018; Katsura 2011; Nishimura and Zaher 2004). Nishimura and Zaher (2004) estimate the direct and indirect cost of COPD separately, using published data between 1990 and 2002. The results show that the direct cost, including inpatient and outpatient care, and the indirect cost, which includes the costs associated with work absence due to COPD symptoms, are estimated to be US$5.5 billion and $1.4 billion, respectively. The indirect cost does not include costs related to disability and premature death, due to limitations on data availability and accuracy. Foo et al. (2016) estimate the average annual cost per patient with moderate-to-severe COPD for Japan to be US$9,893, which is much higher than the $3,694 estimate

---

13 "Advanced medical care" (*senshin iryo*) is sometimes translated as "advanced medicine." Sho (2013) explains that "advanced medicine" commonly refers to the use of newly developed medical devices, drugs, or technologies that have been authorized by the government, but are not yet covered by health insurance.

by Nishimura and Zaher (2004). Foo et al. (2016) point out that Japan had the second highest direct costs, with a high proportion of patients whose self-perceived severity of COPD is mild, mainly due to easier patient access to healthcare, compared with other countries. Also, they find that Japanese patients, even those with the lowest level of self-perceived severity, received among the highest proportions of treatment by specialists.

Many studies report that cancer is associated with diabetes in Japan (Saito et al. 2016; Sasazuki et al. 2013; Noto et al. 2011; Inoue et al. 2006; Kasuga et al. 2013). For example, Sasazuki et al. (2013) show diabetes mellitus was associated with a 20 percent increase in the risk of total cancer incidence in the Japanese population, using the data of eight cohort studies in Japan. The burden of cancer associated with type 2 diabetes is projected to increase in the future with aging. Saito et al. (2016) estimate that cancer incidence and mortality are expected to increase by 38.9% and 10.5% for those aged 20 and over, respectively, and that the number of incident cancer cases associated with type 2 diabetes is also projected to increase by 26.5% in men and 53.2% in women, during the period 2010–30. Haga et al. (2013) estimate that the economic burden of stomach cancer will decrease, mainly due to the decreasing of human capital value with aging. On the other hand, the economic burden of breast cancer is projected to increase, though Matsumoto et al. (2015) expect the number of deaths from breast cancer to decrease. The authors claim the younger average age of death for breast cancer will lead to a higher foregone economic cost per death, which will increase the total economic burden of breast cancer. The economic burden of prostate cancer is projected to increase steadily with aging, but it will still remain low compared with that of other cancers, because the average age of patients with prostate cancer is expected to remain high in the future (Kitazawa et al. 2015). Medical spending on CVDs represented the highest proportion of total medical spending in FY2016. Gochi et al. (2018) find that the cost of heart disease is projected to decrease from ¥1,619.0 billion in 2017 to ¥1,220.5 billion in 2029, mainly due to aging. Murakami et al. (2013) investigate the sex- and age-specific effects of CVD risk factors on medical expenditure, using National Health Insurance data from Shiga Prefecture. They find people with one or two CVD risk factors, especially among non-elderly women, had a higher impact on medical cost than those with three or four CVD risk factors, though the number of people with three or four CVD risk factors increased over the study period of 2000–06. Nakamura (2014), also using National Health Insurance data from Shiga Prefecture, finds medical expenditures increase with the number of concomitant risk factors at the individual level, while at a population level the economic burden related to CVD risk factors results largely from a single, particularly prevalent risk factor.

Regarding net value of care, Eggleston et al. (2019) study this for patients with type 2 diabetes in Japan between 2010 and 2014, using data from medical claims and mandatory annual health checkups. More details about the net value methods are available in the appendix of this book. The authors find that the economic value of improvements in survival and health status for patients with diabetes was approximately equal to increases in healthcare spending in health systems as different as those of Japan (in the study) and the United States (Eggleston et al. 2009). In related analyses, Chen, Eggleston, and Iizuka (2019) study the net value associated with the separation of prescribing and dispensing in Japan. They hypothesize that integrated prescribing and dispensing gave physicians financial incentive to promote medication adherence among their patients. This kind of physician "nudge" can offset patient behavioral hazard from the tendency to forget medication (imperfect adherence to pharmaceutical therapy). To provide some empirical evidence on this trade-off, they analyze data on medical utilization, spending, and health screening for over 500,000 Japanese employees for 2008–14, focusing on individuals with diabetes. Preliminary results suggest heterogeneous effects. Japanese patients can be sophisticated about physician incentives, leading to less differentiation in adherence according to physician "nudges" than would otherwise occur. Overall, Chen, Eggleston, and Iizuka (2019) find that adherence was not higher when physicians gained net revenues from dispensing medications directly to their patients, a finding that reinforces the positive welfare implications of Japan's policy of incrementally separating prescribing and dispensing.

Japan's policies for healthy aging include an emphasis on mandatory health checkups and screening, but there has been relatively little empirical evidence on the effectiveness of that policy. Focusing on the economics of preventive care, Iizuka et al. (2017) study whether preventive care triggered by health checkups is worth the cost. They utilize the fact that the health of individuals just below and above a clinical threshold (such as for pre-diabetes) is similar, whereas treatments differ according to the checkup signals they receive. They use Japanese individual-level panel data for a relatively large sample covered by corporate insurance. They find that people do receive more healthcare if their fasting blood sugar is just slightly above the cutoff for pre-diabetes, compared to those with a value just below the cutoff. However, they find no evidence that the additional care is cost-effective, because none of the measured health indicators are clearly better for the individuals who received the additional care, compared to otherwise similar individuals who did not receive the additional care. Because neither physical measures nor predicted risks of diabetes complications improve in the 3–5 years after the index checkup, one may wonder whether all the time and effort devoted to mandatory annual health checkups could be better spent if the clinical thresholds and follow-up were targeted on those at highest risk.

In a related study, Gao et al. (2014) find that prevention does have some promise. They examine the relationship between expenditures for preventive healthcare services and overall healthcare costs, using data on Japanese individuals insured under Japan's National Federation of Health Insurance Societies between 2003 and 2007. They find a negative correlation between overall medical spending and expenditures for preventive healthcare services, which they take as an encouraging indication that investment in preventive health activities could causally reduce healthcare costs. Other studies examine the cost-effectiveness of specific alternative therapies, another fruitful arena for economics research.[14]

In a comparative study, Quan et al. (2017) also focus on diabetes management in Japan, compared to Singapore, Hong Kong, and rural and peri-urban Beijing, China. Their focus is on avoidable admission rates and spending for diabetes-related complications in the period 2008–14. For Japan, they find that there was a large decrease in the rate of avoidable admissions from 2006–08 (58.9) to 2012–14 (23.3), another encouraging finding. However, if Japan has already embraced approaches that squeeze out inefficiencies, then achieving additional improvements and cost savings may be increasingly difficult, if there are increasing marginal costs to further improvements.

Conclusions

Japan is leading the world in developing social institutions and policies for the oldest population age structure on the globe. While some policies for healthy aging, such as mandatory annual checkups, appear logical and promising for prevention, their value in spurring behavioral change remains unproven, and might benefit from considering additional behavioral economics insights about how to "nudge" people to pay attention to important health signals and change behavior, if the clinical thresholds are carefully chosen.

Cancer has been the leading cause of death in Japan since 1981. While the mortality from cancer has been decreasing, the incidence has been increasing in recent years. Increasing participation in cancer screenings and developing

---

14 For example, Wake et al. (2000) "evaluate the cost and effectiveness of intensive insulin therapy for type 2 diabetes on the prevention of diabetes complications in Japan." The results show that multiple insulin injection therapy is more beneficial than conventional insulin injection therapy in both cost and effectiveness.

localized cancer control policies are important for cancer control. Moreover, tobacco control can play a primary role in the prevention of NCDs, extending survival—and potentially also reducing the gap in life expectancy between men and women in Japan.

However, longer lives almost inevitably mean that Japan will face growing numbers of people with chronic disease, even if compressed into later years of life. Therefore, assessing the net value of different chronic disease management programs represents one promising area for identifying and scaling up best practices for healthy aging.

References

Akter, Shamima, Atsushi Goto, and Tetsuya Mizoue. 2017. "Smoking and the Risk of Type 2 Diabetes in Japan: A Systematic Review and Meta-Analysis." *Journal of Epidemiology* 27 (12): 553–61.

Asano, Hokuto. 2017. "Personalized and Precision Medicine in Japan." Working paper 43, Asia Health Policy Program, Shorenstein Asia-Pacific Research Center, Stanford University.

Asia Insurance Review. 2018. "Japan: 40% of Health Insurance Societies Anticipate Losses for Latest Financial Year." *Asia Insurance Review,* September 20, 2018. http://www3.asiainsurancereview.com/News/ View-NewsLetter-Article/id/44244/Type/eDaily/Japan-40-of-health-in-surance-societies-anticipate-losses-for-latest-financial-year.

Bloom, David E, Simiao Chen, Michael Kuhn, Mark E McGovern, Les Oxley, and Klaus Prettner. 2017. "The Economic Burden of Chronic Diseases: Estimates and Projections for China, Japan, and South Korea." National Bureau of Economic Research, Cambridge, MA.

Cabinet Office, Government of Japan. 2018. *Annual Report on the Aging Society FY2017.* http://www8.cao.go.jp/kourei/whitepaper/w-2018/ html/zenbun/index.html.

Charvat, Hadrien, Atsushi Goto, Maki Goto, Machiko Inoue, Yoriko Heianza, Yasuji Arase, Hirohito Sone, Tomoko Nakagami, Xin Song, and Qing Qiao. 2015. "Impact of Population Aging on Trends in Diabetes Prevalence: A Meta-Regression Analysis of 160,000 Japanese Adults." *Journal of Diabetes Investigation* 6 (5): 533–42.

Chen, Brian K, Hawre Jalal, Hideki Hashimoto, Sze-Chuan Suen, Karen Eggleston, Michael Hurley, Lena Schoemaker, and Jay Bhattacharya. 2016. "Forecasting Trends in Disability in a Super-Aging Society: Adapting the Future Elderly Model to Japan." *Journal of the Economics of Ageing* 8: 42–51.

Chen, Brian, Karen Eggleston, and T. Iizuka. 2019. "Adherence, Vertical Integration, and Behavioral Hazard." Working paper, Asia Health Policy Program, Shorenstein Asia-Pacific Research Center, Stanford University.

Eggleston, Karen, Brian K. Chen, Ying Isabel Chen, Talitha Feenstra, Toshiaki Iizuka, Janet Tinkei Lam, Gabriel M. Leung, Jui-fen Rachel Lu, Joseph P. Newhouse, Jianchao Quan, Beatriz Rodriguez-Sanchez, and Jeroen Struijs. 2019. "Are Quality-Adjusted Medical Prices Declining for Chronic Disease? Evidence from Diabetes Care in Four Health Systems." Working paper 25971, National Bureau of Economic Research, Cambridge, MA.

Ezoe, Satoshi, Hiroyuki Noda, Naoki Akahane, Osamu Sato, Takashi Hama, Tatsunori Miyata, Tomohiro Terahara, Manami Fujishita, Haruka Sakamoto, Sarah Krull Abe, Stuart Gilmour, and Tokuaki Shoobayashi. 2017. "Trends in Policy on the Prevention and Control of Non-Communicable Diseases in Japan." *Health Systems & Reform* 3 (4): 268–77.

Foo, Jason, Sarah H Landis, Joe Maskell, Yeon-Mok Oh, Thys van der Molen, MeiLan K Han, David M Mannino, Masakazu Ichinose, and Yogesh Punekar. 2016. "Continuing to Confront COPD International Patient Survey: Economic Impact of COPD in 12 Countries." *PLOS One* 11 (4): e0152618.

Foundation for Promotion of Cancer Research. 2018. "Cancer Statistics in Japan 2017." Foundation for Promotion of Cancer Research. https://ganjoho.jp/data/reg_stat/statistics/brochure/2017/cancer_statistics_2017.pdf.

Fukui, Tadashi, and Yasushi Iwamoto. 2007. "Policy Options for Financing Future Health and Long-Term Care Costs in Japan." In *Fiscal Policy and Management in East Asia, NBER-EASE, Volume 16*, 415–42. University of Chicago Press.

Fullman, Nancy, Jamal Yearwood, Solomon M Abay, Cristiana Abbafati, Foad Abd-Allah, Jemal Abdela, Ahmed Abdelalim, Zegeye Abebe, Teshome Abuka Abebo, and Victor Aboyans. 2018. "Measuring Performance on the Healthcare Access and Quality Index for 195 Countries and Territories and Selected Subnational Locations: A Systematic Analysis from the Global Burden of Disease Study 2016." *The Lancet* 391 (10136): 2236–71.

Gao, Yan, Akira Babazono, Takumi Nishi, Toshiki Maeda, and Dulamsuren Lkhagva. 2014. "Could Investment in Preventive Health Care Services Reduce Health Care Costs among Those Insured with Health

Insurance Societies in Japan?" *Population Health Management* 17 (1): 42–47.

Gilmour, Stuart, Yi Liao, Ver Bilano, and Kenji Shibuya. 2014. "Burden of Disease in Japan: Using National and Subnational Data to Inform Local Health Policy." *Journal of Preventive Medicine and Public Health* 47 (3): 136.

Gochi, Toshiharu, Kunichika Matsumoto, Rebeka Amin, Takefumi Kitazawa, Kanako Seto, and Tomonori Hasegawa. 2018. "Cost of Illness of Ischemic Heart Disease in Japan: A Time Trend and Future Projections." *Environmental Health and Preventive Medicine* 23 (1): 21.

Goto, Maki, Atsushi Goto, Nayu Ikeda, Hiroyuki Noda, Kenji Shibuya, and Mitsuhiko Noda. 2015. "Factors Associated with Untreated Diabetes: Analysis of Data from 20,496 Participants in the Japanese National Health and Nutrition Survey." *PlOS One* 10 (3): e0118749.

Haga, Kayoko, Kunichika Matsumoto, Takefumi Kitazawa, Kanako Seto, Shigeru Fujita, and Tomonori Hasegawa. 2013. "Cost of Illness of the Stomach Cancer in Japan-A Time Trend and Future Projections." *BMC Health Services Research* 13 (1): 283.

Hirakawa, Yoshihisa, and Kazumasa Uemura. 2013. "No Improvement in Metabolic Health Condition of 40-74-Year-Old Rural Residents One Year after Screening." *Journal of Rural Medicine* 8 (2): 193–97.

Igarashi, Ataru, Yoshinosuke Fukuchi, Kazuto Hirata, Masakazu Ichinose, Atsushi Nagai, Masaharu Nishimura, Hajime Yoshisue, Kenichi Ohara, and Jean-Bernard Gruenberger. 2018. "COPD Uncovered: A Cross-Sectional Study to Assess the Socioeconomic Burden of COPD in Japan." *International Journal of Chronic Obstructive Pulmonary Disease* 13: 2629.

Iizuka, Toshiaki, Katsuhiko Nishiyama, Brian Chen, and Karen Eggleston. 2017. *Is Preventive Care Worth the Cost? Evidence from Mandatory Checkups in Japan*. National Bureau of Economic Research, Cambridge, MA.

Ikeda, Nayu, Nobuo Nishi, Hiroyuki Noda, and Mitsuhiko Noda. 2017. "Trends in Prevalence and Management of Diabetes and Related Vascular Risks in Japanese Adults: Japan National Health and Nutrition Surveys 2003–2012." *Diabetes Research and Clinical Practice* 127: 115–22.

Ikeda, Nayu, Eiko Saito, Naoki Kondo, Manami Inoue, Shunya Ikeda, Toshihiko Satoh, Koji Wada, Andrew Stickley, Kota Katanoda, and Tetsuya Mizoue. 2011. "What Has Made the Population of Japan

Healthy?" *The Lancet* 378 (9796): 1094–105.

Inoue, Manami, Motoki Iwasaki, Tetsuya Otani, Shizuka Sasazuki, Mitsuhiko Noda, and Shoichiro Tsugane. 2006. "Diabetes Mellitus and the Risk of Cancer: Results From a Large-Scale Population-Based Cohort Study in Japan." *Archives of Internal Medicine* 166 (17): 1871–77.

International Diabetes Federation. 2017. "The IDF Diabetes Atlas, 8th Edition—Japan Country Report 2017 & 2045-." https://reports.instantatlas.com/report/view/704eee0e6475b4af885051bcec15f0e2c/JPN.

Inui, Tomohiko, Yukiko Ito, Atsushi Kawakami, Xin Xin Ma, Masaru Nagashima, and Meng Zhao. 2017. *Empirical Study on the Utilization and Effects of Health Checkups in Japan*. Research Institute of Economy, Trade and Industry (RIETI), Tokyo, Japan.

Iso, Hiroyasu. 2011. "A Japanese Health Success Story: Trends in Cardiovascular Diseases, Their Risk Factors, and the Contribution of Public Health and Personalized Approaches." *Epma Journal* 2 (1): 49–57.

Japan Times. 2018. "Male Smoking Rate in Japan Falls Below 30% for First Time." *Japan Times*, September 12, 2018. https://www.japantimes.co.jp/news/2018/09/12/national/male-smoking-rate-japan-falls-30-first-time/#.W73BzmhKjIV.

JDS (Japan Diabetes Society). 2016. "Treatment Guide for Diabetes 2016–2017." Tokyo: Bunkodo Co., Ltd. http://www.fa.kyorin.co.jp/jds/uploads/Treatment_Guide_for_Diabetes_2016-2017.pdf.

Kasajima, Megumi, Hideki Hashimoto, Sze-Chuan Suen, Brian Chen, Karen Eggleston, and Jay Bhattacharya. 2019. "Future Projection of the Health and Functional Status of Older People in Japan: A Pseudopanel Microsimulation Model." Working paper 55, Asia Health Policy Program, Shorenstein Asia-Pacific Research Center, Stanford University. Revised version forthcoming in *Health Economics*.

Kasuga, Masato, Kohjiro Ueki, Naoko Tajima, Mitsuhiko Noda, Ken Ohashi, Hiroshi Noto, Atsushi Goto, Wataru Ogawa, Ryuichi Sakai, and Shoichiro Tsugane. 2013. "Report of the JDS/JCA Joint Committee on Diabetes and Cancer." *Diabetology International* 4 (2): 81–96.

Katsura, Hideki. 2011. "Economic Burden of COPD in Japan." *Japan Medical Association Journal* 54 (2): 110–11.

Kitazawa, Takefumi, Kunichika Matsumoto, Shigeru Fujita, Kanako Seto, Shimpei Hanaoka, and Tomonori Hasegawa. 2015. "Cost of Illness of the Prostate Cancer in Japan—A Time-Trend Analysis and Future Projections." *BMC Health Services Research* 15 (1): 453.

Kohro, Takahide, Yuji Furui, Naohiro Mitsutake, Ryo Fujii, Hiroyuki Morita, Shinya Oku, Kazuhiko Ohe, and Ryozo Nagai. 2008. "The

Japanese National Health Screening and Intervention Program Aimed at Preventing Worsening of the Metabolic Syndrome." *International Heart Journal* 49 (2): 193–203.

Kyodo News. 2018. "Smoking-Linked Losses in Japan Estimated at Over 2 Trillion Yen." *Kyodo News*, August 8, 2018. https://english.kyodonews.net/news/2018/08/bb56e41768a6-smoking-linked-losses-in-japan-estimated-at-over-2-trillion-yen.html.

Matsuda, Tomohiro, and Kumiko Saika. 2018. "Cancer Burden in Japan Based on the Latest Cancer Statistics: Need for Evidence-Based Cancer Control Programs." *Annals of Cancer Epidemiology* 2 (September 5). doi: 10.21037/ace.2018.08.01.

Matsumoto, Kunichika, Kayoko Haga, Takefumi Kitazawa, Kanako Seto, Shigeru Fujita, and Tomonori Hasegawa. 2015. "Cost of Illness of Breast Cancer in Japan: Trends and Future Projections." *BMC Research Notes* 8 (1): 539.

MHLW (Ministry of Health, Labor and Welfare). 2016. "Tobacco Smoking and Health." Ministry of Health, Labor and Welfare. https://www.mhlw.go.jp/file/05-Shingikai-10901000-Kenkoukyoku-Soumuka/0000172687.pdf.

MHLW. 2017. "The Third-Term Basic Plan to Promote Cancer Control Programs." Ministry of Health, Labor and Welfare. https://www.mhlw.go.jp/file/06-Seisakujouhou-10900000-Kenkoukyoku/0000196973.pdf.

MHLW. 2018a. "Draft of Mid-Term Evaluation Report of Health Japan 21 (second term)." Ministry of Health, Labor and Welfare. https://www.mhlw.go.jp/content/10904750/000344232.pdf.

MHLW. 2018b. "Projection of Social Security Cost for 2040." Ministry of Health, Labor and Welfare. https://www.kantei.go.jp/jp/singi/syakaihosyou_kaikaku/dai8/shiryou8-1.pdf.

MHLW. 2018c. "Review of Specific Health Checkups and Specific Health Guidance and Incentives for Insurers." Ministry of Health, Labor and Welfare. https://kenko-keiei.org/document_dl/symposium0402.pdf.

MHLW. 2018d. "Summary of National Medical Expenditure FY 2016." Ministry of Health, Labor and Welfare. https://www.mhlw.go.jp/toukei/saikin/hw/k-iryohi/16/dl/kekka.pdf.

MHLW. 2018e. "Summary of Specific Health Checkups and Specific Health Guidance FY 2017." Ministry of Health, Labor and Welfare. https://www.mhlw.go.jp/content/12400000/000489840.pdf.

Murakami, Yoshitaka, Tomonori Okamura, Koshi Nakamura, Katsuyuki Miura, and Hirotsugu Ueshima. 2013. "The Clustering of Cardiovascular Disease Risk Factors and Their Impacts on Annual Medical

Expenditure in Japan: Community-Based Cost Analysis Using Gamma Regression Models." *BMJ Open* 3 (3): e002234.

Nakamura, Koshi. 2014. "Impact of Cardiovascular Risk Factors on Medical Expenditure: Evidence From Epidemiological Studies Analysing Data on Health Checkups and Medical Insurance." *Journal of Epidemiology* 24 (6): 437–43.

National Institute of Population and Social Security Research. 2017. "Population Projections for Japan: 2016 to 2065 (Appendix: Auxiliary Projections 2066 to 2115)." National Institute of Population and Social Security Research. http://www.ipss.go.jp/pp-zenkoku/e/zenkoku_e2017/pp29_summary.pdf.

Nishimura, Shuzo, and Carol Zaher. 2004. "Cost Impact of COPD in Japan: Opportunities and Challenges?" *Respirology* 9 (4): 466–73.

Nomura, Shuhei, Haruka Sakamoto, Scott Glenn, Yusuke Tsugawa, Sarah K. Abe, Md M. Rahman, Jonathan C. Brown, Satoshi Ezoe, Christina Fitzmaurice, and Tsuyoshi Inokuchi. 2017. "Population Health and Regional Variations of Disease Burden in Japan, 1990–2015: A Systematic Subnational Analysis for the Global Burden of Disease Study 2015." *The Lancet* 390 (10101): 1521–38.

Noto, Hiroshi, Tetsuro Tsujimoto, Takehiko Sasazuki, and Mitsuhiko Noda. 2011. "Significantly Increased Risk of Cancer in Patients with Diabetes Mellitus: A Systematic Review and Meta-Analysis." *Endocrine Practice* 17 (4): 616–28.

Nozaki, Masahiro, Kenichiro Kashiwase, and Ikuo Saito. 2014. *Health Spending in Japan: Macro-Fiscal Implications and Reform Options.* IMF working paper 14/142: International Monetary Fund, Washington, DC.

OECD (Organisation for Economic Co-operation and Development). 2015. "How Does Health Spending in Japan Compare? " https://www.oecd.org/els/health-systems/Country-Note-JAPAN-OECD-Health-Statistics-2015.pdf.

OECD. 2016. "Health Spending—Expenditure by Disease, Age and Gender." http://www.oecd.org/els/health-systems/Expenditure-by-disease-age-and-gender-FOCUS-April2016.pdf.

OECD. 2017a. "Health at a Glance 2017: OECD Indicators." OECD Publishing, Paris.

OECD. 2017b. "Health at a Glance 2017: OECD Indicators How Does Japan Compare?" https://www.oecd.org/japan/Health-at-a-Glance-2017-Key-Findings-JAPAN-in-English.pdf.

OECD. 2017c. "Health Policy in Japan." http://www.oecd.org/health/health-systems/Health-Policy-in-Japan-March-2017.pdf.

OECD. 2018. "OECD Health Statistics 2018." http://www.oecd.org/els/health-systems/health-data.htm.

Osaki, Tomohiro. 2018a. "Japan's Watered-Down Smoking Ban Clears Diet." *Japan Times*, July 18, 2018. https://www.japantimes.co.jp/news/2018/07/18/national/crime-legal/japans-watered-smoking-ban-clears-diet/#.W6SUbehKjIW.

Osaki, Tomohiro. 2018b. "Tokyo Lawmakers Approve Anti-Smoking Ordinance as Capital Gears Up for 2020 Olympics." *Japan Times*, June 27, 2018. https://www.japantimes.co.jp/news/2018/06/27/national/tokyo-lawmakers-approve-anti-smoking-ordinance-capital-gears-2020-olympics/#.W6SVFOhKjIW.

Quan, Jianchao, Huyang Zhang, Deanette Pang, Brian K. Chen, Janice M Johnston, Weiyan Jian, Zheng Yi Lau, Toshiaki Iizuka, Gabriel M. Leung, and Hai Fang. 2017. "Avoidable Hospital Admissions from Diabetes Complications in Japan, Singapore, Hong Kong, and Communities outside Beijing." *Health Affairs* 36 (11): 1896–903.

Saito, Eiko, Hadrien Charvat, Atsushi Goto, Tomohiro Matsuda, Mitsuhiko Noda, Shizuka Sasazuki, and Manami Inoue. 2016. "Burden of Cancer Associated with Type 2 Diabetes Mellitus in Japan, 2010–2030." *Cancer Science* 107 (4): 521–27.

Sakamoto, Haruka, Md. Mizanur Rahman, Shuhei Nomura, Etsuji Okamoto, Soichi Koike, Hideo Yasunaga, Norito Kawakami, Hideki Hashimoto, Naoki Kondo, Sarah Krull Abe, Matthew Palmer, and Cyrus Ghaznavi. 2018. *Japan Health System Review*. Vol. 8, no. 1. World Health Organization, Regional Office for South-East Asia.

Sano, Hiroshi, Rei Goto, and Chisato Hamashima. 2014. "What Is the Most Effective Strategy for Improving the Cancer Screening Rate in Japan." *Asian Pacific Journal of Cancer Prevention* 15 (6): 2607–12.

Sasazuki, Shizuka, Hadrien Charvat, Azusa Hara, Kenji Wakai, Chisato Nagata, Kozue Nakamura, Ichiro Tsuji, Yumi Sugawara, Akiko Tamakoshi, and Keitaro Matsuo. 2013. "Diabetes Mellitus and Cancer Risk: Pooled Analysis of Eight Cohort Studies in Japan." *Cancer Science* 104 (11): 1499–507.

Sauvaget, Catherine, Yoshikazu Nishino, Ryo Konno, Toru Tase, Tadaoki Morimoto, and Shigeru Hisamichi. 2016. "Challenges in Breast and Cervical Cancer Control in Japan." *Lancet Oncology* 17 (7): e305–12.

Sho, Ri, Hiroto Narimatsu, and Masayasu Murakami. 2013. "Japan's Advanced Medicine." *Bioscience Trends* 7 (5): 245–49.

Suzuki, Wataru, Minoru Masujima, Kousuke Shiraishi, and Akihiro Morishige. 2012. "Intergenerational Inequality Caused by the Social Security System." ESRI Discussion Paper Series 281, Economic and Social Research Institute, Tokyo, Japan.

Tabuchi, Takahiro, Takeo Fujiwara, and Tomohiro Shinozaki. 2016. "Tobacco Price Increase and Smoking Behaviour Changes in Various Subgroups: A Nationwide Longitudinal 7-Year Follow-Up Study among a Middle-Aged Japanese Population." *Tobacco Control* 26 (1): 69–77.

Tajika, Eiji, and Jun Kikuchi. 2004. "A Projection of Total Cost of Long-Term Care and the Ratio of Benefits and Burdens by Year of Birth." *Financial Review,* 147–63.

Terahara, Tomohiro. 2015. "The Japanese Ministry of Health, Labour and Welfare's Measures on Tobacco Control." *Journal of the National Institute of Public Health* 64: 5.

Tsugawa, Yusuke, Ken Hashimoto, Takahiro Tabuchi, and Kenji Shibuya. 2017. "What Can Japan Learn from Tobacco Control in the UK?" *The Lancet* 390 (10098): 933–34.

Tsushita, Kazuyo, Akiko S Hosler, Katsuyuki Miura, Yukiko Ito, Takashi Fukuda, Akihiko Kitamura, and Kozo Tatara. 2018. "Rationale and Descriptive Analysis of Specific Health Guidance: The Nationwide Lifestyle Intervention Program Targeting Metabolic Syndrome in Japan." *Journal of Atherosclerosis and Thrombosis* 25 (4): 308–22.

Ueda, Junji, Yohihiro Horiuchi, and Tadashi Tsutui. 2011. "Long-Term Projections of Health and Long-Term Care Spending and Labor Demand in Future." KIER Discussion Paper 1017, Kyoto Institute of Economic Research, Japan.

Unami, Hirotaka. 2018. "The Policy Challenges of Financing Longevity—A Perspective from Japan." *Journal of the Economics of Ageing* 13 (C): 10–13.

Wake, Nakayasu, Akinori Hisashige, Takafumi Katayama, Hideki Kishikawa, Yasuo Ohkubo, Masakazu Sakai, Eiichi Araki, and Motoaki Shichiri. 2000. "Cost-Effectiveness of Intensive Insulin Therapy for Type 2 Diabetes: A 10-Year Follow-Up of the Kumamoto Study." *Diabetes Research and Clinical Practice* 48 (3): 201–10.

WHO (World Health Organization). 2015. *WHO Global Report on Trends in Prevalence of Tobacco Smoking 2015.* World Health Organization, Geneva.

Yuda, Michio. 2013. "The Impacts of Recent Smoking Control Policies on Individual Smoking Choice: The Case of Japan." *Health Economics Review* 3 (1): 4.

4 The Political Economy of Precision Health

The Case of Japan

Minori Ito

In the past two years, "precision health" has gained forward momentum as a transformative approach in medicine for a long, healthy life. Precision health is a population-based strategy to prevent and detect diseases before they strike patients, using technology along with big data on health, lifestyle, and environmental factors that influence a population's health. Precision health aims to prevent and detect diseases early, at the population level, with an integrated health portal analyzing vast quantities of data at the individual level from various sources, including electronic medical records, genomic sequences, insurance and pharmaceutical records, wearable sensors, and social and environmental information. Given its focus on the prevention and early detection of diseases, precision health plays an important role in promoting healthy living and aging.

The concept of precision health goes beyond "precision medicine." Since U.S. president Barack Obama's 2015 launch of an initiative to promote and extend precision medicine (White House 2015), the approach has led to the development of therapies to cure disease that are tailored to individual patients. Discussions on precision health date back to 2016, including a commentary by Stanford Medicine dean Dr. Lloyd Minor (2016), "We Don't Just Need Precision Medicine, We Need Precision Health." Precision health empowers individuals to monitor their health and uses collective data to better predict and detect diseases at the population level. While precision medicine is about providing "the right treatment to the right patient at the right time," precision health is concerned with "the right intervention to the right population at the right time" (Khoury 2016). Precision health provides positive impacts both for patients and doctors: increased health monitoring enables patients to proactively monitor their own health in real time and to

FIGURE 4.1 The precision health cycle

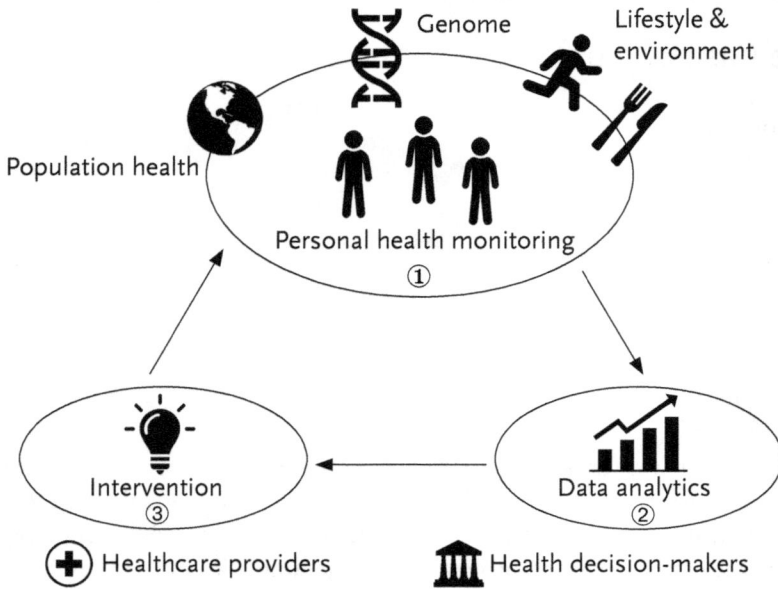

Precision health uses collective information to enable early detection of and intervention in diseases. (1) An integrated secure health portal collects health data, including genetic information, population health data, individual health records, and behavioral and environmental information through wearable and smart devices at home. (2) The portal and collected data enable health decision-makers to analyze and identify appropriate interventions. While simple interventions can be presented directly to patients with guidance, (3) other interventions for disease detection and management may require the engagement of healthcare providers. Precision health empowers individuals to proactively monitor their health and prevent and detect diseases at the earliest stages.

SOURCES: Author. Icons from the Noun Project: DNA by Dmitry Mirolyubov; globe by Ico-Moon; person by Adrien Coquet; runner by Centis MENANT; fork and knife by Adrien Coquet; innovation by Numero Uno; cross by Untashable; government by Marco Livolsi; graph by iconmarketpk.

visit physicians only when needed; the approach of precision health enables doctors to provide engagement and treatments of diseases at the earliest stage and to be more focused on how to treat patients (see figure 4.1).

Additionally, precision health can contribute to reducing healthcare costs in an era of increased longevity. As life expectancy improves, financing increased healthcare costs is a pressing issue for both individuals and governments. By making preventive care and health checkups more effective based on big data, precision health can reduce unnecessary treatments or hospital visits and thus have a significant impact on reducing healthcare costs.

When introducing the precision health approach, it is essential to consider various factors that could be associated with people's health. In addition to an individual's health information, for example, the socioeconomic determinants of disease incidence, such as household income, unemployment rates, and educational attainment, can also help in the observation of a population's health, and thus should be considered in the implementation of precision health.

Putting precision health into practice requires a transformation of health policies. Precision health necessitates data collection and data analytics of all factors unique to people's lives (health, environmental, etc.), risk assessment at all stages of life, customized monitoring, and intervention. The entire cycle of precision health cannot be achieved by a single institution; it needs a nationwide initiative to transform health policies, build an effective platform, and enable collaboration among relevant stakeholders.

This chapter aims to provide an overview of the health policy transformations necessary to introduce precision health by looking at the case of Japan. Japan is facing an increase both in life expectancy and healthcare costs, which poses significant challenges for the society. In 2017, Japan had the highest life expectancy in the world at 83.7 years. On the other hand, the number of noncommunicable diseases (NCDs), such as cancer and diabetes, has been growing in recent decades. Furthermore, rapid aging of the population puts severe pressure on public finance, with ballooning social security costs, helping to push up the public debt to 253 percent of gross domestic product (GDP) in 2017. This scenario, combined with the nation's economic slowdown over the past two decades, means that Japan needs health policies that balance universal coverage, support for the elderly, and financial sustainability. One potential solution is to introduce the approach of precision health. Japan historically has had universal health coverage and mandatory annual healthcare checkups, but there may be room for improvement in current health policies and healthcare checkups through the use of nascent technologies. This chapter aims to determine the health policies necessary to introduce precision health to Japan, and what the use of precision health might mean for healthy aging in Japan.

The rest of the chapter is structured as follows. It begins with an overview of Japan's health policies and health insurance, including the historical context and current major stakeholders. It then continues to discuss Japan's current healthcare status, the potential impacts of introducing precision health, and the health policy transformations necessary to put precision health in place. Next is a comparative analysis with Australia's precision health policies and a discussion of future implementation challenges for Japan. The chapter concludes with a summary of proposed policies.

Overview of Current Health Policies and Health Insurance in Japan

Japan's healthcare system is characterized by its universal insurance coverage, which began in 1961 and has been maintained for over 50 years. All residents in Japan, including foreign nationals with resident cards, are required by law to be enrolled in health insurance. The Japanese healthcare system has achieved excellent health outcomes at a relatively low cost. It is unique in having achieved both depth and breadth: Japan has both Employees' Health Insurance (EHI) and National Health Insurance (NHI), two programs that over time extended coverage to the entire population. EHI, which originated in the German Bismarck system of social health insurance, is provided to company employees and their dependents and covers 58.7 percent of the population (Sakamoto et al. 2018). NHI is for self-employed and unemployed persons, covering 28.3 percent of the population (Sakamoto et al. 2018), and is administered by municipalities. Most healthcare procedures and products, including drugs, are administered using a nationally uniform fee schedule. Health insurance covers 70–90 percent of the cost and the rest is paid by the insured as copayment (Ishii 2012).[1]

Additionally, in 2008, Japan introduced a late-stage medical care system for the elderly, a program for those who are 75 years old and above, covering 12.4 percent of the population (Sakamoto et al. 2018). In recent decades, the number of retired elderly has increased, adding to the population covered by NHI and increasing its financial burden. The late-stage system was introduced in an effort to improve financial equity between the NHI and the EHI.

In Japan, consumers have the freedom to choose healthcare facilities. In 2006, there were 8,442 hospitals, 101,529 clinics, and 68,940 dental clinics, and the majority (81.1 percent) were privately owned (70 percent of hospitals and 94 percent of clinics are provided by the private sector) (Sakamoto et al. 2018). While most aspects of healthcare, including the nationally uniform fee schedule, are administered by the government, there are no limitations on the purchase of equipment and technologies by private-sector healthcare

---

1   As of March 2017, the copayment rate is based on the patient's age, as follows: for those prior to the start of compulsory education (the age of six), it is 20%; from the age of six to 69 it is 30%; from 70 to 74 it is 20%, and the copayment is 10% for those 75 and over.

facilities, including advanced, expensive, and new technologies. Combined with the rapid aging of the population, growing expenditures for expensive new technologies contribute to Japan's high total medical expenditure, which stands at 10.9 percent of GDP, the third highest among member countries of the Organisation for Economic Cooperation and Development (OECD) in 2015 (Sakamoto et al. 2018).[2] Moreover, Japan's economy has been stagnating for decades; declining tax revenue for universal health insurance has resulted in Japan's growing health expenditure per GDP.

The historical context of Japan's healthcare policies and health insurance

The landscape of Japan's healthcare and health insurance has been shaped by the country's political economy dynamics. Besides public opinion, healthcare interest groups have often influenced political discussions, especially during national elections. Understanding the historical context of Japanese healthcare policies provides a critical background for the current challenges the society is facing.

The development of national health insurance after the Second World War was achieved by political leadership amid conflicts among parties. Nobusuke Kishi, the Liberal Democratic Party (LDP) prime minister, promoted the expansion of health insurance coverage to relatively vulnerable groups in a bid to take away a platform from other competing parties. He announced his plan to pursue universal insurance coverage in the Diet in 1957 and enacted the National Health Insurance Act in 1958 (Sakamoto et al. 2018). The legislation went into force in 1959, requiring all municipalities to change voluntary-basis Community Health Insurance to mandatory National Health Insurance, which led to the official achievement of universal health insurance coverage in 1961.

During the 1960s—the time of Japan's "economic miracle," characterized by an unprecedented 10 percent annual economic growth—LDP prime ministers Hayato Ikeda and Kakuei Tanaka expanded both the breadth and depth of universal insurance coverage. The copayment rate was reduced from 50 percent to 30 percent by the 1980s (Sakamoto et al. 2018). There was growing pressure from the Socialist Party to expand coverage to the elderly; they argued the elderly had lower income and did not proportionately benefit from economic growth. The ruling LDP decided to provide free healthcare for the elderly over the age of 70, which would later lead to severe financial stress on the health system.

2   Another reason for Japan's high health expenditure is a recent change in the rules that includes expenditure on long-term care in total healthcare expenditure.

In the early 1980s, facing slower economic growth and increasing political tension over limited fiscal space and increasing health expenditures since the 1970s, LDP prime minister Yasuhiro Nakasone started a contractional fiscal policy, known as "small government." Free healthcare for the elderly was terminated and a fee-control schedule was introduced that determined nationally uniform costs of medicine and care. Meanwhile, the issue of fragmented insurance plans with various premium levels remained in the healthcare system.

In 2001, LDP candidate Junichiro Koizumi won the national election with his promise of achieving more "progressive" healthcare policies with an austere fiscal policy and increased out-of-pocket payments and insurance premiums. His proposed policies encountered opposition, including from the Japan Medical Association (JMA), and were not enacted (Sakamoto et al. 2018). However, Koizumi's overwhelming victory in the 2005 general election increased the momentum; Koizumi put in place an austere fiscal policy for social security, reducing the social security budget by ¥1.1 trillion over five years (Sakamoto et al. 2018). This policy shed light on the balance between the cost and quality of healthcare.

In 2015, "Japan Vision: Health Care 2035," a forward-looking proposal for healthcare policies through 2035, was presented by an advisory panel commissioned by Yasuhisa Shiozaki, a former health minister. The plan's goal is to build a "sustainable [healthcare] system that delivers unmatched health outcomes through care that is responsive and equitable to each member of the society and that contributes to prosperity in Japan and around the world" (Health Care 2035 Advisory Panel 2015).

Japan's national screening programs

There are three types of health checkups that cover the entire population under Japan's "checkup for all" policy: general health checkups, specific health checkups and specific health guidance (SHCSHG), and cancer screening. The Japanese government introduced the SHCSHG policy in 2008 to conduct screening for early detection and intervention for chronic conditions, such as metabolic syndrome. All healthcare insurers are required to conduct SHCSHG for enrollees aged 40 to 74. Based on checkup results, specific guidance is provided to those participants identified as having risk factors for lifestyle-related diseases.

However, no general consensus has been reached on whether the SHCSHG has contributed to advancing health (Matsuda and Sobue 2015; Iizuka et al. 2017). There is a significant discrepancy in SHCSHG coverage across healthcare plans that are linked to employment status. In 2017, the coverage of checkups was 53.1%, with a higher rate of checkups among full-time employees than part-time employees, while the government's target for checkup coverage is 70% in 2023 (MHLW 2019). Furthermore, cancer screening rates also leave room for improvement. The national government subsidizes voluntary screening for cancer for those aged 40 to 69, with varying copayment rates. However, the screening rates remain low, at 45.8% for stomach cancer, 41.4% for colon cancer, and 47.5% for lung cancer in 2013.

Japan's national screening programs play an important role in the prevention and early detection of certain diseases, but there is room for a more efficient use of health resources by making the screenings more tailored to the Japanese population and to each individual. Improving SHCSHG checkup rates regardless of employment status and directing cancer screening at high-risk individuals would be an important step in the early detection and prevention of targeted diseases. Additionally, the SHCSHG targets chronic conditions, such as metabolic syndrome, and cancer screening is aimed at detecting various cancers; however, the current national screening programs do not necessarily address other growing diseases in Japan's aging population, including neurodegenerative ones, especially Alzheimer's-related diseases.

Major stakeholders in Japan's healthcare

Since the approach of precision health requires collaboration among all healthcare stakeholders, understanding stakeholder dynamics is essential to its successful introduction. The following institutions and groups play a role in the political economy of Japan's healthcare.

Ministry of Health, Labor, and Welfare (MHLW): The MHLW is the central organization in Japan's healthcare system, regulating and controlling all aspects of the health system, including the health insurance system. The ministry sets the national uniform fee schedule for insurance reimbursement, and subsidizes and supervises local governments, insurers, and healthcare providers at the prefecture level. The bureaus that are relevant to precision health include the Health Policy Bureau, Health Services Bureau, Pharmaceutical Safety and Environmental Health Bureau, Labor Standards Bureau, Health and Welfare for the Elderly Bureau, Health Insurance Bureau, and Pension Bureau. The Medical Economics Division (under the Health Policy Bureau) plays a role in health technology assessment (HTA), as it oversees the development and revision of the fee schedule and drug price list (details are discussed below in the section on health technology assessment). Under the MHLW, the Pharmaceutical and Medical Device Agency (PMDA) evaluates new drugs and medical devices.

Central Social Insurance Medical Council ("Chuikyou"): The council is run by MHLW staff and advises the health minister on health insurance policy. The council has representatives from the payer side, provider side, and those representing public interest. The council plays a central role in conducting debates for fee schedule revisions every two years.

Ministry of Finance (MOF): The MOF's Budget Bureau oversees the government's budget for social security, including medical expenditures.

Ministry of Economy, Trade, and Industry (METI): METI oversees Japan's economic and industry policies, including developing national economic strategies related to healthcare, in partnership with medical and pharmaceutical companies.

Liberal Democratic Party (LDP): The LDP is the current ruling party of Japan and has held the majority of the Diet almost the entire time, except for 11 months between 1992 and 1994 and three years between 2009 and 2011 (Health and Global Policy Institute n.d.). As discussed earlier regarding the historical context of Japan's healthcare policies, healthcare and health insurance are among the main topics in public debates. LDP leaders have often played a leading role in shaping Japan's healthcare policies.

Japan Medical Association (JMA): The JMA is a health policy interest group, with about 55 percent of Japanese physicians belonging to it (Health and Global Policy Institute n.d.), the majority of them private practice physicians. The JMA has seats on the Central Social Insurance Medical Council. JMA opposes HTA due to its potential negative impacts on innovation and care provision (Health and Global Policy Institute n.d.).

Other professional organizations: Japan has more than 50 other professional organizations related to healthcare. In addition to the JMA, the Japan Dental Association and Japan Pharmaceutical Association are among the largest doctors' organizations (Health and Global Policy Institute n.d.).

Prefectural governments: Japan has 47 prefectures and each prefectural government oversees medical facilities and providers at the local level. Prefectural governments manage and regulate facilities, workforce, and suppliers, while managing public health centers for sanitation, disease control, and health environments.

Municipal governments: Municipal governments, such as city, town, and village governments, oversee disease prevention and family health through community health centers.

Consumer groups and patient organizations: There are over 3,000 patient organizations in Japan, which appear to be fragmented compared with those in the United States and Europe (Health and Global Policy Institute n.d.).

Introducing Precision Health to Japan

As of 2017, Japan had a relatively long life expectancy of 80.5 years for men and 86.8 years for women, as well as a long healthy life expectancy of 71.5 years for men and 76.3 years for women (Sakamoto et al. 2018). Japan's relatively long life expectancy may be attributed to universal and equitable health coverage, healthy lifestyle, diets, sanitation and hygiene, and socioeconomic determinants. Like other developed countries, the burden of communicable diseases has significantly decreased over the past several decades, while NCDs are the leading causes of mortality and morbidity in Japan. Table 4.1 shows the leading causes of death in Japan in 1990, 2005, and 2015, based on the number of deaths from each cause. The top three leading causes of death in 1990, cerebrovascular disease, ischemic heart disease, and lower respiratory infection, remain the top three causes of death in 2005 and 2015, while their age-standardized death rates significantly declined by 39.6 percent from 1990 to 2005 and by 19.3 percent from 2005 to 2015. On the other hand, Alzheimer's disease remains the fourth leading cause of death in Japan in 2015 with the constantly increasing age-standardized death rate from 1990 through 2015.

Although the quality of population health in Japan is broadly high, there remains a discrepancy in life expectancy across prefectures. The discrepancy in life expectancy narrowed until the 1990s but widened again between 1990 and 2015 from 2.5 years to 3.1 years (Nomura et al. 2017). Among the causes may be social determinants of health. There is a substantial difference across prefectures in the risk factors, such as smoking, as well as in socioeconomic indicators, such as household income, educational attainment, and unemployment rates.

The potential impact of introducing precision health to Japan

By introducing the precision health approach, Japan would be able to prevent and detect diseases at the earliest stages with a population-based strategy to promote healthy aging. Precision health can empower patients to proactively monitor their own health, visiting physicians only when necessary. Precision health can help doctors become more focused on engagement and treatment of diseases. Additionally, precision health can play an important role in allocating limited resources efficiently and managing healthcare costs in the era of longevity.

Moreover, given that precision health aims to provide "the right intervention to the right population at the right time" (Khoury, Iademarco, and

TABLE 4.1 Leading causes of death in Japan (1990, 2005, 2015)

Rank	1990	2005	Percent change in age-standardized death rate from 1990	2015	Percent change in age-standardized death rate from 2005
1	Cerebrovascular disease	Cerebrovascular disease	−39.6	Cerebrovascular disease	−19.3
2	Ischemic heart disease	Ischemic heart disease	−38.4	Ischemic heart disease	−11.6
3	Lower respiratory infection	Lower respiratory infection	−17.5	Lower respiratory infection	−6.5
4	Stomach cancer	Alzheimer's disease	3.7	Alzheimer's disease	3.7
5	Alzheimer's disease	Lung cancer	2.8	Lung cancer	−8.7
6	Lung cancer	Stomach cancer	−9.5	Stomach cancer	−11.2
7	Colorectal cancer	Colorectal cancer	3.0	Colorectal cancer	−6.4
8	Liver cancer	Liver cancer	−9.5	Chronic kidney disease	−11.2
9	Self-harm	Self-harm	21.7	Liver cancer	4.1
10	COPD	Chronic kidney disease	−23.3	COPD	−16.0

SOURCE: Sakamoto et al. 2018.
NOTE: COPD = chronic obstructive pulmonary disease.

Riley 2016), this approach can contribute to the prevention and detection of diseases that are currently growing in the Japanese population, which is rapidly aging: the number of the elderly is estimated to increase from the current 16 million to 20 million by 2020, and simultaneously, the working-age population is expected to decrease from 109 million to 100 million (Sakamoto et al. 2018). This demographic change will necessitate a transformation of the nation's healthcare systems. Rapid aging can impose an increasing burden on the healthcare system, including the universal health insurance program, as in 2016 more than 50 percent of medical care expenditure was spent on the elderly population aged 65 years and above, while the expenditure on the population aged 0–14 was only 8 percent (Sakamoto et al. 2018).

Specifically, in the case of Japan, the precision health approach can be introduced to target the growing neurodegenerative diseases in the population, especially Alzheimer's disease. Alzheimer's disease, the fourth leading cause of death in Japan, is expected to further grow. The MHLW predicts that one in five persons over the age of 65 will have Alzheimer's disease in 2025 (MHLW 2017). Precision health is an effective approach for those diseases that (1) can be attributed to a combination of lifestyle, environments, health, and other factors and for which (2) early detection and prevention can make an important difference. Thus Alzheimer's could be a good match for precision health, as it is impacted by health, lifestyle, and environmental factors, including metabolism; moreover, since it is incurable and irreversible, early detection and prevention is crucial, and early detection could manage or mitigate or slow the disease's impact before irreversible brain damage and mental decline occurs. The current method of diagnosing Alzheimer's depends on an evaluation of mental decline, at which time severe brain damage has already taken place (Alzheimer's Association 2018). However, recently, several genes have been identified as being associated with increased risk of the disease with age (Alzheimer's Association 2018). Early intervention for asymptomatic individuals at high risk could prevent or delay onset and increase healthy life years (Prince, Bryce, and Ferri 2011).

Prevention and early detection of Alzheimer's disease with precision health can have an important impact on the reduction of associated healthcare costs. The national medical care expenditure for Alzheimer's disease increased by approximately 39.7 percent over the five years 2011–16, from ¥219.6 billion (~ US$2 billion) (MHLW 2013) to ¥306.7 billion (~ $2.8 billion) (MHLW 2018), which accounted for about 1 percent of total medical care expenditures (MHLW 2018). Furthermore, the social cost of Alzheimer's disease was estimated to be ¥14.5 trillion (~$145 billion) annually in 2014, which consisted of medical care expenditure (¥1.9 trillion), nursing care costs (¥6.4 trillion), and informal care costs[3] (¥6.2 trillion) (Sado 2015). The social cost of Alzheimer's disease is projected to be ¥24.3 trillion in 2060 (Sado 2015). The medical cost of Alzheimer's disease has been increasing not only in Japan, but also in other countries, including the United States, where the 2017 total medical expenditure for Alzheimer's disease was $277 billion (Alzheimer's Association 2018). However, significant cost savings can be achieved by early diagnosis; diagnosis of Alzheimer's disease during the mild cognitive impairment (MCI) stage[4] could save $7.9 trillion in health and long-term care expenditures in the United States (Alzheimer's Association 2018). Early diagnosis of Alzheimer's also provides benefits for patients and families (Alzheimer's Association 2018); early detection of the disease at the MCI stage can allow patients to continue to work for another 10 years (in some cases, the disease can be fully prevented), compared to 3–5 years without early detection (Alzheimer's Association n.d.). In the case of Japan, with the intervention of primary prevention for dementia, healthcare expenditures and nursing care costs for those over 60 are estimated to decline by ¥3.2 billion and ¥3.2 trillion by 2034, respectively (METI 2018). Furthermore, as part of the indirect impact of promoting healthy aging in Japan, it is estimated that the nation's workforce will increase by 8.4 million people and consumption will grow by ¥1.8 trillion by 2025 (METI 2018).

The health policy transformations necessary to introduce precision health to Japan

To achieve the potential positive impacts of introducing precision health to Japan, a nationwide policy infrastructure needs to be developed in the following three areas: (1) health data network, (2) research platform, and (3) intervention. The Japanese government has developed the "Integrated Community Care System for Dementia" (a.k.a. "New Orange Plan")[5] with a focus on promoting community support for people with dementia (MHLW 2018). However, the announced measures mostly emphasize providing the

---

3   Informal care costs are care that patients' families provide at no charge.

4   People at the MCI stage have a slight but noticeable decline in cognitive and thinking abilities and have an increased risk of developing Alzheimer's disease or other dementia.

5   The plan has seven focus areas: (1) raise awareness and promote understanding of dementia, (2) provide healthcare services in a timely and appropriate manner as dementia progresses, (3) reinforce measures to counter younger-onset dementia, (4) provide support for people who look after patients with dementia, (5) create dementia-friendly communities, (6) promote research on the prevention, diagnosis, cure, and care of dementia, and (7) promote understanding of people with dementia and their families.

appropriate care and treatment for patients, rather than early prevention and detection. With the approach of precision health, Japan can focus on the prevention and early detection of the disease, using big data ranging from health to environmental factors.

Health data network

The introduction of precision health to Japan necessitates the construction of a nationwide health data network. Precision health collects and analyzes data to identify an appropriate population-based intervention. The Japanese government has slowly but steadily changed its policies to make government data available for data-driven policymaking. However, health databases remain fragmented and the organizational infrastructure needs to be improved for better-quality data and for wider use. For example, Japan has a number of health databases and disease registries, such as the National Insurance Claim and Health Checkup Database (NDB), Kokuho Database (KDB),[6] Long-term Care Insurance Database, National Clinical Database, and Japan Cancer Registry. However, these were established by individual medical or research institutions and are not fully interlinked. In the NDB and KDB, data are not continuously tracked when individuals change insurers. Furthermore, the NDB mainly exists for reimbursement and not for research or analysis; it does not include detailed procedure or outcome data, which are critical for the precision health approach and for analysis of the effectiveness of healthcare. This lack of empirical evidence on procedures or outcomes could impede a transparent discussion of efficient resource allocation. The development of a nationwide healthcare data network would enable comprehensive analysis of the links among individuals' risk factors, health status, previous treatments, and treatment outcomes, while preventing unnecessary diagnosis, treatment, and prescription of medications. In order to establish a nationwide healthcare data network, the Japanese government needs to first enhance its organizational capacity and expertise, given the current MHLW's limited resources.

Additionally, the introduction of precision health means that the digitization of health records will be an important area of focus. The MHLW has developed standards of medical-information sharing and subsidizes regional healthcare providers to implement web-based electronic health record systems. The digitization process remains slow, and it is essential to further

---

6   The NCD is a database of national health insurance claims and specific screening information; KDB is a database on national health insurance, including health checkups, medical costs, and nursing insurance.

accelerate the promotion of electronic health records.

Research platform

Japan also will need a research platform dedicated to precision health research, focused on prevention and early detection of diseases. The nation-wide database discussed above needs to be accessible for precision research purposes while securing privacy and access controls. Currently, individual research institutions lead research on specific diseases; for example, the Center for Development of Advanced Medicine for Dementia currently plays a central role in developing treatments and care for dementia under the New Orange Plan, while the National Cancer Center takes the lead in research on cancer. However, some institutions may put more emphasis on treatment rather than prevention and early detection, and may not have expertise in the population health approach and data analytics, which are essential to put precision health in place. Thus, it may be most effective to establish a public program dedicated to precision health research and have that program collaborate with public and private research institutions with expertise in specific diseases.

Intervention

Japan should develop an organization that can identify specific populations with tailored interventions for prevention and early detection based on data analysis and research outcomes, targeting people with high-risk profiles for a specific disease. For example, once a specific population is identified as being at high risk for Alzheimer's disease, one potential intervention could be to highlight the importance of preventative efforts, such as improvements in diet, lifestyle, and exercise. Another intervention could be to pursue early diagnosis by encouraging those over a certain age with high-risk profiles to undergo periodical mental assessments with memory evaluation tests, mood evaluations for depression detection, and blood tests and brain structure imaging. These assessments of mental status and mood evaluation can be conducted by trained public health workers, nurses, occupational therapists, and speech-hearing therapists, instead of doctors (MHLW 2009). Given that Japan has national health checkup programs with high coverage, the government can consider integrating some forms of intervention for those with high-risk profiles into the existing health checkup systems. As a caveat, given Japan's fiscal situation, the government should carefully examine which intervention should be covered by national insurance or public finances, based on the cost-effectiveness of interventions.

Health technology assessment

In addition to the three areas above, health technology assessment (HTA) is another area to consider in discussing the introduction of precision health. HTA is an evidence-based evaluation of healthcare technologies' cost-effectiveness to help governments efficiently allocate their limited resources. Some countries have adopted HTA to guide their health technology policy decisions.[7] Given Japan's tight public finance situation, interventions based on the approach of precision health should be cost-effective by targeting people with risk profiles for prevention and early detection, which HTA may be able to help identify.

Currently in Japan, the MHLW's Medical Economics Division decides all the prices of healthcare, medical devices, and pharmaceuticals and revises these every two years, based on input from the Pharmaceutical and Medical Device Agency's evaluation of new drugs and medical devices, as well as through discussions at the Central Social Insurance Medical Council with representatives from the payer side, provider side, and public interest. In 2012, the first Special Committee on Cost-Effectiveness was established under the Central Social Insurance Medical Council; it conducted the pilot HTA project from 2016 to 2018. The committee's plan to carry out re-pricing in 2018 was postponed.

The official introduction of HTA, especially for precision-health interventions, may face several hurdles. Japan has a dearth of HTA experts, so the MHLW would need to provide training. Additionally, the MHLW would need to develop its administrative capacity to oversee HTA, including through creating an HTA-focused agency or bureau. Furthermore, the motivations of all stakeholders would need to be aligned, especially since some stakeholders may be concerned that HTA could reduce resources for medical innovation and research.

Comparative Analysis with Australia

As we consider the implications of introducing a precision-health approach to Japan, a comparative analysis with Australia may provide important insights, especially for establishing health data networks, research platforms, and interventions. Australia is one of the countries to lead the introduction

---

7   Countries such as the United Kingdom, France, Australia, and Canada have adopted HTA to allocate public resources for healthcare based on cost-effectiveness.

of precision health and associated health policy transformations. Australia announced its national mission for precision health policies in 2017 in "Australia 2030: Prosperity through Innovation" (MISI 2017) and "Australia's National Digital Health Strategy 2018–2022" (Australian Digital Health Agency n.d.). The country started its focused genomic research and "one health" approach with stronger partnerships among government, industry, and research institutions. Toward this end, Australia established the Australian Digital Health Agency in July 2016 to reform its health policies and introduce the precision health approach.

The Australian Digital Health Agency manages Australia's nationwide health data platform, known as "My Health Record," an individualized digital clinic record system using single individual health identification. This shared digital health platform links patients' healthcare data across multiple sources and is used to improve the efficiency and quality of healthcare through clinical research, effective public health planning, and the evaluation of health interventions. On the platform, patients can have access to and securely control their own health information, including privacy and access controls. The data are connected through and can be shared with hospitals, pharmacies, general practices, pathology providers, and other healthcare providers, as well as with the Immunization Registry and the Organ Donor Registry.[8] Given its lack of such a data platform, as discussed earlier, Japan can learn from Australia's experience in integrating various healthcare databases with a single individual health identification.

Furthermore, Australia has led the initiation of international collaboration on digital health. In February 2018, the Australian Digital Health Agency initiated the Global Digital Health Partnership (GDHP), an informal framework for the international collaboration of governments and government agencies, as well as for the World Health Organization (WHO). The aim of the GDHP is to facilitate global cooperation in implementing digital health services by sharing insights, evidence, and policy considerations. Currently, 18 countries and WHO participate in the GDHP; the participants include senior digital health officials from Argentina, Australia, Austria, Brazil, Canada, Hong Kong, India, Indonesia, Italy, Saudi Arabia, New Zealand, the Republic of Korea, Singapore, Sweden, Ukraine, the United Kingdom, the United States, Uruguay, and WHO (Global Digital Health Partnership n.d.). The Australian Digital Health Agency noted that successful implementation of a digital health platform requires "the commitment and involvement of all stakeholders, good organizational management, and interdisciplinary teams

8   Countries that have established similar health data networks include Austria, Denmark, the United Kingdom, Estonia, Singapore, Sweden, and the United States.

with information technology experience" (Australian Digital Health Agency, n.d., "International Overview."). This initiative can also inform Japan in how to implement a nationwide health data platform.

Additionally, Australia's Commonwealth Scientific and Industrial Research Organization (CSIRO), a publicly funded government research institution, announced its "Precision Health Project" to promote healthy aging. Precision health is now one of eight investment areas under CSIRO's Future Science Platforms (CSIRO 2019). The project focuses on the research of tailored public health interventions, using big data about lifestyles, genes, and environment, as well as on the development of wearable sensors for real-time health monitoring. CSIRO has the highest concentration of data scientists in Australia and a track record for industry engagement and translation of digitally based research (CSIRO 2019). Such a research platform focused on precision health—which Japan has not yet developed—may help promote research for the prevention and early detection of growing diseases in the era of longevity.

Australia is furthermore considering providing early interventions for those with high-risk profiles for dementia in order to delay onset and enable them to lead longer healthy lives, although the details of such interventions are yet to be announced (Finkel et al. 2018). Based on genomic research outcomes, a potential next step for Australia is to enable asymptomatic individuals at high risk for dementia to be recruited for clinical trials to accelerate the discovery of effective therapies and treatments (Finkel et al. 2018).

Future implementation challenges for Japan

In implementing these suggested health policies in Japan, health decision-makers should be aware of the political economy and dynamics of Japanese healthcare. As discussed earlier, there are various stakeholders in Japan's healthcare, and the concept of precision health can be achieved only with all their support and engagement. It is essential for the government to align each stakeholder's motivation and incentives for the introduction of precision health. It is especially important—given the potential sensitivity of sharing and using the data that each institution collects and manages—that the government emphasize that the nationwide data and research platform is critical for the population's healthy aging and for efficient allocation of limited resources under the concept of precision health. Moreover, decision-makers using the precision health approach should also consider the socioeconomic determinants of health. With regional disparities in health and in checkup rates across work statuses still significant in Japan, the nation's precision health approach should encompass not only health and environmental factors, but also socioeconomic indicators, such as income level, educational attainment, and work status.

Conclusion

Precision health is an increasingly important approach in medicine in the era of longevity and advanced technologies. It empowers individuals to lead longer healthy lives by preventing and detecting diseases before they strike, while also helping reduce healthcare costs. Introducing precision health requires a nationwide initiative to transform health policies and necessitates all stakeholders' engagement. This chapter has examined how the precision health approach can help improve health in Japan and what health policy transformations would be necessary to introduce it. In Japan, the rapid aging of the population is putting severe pressure on public finances; rising social security costs have helped push up the public debt to 253 percent of GDP in 2017. Although Japan has had universal health coverage since 1961 and has national health checkup programs for its whole population, the evidence on their effectiveness is limited. There is room to improve health checkup systems by better tailoring them to the current population health of Japan, using big data and technologies based on the approach of precision health. Specifically, Japan can use precision health to target growing diseases in the aging population, especially Alzheimer's disease. The prevention and early detection of Alzheimer's disease can have a significant impact on national medical expenditures and social costs, including of nursing and informal care. Early diagnosis of Alzheimer's disease during the MCI stage can reduce medical and long-term care expenditures, while also providing benefits for patients and families by enabling them to have longer healthy lives. Given the primary prevention of dementia, Japanese national medical expenditures and nursing care costs for those over 60 are estimated to decline by ¥3.2 billion and ¥3.2 trillion by 2034, respectively (METI 2018). To put precision health in place, Japan should (1) transform its fragmented health databases into a single, secure, individualized health data network that includes detailed procedure and outcome data for precision health research purposes, (2) develop a research platform focused on health research and data analysis for precision health that collaborates with other leading research institutions, and (3) identify effective interventions that target patients with high-risk profiles and provide those interventions, including through existing programs, such as health checkups. In this regard, comparative analysis with Australia provides insights for Japan. Australia provides a leading case study of the implementation of precision health policies. It has established a nationwide digital health database; played a major role in international collaboration in digital health; strengthened publicly funded research programs for precision health; and sought to detect and prevent diseases early on by targeting people with high risk profiles. To implement these policies in Japan, healthcare decision-makers should align all stakeholders' motivations and incentives to ensure their support and engagement in improving Japan's healthcare through precision health.

References

Alzheimer's Association. 2018. "New Alzheimer's Association Report Reveals Sharp Increase in Alzheimer's Prevalence, Deaths and Cost of Care." Alzheimer's Association, March 20, 2018. https://www.alz.org/news/2018/new_alzheimer_s_association_report_reveals_sharp_i.

Alzheimer's Association. n.d. "Earlier Diagnosis." Accessed January 25, 2019. https://www.alz.org/alzheimers-dementia/research_progress/earlier-diagnosis.

Australian Digital Health Agency. n.d. *Australia's National Digital Health Strategy.* https://conversation.digitalhealth.gov.au/sites/default/files/adha-strategy-doc-2ndaug_0_1.pdf.

Australian Digital Health Agency. n.d. "International Overview of Digital Health Record System." https://www.digitalhealth.gov.au/get-started-with-digital-health/digital-health-evidence-review/international-overview-of-digital-health-record-systems.

MISI (Ministry of Industry, Science, and Innovation [Australia]). 2017. *Australia 2030: Prosperity through Innovation.* https://www.industry.gov.au/data-and-publications/australia-2030-prosperity-through-innovation.

CSIRO (Commonwealth Scientific and Industrial Research Organization). 2019. *Precision Health Project.* https://www.csiro.au/en/Research/Health/Future-Science/Precision-Health.

Finkel, Alan, Adam Wright, Shafique Pineda, and Robert Williamson. 2018. "Precision Medicine." Australian Government Office of the Chief Scientist. https://www.chiefscientist.gov.au/wp-content/uploads/Precision-medicine-final.pdf.

Global Digital Health Partnership. n.d.. *Who Is Involved.* https://www.gdhp.org/whos-involved.

Health and Global Policy Institute. n.d. "Players in Health Policy Making in Japan." *Japan Health Policy NOW.* http://japanhpn.org/ja/section2-3/.

Health Care 2035 Advisory Panel. 2015. "Japan 2035: Leading the World through Health." Presentation, Ministry of Health, Labour and Welfare. https://www.mhlw.go.jp/seisakunitsuite/bunya/hokabunya/shakaihoshou/hokeniryou2035/assets/file/healthcare2035_proposal_150703_slide_en.pdf.

Iizuka, Toshiaki, Katsuhiko Nishiyama, Brian Chen, and Karen Eggleston. 2017. "Is Preventive Care Worth the Cost? Evidence from Mandatory Checkups in Japan." NBER Working Paper 23413,

National Bureau of Economic Research, Cambridge, MA.

Ishii, Masami. 2012. "DRG/PPS and DPC/PDPS as Prospective Payment Systems." *JMA Policies* 55 (4): 279–91.

Khoury, Muin J., Michael F. Iademarco, and William T. Riley. 2016. "Precision Public Health for the Era of Precision Medicine." *American Journal of Preventive Medicine* 50 (3): 398.

Matsuda, Tomohiro, and Tomotaka Sobue. 2015. "Recent Trends in Population-Based Cancer Registries in Japan: The Act on Promotion of Cancer Registries and Drastic Changes in the Historical Registry." *International Journal of Clinical Oncology* 20 (1): 11–20.

METI (Ministry of Economy, Trade and Industry of Japan). 2018. *Keizaisangyosho ni okeru healthcare sangyo seisaku ni tsuite* [Ministry of Economy, Trade and Industry's healthcare industry policy]. http://www.meti.go.jp/policy/mono_info_service/healthcare/01metihealth-carepolicy.pdf.

MHLW (Ministry of Health, Labour, and Welfare of Japan). 2009. *Ninchisho yobo shien manual kaiteiban* [Revised manual for prevention and support for dementia]. https://www.mhlw.go.jp/topics/2009/05/dl/tp0501-1h_0001.pdf.

MHLW. 2013. *Heisei 23 nendo Kokumin Iryohi no Gaikyo* [Overview of national health expenditure in 2011]. https://www.mhlw.go.jp/toukei/saikin/hw/k-iryohi/11/dl/toukei.pdf.

MHLW. 2017. *Ninchisho shisaku suishin sogo senryaku* [Comprehensive strategy for promoting measures regarding dementia]. Ministry of Health, Labour, and Welfare. https://www.mhlw.go.jp/stf/seisakunit-suite/bunya/0000064084.html.

MHLW. 2018. *Heisei 28 nendo Kokumin iryohi no gaikyo* [Overview of national health expenditure in 2016]. https://www.mhlw.go.jp/toukei/saikin/hw/k-iryohi/16/dl/data.pdf.

MHLW. 2019. *2017 nendo tokutei kenko shinsa tokutei hoken shido no jisshi jyokyo* [Overview of implementation of special health check-ups and specific health guidance in 2017]. https://www.mhlw.go.jp/stf/houdou/0000173038_00004.html.

Minor, Lloyd. 2016. "We Don't Just Need Precision Medicine, We Need Precision Health." Stanford School of Medicine. http://med.stanford.edu/school/leadership/dean/dean-minor-on-precision-health.html.

Nomura, Shuhei, Haruka Sakamoto, Scott Glenn, Yusuke Tsugawa, Sara K. Abe, Md M. Rahman, Jonathan C. Brown et al. 2017. "Population Health and Regional Variations of Disease Burden in Japan, 1990-2015: A Systemic Subnational Analysis for the Global Burden of

Disease Study 2015. *Lancet* 390 (10101): 1521–38.

Prince, Martin, Renata Bryce, and Cleusa Ferri. 2011. *World Alzheimer Report 2011: The Benefits of Early Diagnosis and Intervention*. Alzheimer's Disease International.

Sado, Mitsuhiro. 2015. Wagakuni ni okeru ninchisho no keizaiteki eikyo ni kansuru kenkyu Heisei 26 nendo soukatsu buntan kenkyu hokokusho [Study on the economic impact of dementia in Japan 2014 summary: shared research report]. http://csr.keio.ac.jp/pdf/2014年度認知症社会的コスト総括分担報告書.pdf.

Sakamoto, Haruka, Md. Mizanur Rahman, Shuhei Nomura, Etsuji Okamoto, Soichi Koike, Hideo Yasunaga, Norito Kawakami, Hideki Hashimoto, Naoki Kondo, Sarah Krull Abe, Matthew Palmer, and Cyrus Ghaznavi. 2018. *Japan Health System Review*. Health Systems in Transition vol. 8, no. 1. World Health Organization, Regional Office for South-East Asia.

White House, President Barack Obama Archives. 2015. "The Precision Medicine Initiative." https://obamawhitehouse.archives.gov/precision-medicine.

Personalized and Precision Medicine in Japan

Hokuto Asano

As advanced technologies reduce the involved cost and time, genome analysis is starting to be used for the development of personalized and precision medicine (PPM) and its accompanying diagnostics. Many countries are working to develop PPM. The United States has the Precision Medicine Initiative and Million Veteran Program; the United Kingdom has Genomics England; China, South Korea, and Saudi Arabia have all started their own projects; and Japan is also working to develop PPM. In all these countries, though, the development of PPM may be hampered by insurance issues. Governments may be reluctant to cover PPM and its accompanying tests with public insurance because they are expensive and may increase healthcare expenditures. This chapter looks at Japan's PPM policies, as well as the country's experience covering PPM and its companion tests with public insurance. For the sake of comparison, the chapter also considers the development of PPM in the United Kingdom.

Personalized and Precision Medicine: Strategy

The Japanese government supports the development of PPM, as clearly stated in the Japan Revitalization Strategy 2016 and the Healthcare Policy Strategy (Government of Japan 2016, 2014). Based on these strategies, the Cabinet Office; the Ministry of Health, Labour and Welfare (MHLW); the Ministry of Education, Culture, Sports, Science, and Technology (MEXT);

and the Ministry of Economy, Trade and Industry (METI) have all set goals[1] and have worked on PPM-related policies. Similar to the UK Department of Health, which leads Genomics England, the MHLW plays a significant role in PPM in Japan. The MHLW has established a task force for using genome information for medical services and focuses on PPM development, while the Japan Agency for Medical Research and Development (AMED), under the MHLW, focuses on PPM research.

In accordance with the accumulated biodata, Japan plans to initially target rare diseases, incurable diseases, cancer, infectious diseases, dementia, undiagnosed diseases, and pharmacogenomics (Headquarters for Health Policy 2017). The MHLW, focusing its efforts on PPM for cancer, established a study group for a consortium of genomic medical care for cancer in March 2017. The second target would be lifestyle-related diseases, such as diabetes and circulatory diseases (Headquarters for Health Policy 2017). In addition, according to the goals of the Healthcare Policy Strategy, the government will also encourage genomic therapy for depression and dementia. Similarly, the United Kingdom focuses on rare diseases and cancer (NHS England 2016).

Related Policies

The development of PPM heavily depends on the amount of genome data available. Japan is collecting genome data mainly through its three largest biobanks—Bio Bank Japan, Tohoku Medical Megabank, and National Center Bio Bank Network—which work together. Bio Bank Japan, the largest of the three, plans to collect data from 300,000 people. Japan supports clinical trials and clinical research on genomic medical care and plans to select seven core hospitals in 2017 where it will support the provision of genomic medical treatment (MHLW 2017a). In 2016, the total budget for these plans was ¥11.36 billion (US$103 million) (MHLW 2016b). The National Cancer Center started the SCRUM-Japan Project, which helps hospitals and pharmaceutical companies develop PPM for cancer. There are no government regulations on genetic testing.

In the United Kingdom, the Department of Health started the 100,000 Genomes Project in 2012, which targeted 70,000 patients in the National Health Service (NHS) who suffer from rare diseases or cancer, along with

---

1   Goals include (1) dramatically improving therapies for lifestyle-related diseases (diabetes, stroke, myocardial infarction, etc.); (2) establishing predictive diagnosis of cancer incidence, and of reactions to and adverse side effects from anti-cancer drugs; (3) starting clinical research concerning genomic therapy for depression and dementia; and (4) developing innovative methods of diagnosing and treating incurable neuromuscular diseases.

30,000 of their family members. The UK government's budget for this initiative was £310 million (US$403 million) for the period 2013–17 (MHLW 2015). The size of the United Kingdom's biobank and data collection budget is much larger than that of Japan. The United Kingdom also established the Genomics England Clinical Interpretation Partnership (which includes clinicians and researchers) and the Genomics Expert Network for Enterprises (GENE) Consortium (which enables partner companies to access gene data collected under Genomics England and to develop new testing and medication). In 2015, the Precision Medicine Catapult was initiated to accelerate the development of PPM (Innovate UK 2015).

Insurance Coverage

In Japan, based on the Health Insurance Act, public insurance generally covers medication (see figure 5.1). First, the medication's quality, effectiveness, and safety must be approved based on the Law on Securing Quality, Efficacy, and Safety of Products including Pharmaceuticals and Medical Devices, Article 14 (1). To receive public insurance coverage, PPM testing kits and testing equipment also need to be examined. At the same time, drug pricing is decided based on the Director General of Health Insurance Bureau Notification, No. 0210-1, February 10, 2016 (MHLW). The Central Social Insurance Medical Council has the authority to decide whether new medical technology and treatment should be covered by public insurance. Members of this council include insurers, doctors, academics, pharmaceutical companies, and medical equipment companies.

Currently in Japan, cost-effectiveness is not a criterion in decisions regarding which medicines or medical equipment should be covered by public insurance (MLHW 2016d). Although MHLW does test the cost-effectiveness of a few medications, it does not use this criterion when considering whether public insurance can cover PPM testing kits and equipment. However, in the United Kingdom, the National Institute for Health and Care Excellence (NICE) considers the cost-effectiveness of medications to be covered by the national insurance, and therefore restricts the use of some drugs. Among the 169 technology appraisal guidelines published by NICE between 2000 and the end of March 2009, 53 limited the use of drugs and equipment among 169 because of their low cost-effectiveness (Shiroiwa et al. 2009). Thus, while decision-makers in the United Kingdom face an economic obstacle when considering whether PPM should be covered by insurance (Davis et al. 2009), their peers in Japan do not.

Examples of Approved Drugs and Companion Diagnostics in Clinical Practice

In Japan, cancer has been the leading cause of death since 1981. Among patients newly diagnosed with cancer, colorectal cancer is the most common, followed by gastric, lung, prostrate, and breast cancers (National Cancer Center 2016). Since the treatment demands for these are enormous, this chapter

FIGURE 5.1 The process for determining insurance coverage for drugs in Japan

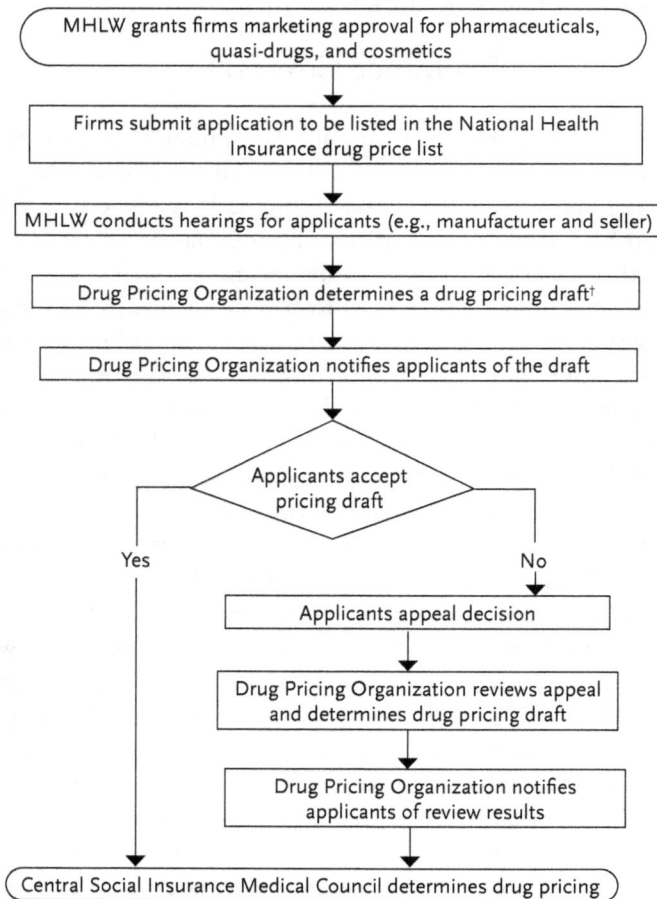

SOURCE: Author.
NOTE: MHLW = Ministry of Labour, Health and Welfare; *In accordance with the Law on Securing Quality, Efficacy and Safety of Products Including Pharmaceuticals and Medical Devices, article 14 (1); †the Drug Pricing Organization is under the Central Social Insurance Medical Council.

considers approved drugs and companion diagnostics for those cancers that are already covered by public insurance in Japan (see table 5.1). For example, Japan approves Herceptin for patients whose HER2 is excessive. Herceptin, Erbitux, and Gleevec were approved in Japan after being approved in the United States and the European Union (EU). Gefitinib was approved first in Japan and then in the United States and EU due to its advanced effectiveness.

TABLE 5.1 Four approved cancer drugs and companion diagnostics in clinical practice

Drug	Companion diagnostic	Target disease
Herceptin (Trastuzumab)	HER2 genetic specimen preparation	Breast cancer
Erbitux (Cetuximab)	EGRF genetic test	Colorectal cancer
Gleevec (Imatinib)	Amp-CML	Gastrointestinal stromal tumor
Gefitinib (Iressa)	EGRF genetic test	Lung cancer

SOURCE: Author.

TABLE 5.2 General information on four approved cancer drugs

Drug	Application[1]	Approval[2]	Japan producer	Japan sales	
				Year	Yen (USD)
Herceptin* (Trastuzumab)	January 2001	Apr. 2001 (U.S. 1998)	Chugai Pharmaceutical Co., Ltd	2016	¥34.1 billion ($310 million)
Erbitux† (Cetuximab)	January 2007	July 2008 (U.S 2004)	Merck Serono Co.	N/A	N/A
Gleevec‡ (Imatinib)	April 2001	November 2001 (U.S.: 2001)	Novartis Pharmaceuticals Corporation	2016	¥27.5 billion ($250 million)
Gefitinib§ (Iressa)	January 2002	July 2002 (U.S.: 2003)	AstraZeneca Plc	2013	¥20.2 billion ($184 million)

SOURCES: *Chugai Pharmaceutical Co., Ltd 2016a, 2016b; †Merck Serono 2015; ‡Novartis Pharmaceuticals Corporation 2016 and Mixonline 2017; §AstraZeneca Corporation 2010.
NOTE: ¹Application: date of application for public insurance coverage in Japan; ²Approval: date of approval for public insurance coverage in Japan (U.S. approval date in parentheses).

Table 5.3 shows the prices—which are quite expensive—of approved drugs in Japan and the United Kingdom. For example, the monthly expenditure of patients who have to take just one Gefitinib a day is more than ¥180,000 ($1,636), and for those who have to take 400 milligrams of Gleevec every day, it is more than ¥295,860 ($2,688). Because there are differing copayment rates, not everyone pays the same: among people 70 years and under, the copayment rate is 30 percent; for those who are 70 to 74 years old it is 20 percent; and for those above 74 years it is 10 percent. In addition, Japan

TABLE 5.3 Price of four approved cancer drugs in Japan and the United Kingdom

| Drug | Japan | | United Kingdom | |
	Price in yen (quantity)	Unit price USD	Price in pounds (quantity)	Unit price USD
Herceptin (Trastuzumab)	¥24,469 (60 mg)	$3.7 mg	£407.40 (150 mg)	$3.5 mg
Erbitux (Cetuximab)	¥36,920 (20 ml/100 mg)	$3.4 mg	£178.10 (20 ml/100 mg)	$2.3 mg
Gleevec (Imatinib)	¥2,465.5 (1 cap/100 mg)	$22.4 cap	£1,442.01 (120 caps, 100 mg ea)	$15.6 cap
Gefitinib (Iressa)	¥6,712.7 (1 tab/250 mg)	$61 tab	£2,167.71 (30 tabs/250 mg)	$93.8 tab

SOURCES: Japan prices from MLHW (2017b). UK prices: Herceptin from NICE (n.d.); Erbitux from NICE (2015); Gleevac from Novartis Korea (2001); Gefitinib from NICE (2014).
NOTE: Cap = capsule; tab = tablet; USD = U.S. dollar. Japan prices are as of March 17, 2017, with exchange rate $1 = ¥110. UK prices are from various years (see sources) with exchange rate $1 = £0.77.

TABLE 5.4 Approval dates and price of companion diagnostics

Diagnostics	Approval date	Price in yen (USD)
HER2 genetic specimen preparation	April 2010	¥27,000 ($245)
EGRF genetic test for colorectal cancer	April 2010	¥36,920*
Amp-CML (TMA method)	November 2004	¥12,000 ($109)
Amp-CML (Real-time RT-PCR method)	April 2015	¥25,200 ($229)
EGRF genetic test for lung cancer	April 2006	¥25,000 ($227)[†] ¥21,000 ($191)[‡]

SOURCES: LSI Medience Corporation, "Molecular Target Drug and Clinical Examination," July 13, 2013, accessed June 3, 2017, http://www.aichi-amt.or.jp/labo/patho/reco/20130713_01.pdf; MLHW listing in the National Health Insurance drug price list (apply from March 17, 2017), accessed May 17, 2017, http://www.mhlw.go.jp/topics/2016/04/tp20160401-01.html.
NOTE: USD = U.S. dollar; *Price is per 100 mg/20ml; [†]using polymerase chain reaction (PCR) method; [‡]using non-PCR method.

has a High-Cost Medical Expense Benefit that has established a cap on the insured's drug expenditures. Except for Gefitinib, drug prices in Japan are more expensive than those in the United Kingdom. These results are similar to that of another research study that showed the average price of a new drug in Japan as 108–204 percent higher than that of the United Kingdom, depending on the exchange rate (MHLW 2013).

Furthermore, although both Japan and the United Kingdom have approved Imatinib, the United Kingdom limits its use because of cost-effectiveness (Shiroiwa et al. 2009). One NICE (2004) guideline states that an increase in the dose of Imatinib is not recommended for patients unresponsive to treatment or for patients who develop a progressive disease.

When we compare tables 5.2 and 5.4 we observe a time lag between the approval of drugs and the approval of the companion diagnostics. For example, although Herceptin was approved in April 2001, the HER2 genetic specimen preparation was approved only in April 2010. Hence, between April 2001 and March 2010, the HER2 genetic specimen preparation tests conducted by medical institutions were not covered by public insurance. According to a research study (Hamburg and Collins 2010), due to this time lag physicians did not have accurate information on which to base decisions regarding treatments, and this also decreased the chances of physicians adopting a new therapeutic-diagnostic approach. In July 2000, soon after Herceptin was approved, the Japanese Society of Pathology published guidelines for an HER2 examination for breast cancer to provide physicians with accurate information.

TABLE 5.5   Genetic tests covered under public insurance and their costs

Test	Price in yen (USD)	Purpose
Genetic testing for targeted 72 diseases	¥38,800 ($353)	Diagnose hereditary diseases.*
Twelve tissue examinations for cancer	¥21,000–¥65,200[†] ($191–$593)	Determine a method of treating and conducting a precise pathological diagnosis.
Hematopoietic tumor genetic testing	¥21,000 ($191)	Determine a method of treating leukemia patients.
Polymorphism of UGT1A1 gene	¥21,000 ($191)	Determine the dosage of irinotecan hydrochloride.[‡]

SOURCES: See sources and notes for tables 5.3 and 5.4, MHLW website, and MHLW (2016c).
NOTE: USD = U.S. dollar; *In principle, hospitals or clinics can claim the fee of this testing through public insurance only once for each patient; [†]depending on the test; [‡]Irinotecan hydrochloride is an anti-cancer drug used to treat lung cancer and metastatic-colorectal-cancer patients.

Other Genetic Testing

Japan's public insurance also covers the genetic testing mentioned in table 5.5. Coverage of the above tests has been expanded. Since MHLW needs to financially support patients who suffer from incurable diseases based on the Act on Medical Care for Rare Disease Patients enacted in 2015, it transformed genetic testing for the targeted 34 diseases to genetic testing for the targeted 72 diseases in 2015 (Genomu jōhō o mochiita iryō-tō no jitsuyō-ka suishin tasukufōsu 2016). Also, in 2017, RET gene testing for medullary thyroid cancer and RB1 gene testing for swollen bud cells of the omentum were included in genetic testing for the targeted 72 diseases. In addition to the above, genetic counseling is also covered by public insurance and costs ¥5,000 (US$45).

Japan's public insurance, however, does not cover some genetic testing (such as BRCA1/2 genetic testing for breast cancer) due to several reasons, such as insufficient patient data.

Conclusion

The Japanese government has not examined the cost-effectiveness of PPM and its impact on healthcare expenditures. One research study examined the cost-effectiveness of Gefitinib and epidermal growth factor receptor (EGFR) testing in Japan by calculating the incremental cost-effectiveness ratio and showing that this combination was more cost-effective than treatment without EGFR testing (Narita et al. 2015). Japan currently covers companion genetic tests. Furthermore, for cancer-related genetic testing, Japan is considering whether public insurance should cover genetic panel testing, which does not specify the target molecule but rather examines multiple genes at the same time (MHLW 2017a). In addition, Japan plans to approve PPM that has been proven effective and safe under certain conditions. However, policies to promote PPM may increase total healthcare expenditures. Since Japan already has extensive public debt and its healthcare expenditures are expected to increase due to its aging population, the Japanese government must consider cost-effectiveness when determining public insurance coverage for PPM.

References

AstraZeneca Corporation. 2010. "Iressa Tablets 250." [In Japanese.] Pharmaceutical interview form. AstraZeneca. http://i250-higainokai.com/2010-11-iressa_if.pdf, accessed June 3, 2017.

Chugai Pharmaceutical Co., Ltd. 2016a. "Herceptin." [In Japanese.] Pharmaceutical interview form. Chugai Pharmaceutical Co., Ltd. https://chugai-pharm.jp/hc/ss/pr/drug/her_via0060_01/if/PDF/her_if.pdf?_back=6,1.

Chugai Pharmaceutical Co., Ltd. 2016b. "Sei shōhin betsu uriagedaka no suii" [Trends in sales by product]. Chugai Pharmaceutical Co., Ltd. https://www.chugai-pharm.co.jp/ir/finance/revenue_product.html.

Davis, Jerel C., Laura Furstenthal, Amar A. Desai, Troy Norris, Saumya Sutaria, Edd Fleming, and Philip Ma. 2009. "The Microeconomics of Personalized Medicine: Today's Challenge and Tomorrow's Promise." *Nature Review Drug Discovery* 8 (4): 279–86.

Government of Japan. 2014. *The Healthcare Policy*. https://www.kantei.go.jp/jp/singi/kenkouiryou/en/pdf/policy.pdf, accessed November 10, 2019.

Government of Japan. 2016. *Japan Revitalization Strategy 2016 (Provisional)*. https://www.kantei.go.jp/jp/singi/keizaisaisei/pdf/zentaihombun_160602_en.pdf, accessed November 10, 2019.

Hamburg, Margaret A., and Francis S. Collins. 2010. "The Path to Personalized Medicine." *New England Journal of Medicine* 363 (4): 301–04.

Headquarters for Healthcare Policy. 2017. "Genomuiryou jitsugen nimuketa taishoushikkan no kangaekata" [The concept of target diseases for genomic medical care]. Cabinet Secretariat, February 15. https://www.kantei.go.jp/jp/singi/kenkouiryou/genome/dai7/siryou3_1.pdf.

Innovate UK. 2015. "Precision Medicine Catapult." Innovate UK, April. https://www.catapult.org.uk/wp-content/uploads/2016/04/Precision-Medicine-Catapult-April-2015.pdf.

Merck Serono. 2019. "Erbitux Injection." [In Japanese.] Pharmaceutical interview form. Merck Serono. https://www.merckgroup.com/content/dam/web/corporate/non-images/country-specifics/japan/buisness/documents_center/product-info/erbitux/190918_erbitux_intvform_JP.pdf.

MHLW (Ministry of Health, Labour and Welfare). 2013. "Shin'yaku no yakka ni okeru Ōshū to no hikaku" [Comparison on price of new drugs with Europe]. Ministry of Health, Labour and Welfare, February 27. http://www.mhlw.go.jp/stf/shingi/2r9852000002w6r3-att/2r-9852000002w6uj.pdf.

MHLW. 2015. "Genomu iryō ni kansuru sho gaikoku no torikumi ni tsuite" [On foreign countries' PPM policies]. Ministry of Health, Labour and Welfare, July 15. http://www.kantei.go.jp/jp/singi/kenkoui-ryou/genome/dai4/siryou02.pdf.

MHLW. 2016a "Standard of Drug Price." [In Japanese.] Director General of Health Insurance Bureau.

MHLW. 2016b. "Genomu kanren shisaku" [Policies related to genomic medical care]. Ministry of Health, Labour and Welfare, January 27. http://www.mhlw.go.jp/file/05-Shingikai-10601000-Daijinkanboukou-seikagakuka-Kouseikagakuka/160127_task_s1.pdf.

MHLW. 2016c. "Genomu jōhō o mochiita iryō-tō no jitsuyō-ka suishin tasukufōsu dai 5-kai gijiroku" [The fifth meeting of the task force for using genomic information for medical services]. Meeting minutes. Ministry of Health, Labour and Welfare, February 18. http://www.mhlw.go.jp/file/05-Shingikai-10601000-Daijinkanboukouseikagaku-ka-Kouseikagakuka/0000125748.pdf.

MHLW. 2016d "Hiyōtaikōka hyōka no shikenteki dōnyū ni tsuite" [Testing cost-effectiveness]. Ministry of Health, Labour and Welfare, April 27. https://www.mhlw.go.jp/file/05-Shingikai-12404000-Hokenkyo-ku-Iryouka/0000122983.pdf.

MHLW. 2017a. "Gan genomu iryō suishin konsōshiamu kondan-kai" [Study group for a consortium of genomic medical care for cancer]. Draft report. Ministry of Health, Labour and Welfare, May 20. http://www.mhlw.go.jp/file/05-Shingikai-10901000-Kenkoukyoku-Sou-muka/0000166310.pdf.

MHLW. 2017b. "Yakka kijun shūsai hinmoku risuto oyobi kōhatsu iyakuhin ni kansuru jōhō ni tsuite" [Listing in the National Health Insurance drug price list]. Ministry of Health, Labour and Welfare. http://www.mhlw.go.jp/topics/2016/04/tp20160401-01.html, accessed May 17, 2017.

Mixonline. 2017. "Nobarutisu Tsunaba shin shachō kongo 10-nen de 'Shakai kara mottomo shinrai sa reru kigyō ni'" [New Novartis president Tsunaba: Within the next ten years "to be the most socially trusted company"]. Mixonline. https://www.mixonline.jp/tabid55.html?artid=57773, accessed November 10, 2019.

Narita, Yusuke, Yukiko Matsushima, Takeru Shiroiwa, Koji Chiba, Yoichi Nakanishi, Tatsuo Kurokawa, and Hisashi Urushihara. 2015.

"Cost-effectiveness Analysis of EGFR Mutation Testing and Gefitinib as First-line Therapy for Non-small Cell Lung Cancer." *Lung Cancer* 90 (1): 71–77.

National Cancer Center. 2016. "Cancer Statistics 2015." National Cancer Center, July 15, Japan.

NHS (National Health Service) England. 2016. "100,000 Genomes Project." NHS England, September. https://www.england.nhs.uk/wp-content/uploads/2016/09/100k-genomes-project-paving-the-way.pdf.

NICE (National Institute for Health and Care Excellence). 2004. "Imatinib for the Treatment of Unresectable and/or Metastatic Gastro-intestinal Stromal Tumours." NICE, October 27. https://www.nice.org.uk/guidance/ta86/documents/appraisal-consultation-document-imatinib-for-the-treatment-of-unresectable-andor-metastatic-gastrointestinal-stromal-tumours.

NICE. 2014. "Erlotinib and Gefitinib for Treating Non-small-cell Lung Cancer that Has Progressed after Prior Chemotherapy." NICE, August 7. https://www.nice.org.uk/guidance/ta374/documents/erlotinib-and-gefitinib-for-treating-nonsmallcell-lung-cancer-that-has-progressed-following-prior-chemotherapy-review-of-ta162-and-ta175-appraisal-consultation-document.

NICE. 2015. "Cetuximab, Bevacizumab, and Panitumumab for the Treatment of Metastatic Colorectal Cancer after First-line Chemotherapy: Cetuximab (Monotherapy or Combination Chemotherapy), Bevacizumab (in Combination with Non-oxaliplatin Chemotherapy), and Panitumumab (Monotherapy) for the Treatment of Metastatic Colorectal Cancer after First-line Chemotherapy." NICE, January 25. https://www.nice.org.uk/guidance/ta242/chapter/3-the-technologies.

NICE. N.d. "Herceptin® (Roche) Report Adverse Reaction(s)." NICE. https://www.evidence.nhs.uk/formulary/bnf/current/8-malignant-disease-and-immunosuppression/81-cytotoxic-drugs/815-other-antineoplastic-drugs/trastuzumab/trastuzumab/herceptin, accessed June 4, 2017.

Novartis Korea. 2001. "Application for Reimbursement Price Adjustment in Korea." Consumer Project on Technology. http://www.cptech.org/ip/health/gleevec/7prices.pdf.

Novartis Pharmaceuticals Corporation. 2016. "Glivec Tablets 100mg." [In Japanese.] Pharmaceutical interview form. Novartis Pharmaceuticals Corporation. https://drs-net.novartis.co.jp/SysSiteAssets/common/pdf/gli/if/if_gli.pdf, accessed June 3, 2017.

Shiroiwa, Takeru, Takashi Fukuda, Shigeru Watanabe, and Kiichiro Tsutani. 2009. "A Review of Technology Appraisal Guidances and Health Technology Assessment by the National Institute for Health and Clinical Excellence in the UK." [In Japanese.] *Japanese Journal of Health Economics and Policy* 21 (2): 155–69.

Genomu jōhō o mochiita iryō-tō no jitsuyō-ka suishin tasukufōsu [Task force for using genomic information for medical services]. 2016. "Genomu iryō-tō no jitsugen hatten no tame no guteiteki hōsaku ni tsuite (iken torimatome)" [Concrete measures for development of genomic medical services (summary of opinions)]. Ministry of Health, Labour and Welfare, October 28. http://www.mhlw.go.jp/file/05-Shingikai-10601000-Daijinkanboukouseikagakuka-Kouseikaga-kuka/0000140440.pdf.

Wakita, Satoshi. 2013. "Bunshi hyōteki kusuri to rinshō kensa" [Molecularly targeted drugs and clinical tests]. LSI Medience Corporation, July 13. http://www.aichi-amt.or.jp/labo/patho/reco/20130713_01.pdf.

6 Diabetes Care Management and Policy toward Healthy Aging in South Korea

Hongsoo Kim

Diabetes mellitus (hereafter diabetes) is a common chronic disease, and the provision of quality diabetes management is high on the public health agenda in most developed countries with aging populations (OECD 2015). South Korea (hereafter Korea) is no exception. Korea experienced rapid industrialization starting in the 1960s, which brought rapid socioeconomic and cultural changes such as urbanization, family nuclearization, and the popularity of Western-style diets (Kwon n.d.; WHO 2015). These changes, along with improved medical technology and access to care, have resulted in a rapid increase in life expectancy and also an epidemic of chronic diseases (WHO 2015). The country's current health system does not respond well to the changing needs of its aging population; it is still oriented toward acute, inpatient care, and fragmented. Reforms toward a health system promoting healthy aging are urgently needed, and, for this, preventing and managing noncommunicable diseases (NCDs) in the aging population are key priorities.

Diabetes, along with hypertension, are the two chronic conditions that Korea's NCD policy has targeted to tackle over the past several decades, with lessons that showcase the challenges, responses, and future agenda of the country's NCD policy. This chapter will begin with a brief overview of Korea's health profile and the burden of diabetes in the context of population aging. It will present major policy efforts toward advanced diabetes management through improving clinical standards and implementing strategies to promote

This work was supported by a 2016 AXA Award from the AXA Research Fund. The author thanks Minji Kim and Seung Yeon Chun at Seoul National University for their support of the chapter's preparation.

quality diabetes care. The chapter will then review existing evidence on the outcomes of such policy efforts and end with a discussion of future research and policy agendas.

Country Health Profile

Korea is an East Asian country located in the southern part of the Korean Peninsula. As shown in table 6.1, its total population was 51.0 million in 2015 (World Bank n.d.), and is projected to reach its peak at 51.9 million in 2028, and then by 2067 decrease to 39.3. million, which was the population in 1982 (Statistics Korea 2019a). The expected shrinking of the population is related to a consistent decrease in the total fertility rate, which was 1.23 in 2015, less than half its rate of 2.82 in 1980 (World Bank n.d.). Over those 35 years, the economy of Korea rapidly improved: the gross domestic product (GDP) per capita (USD 2010 purchasing power parity [PPP]) increased from US$5,087 in 1980 to $34,193 in 2015 (OECD 2019; World Bank n.d.). During that same period the life expectancy also dramatically increased, from 66.0 years in 1980 to 82.0 years in 2015. By sex, the life expectancy at birth was 79.0 years among men and 85.2 years among women in 2015, higher than the average life expectancy in member countries of the Organisation for Economic Co-operation and Development (OECD), which was 77.9 years for men and 83.1 years for women (OECD 2017; World Bank n.d.). Due to the increasing longevity and rapid decrease in fertility, the proportion of people aged 65 or older rapidly tripled over those 35 years (4.1% in 1980 vs. 13.0% in 2015); today, population aging is expected to continue, with these proportions expected to go up to 25.0% by 2030 and even 46.5% by 2067 (Statistics Korea 2019a). Amid rapid population aging, the age dependency ratio (the proportion of the population that is of working age) dropped by almost half, from 61.3 to 36.7, over the 35 years observed (table 6.1). The proportion of single-person households out of total households increased more than five times from 4.8% in 1980 to 27.2% in 2015 (Statistics Korea 2019b).

Table 6.2 shows the top 10 causes of death and their rates between 2000 and 2017 (Statistics Korea 2011, 2016, 2018b). Cancer (malignant neoplasms) is consistently the leading cause of death in Korea over the period, although its rate of increase has slowed recently. This slowdown is partially due to the aggressive policy efforts of the National Cancer Screening Program (NCSP), which screens six common sites of cancer for all citizens when they reach certain ages (Korea National Cancer Center n.d.), and the expansion of cost coverage since 2013 (National Archives of Korea 2014). Cerebrovascular

TABLE 6.1 A health profile of Korea at five points in time, 1980–2015

	1980	1990	2000	2010	2015
Population (million)	38.1	42.9	47.0	49.4	51.0
Birth rate, crude (per 1,000 people)	22.6	15.2	13.3	9.4	8.6
Death rate, crude (per 1,000 people)	7.3	5.6	5.2	5.1	5.4
Total fertility rate (children per woman)	2.82	1.57	1.47	1.23	1.23
Population density (people/km2)	395.2	444.4	487.3	509.8	523.5
GDP (billions, USD)	64.9	279.3	561.6	1,094.0	1,383.0
GDP annual growth (%)	-1.7	7.0	8.9	6.5	2.8
GDP per capita, 2010 PPPs (USD)	5,086.5	11,637.7	20,765.8	30,365.3	34,192.5
Public expenditure (% of GDP)	15.1	13.5	15.8	18.4	24.9
Life expectancy, both sexes (years)	66.0	71.6	75.9	80.1	82.0
Life expectancy, women (years)	70.4	75.9	79.7	83.6	85.2
Life expectancy, men (years)	61.9	67.5	72.3	76.8	79.0
Population aged 65 years or older (%)	4.1	5.2	7.2	10.7	13.0
Age dependency ratio	61.26	44.22	38.51	36.63	36.74
Single-person households rate (%)	4.8	9.0	15.5	23.9	27.2

SOURCE: OECD 2017; Statistics Korea 2019b; World Bank n.d.
NOTE: GDP = gross domestic product; PPP = purchasing power parity.

diseases and heart diseases were the second and third leading causes of death, respectively, until 2010, though the order recently switched. A noticeable change was that intentional self-harm was the eighth leading cause of death in 2000, but it has risen to the fourth or fifth leading cause of death since 2005. On the other hand, transport accidents were the fourth leading cause of death in 2000, but their ranking went down to seventh in 2005 and further down to ninth or tenth in later years. Diabetes mellitus has been the fifth or sixth leading cause of death over the years: 17.9 out of 100,000 people died with diabetes as the principal diagnosis in 2017. The average age-adjusted mortality rate due to diabetes was 28.9 per 100,000 in Korea between 2012 and 2015, higher than the average of OECD countries (22.8) during the same years (KCDC 2017a). Several other NCDs—hypertensive diseases, chronic lower respiratory diseases, and liver diseases—were also in the top 10 list. Among people aged 65 or older, the top causes of death follow a similar pattern. Cancer was the number one cause of death, followed by cardiovascular disease and cerebrovascular disease, in the older population aged 65 or over in 2017 (Korea Statistics 2018a). Diabetes (257.6 per 100,000 older people) and pneumonia are also listed in the top five common causes of death among older people, unlike the general population.

TABLE 6.2 Top ten causes of death in Korea, 2000–17 (per 100,000 people)

	2000		2005		2010		2015		2017	
1	Malignant neoplasms	121.4	Malignant neoplasms	133.8	Malignant neoplasms	144.4	Malignant neoplasms	150.8	Malignant neoplasms	153.9
2	Cerebrovascular diseases	73.1	Cerebrovascular diseases	64.1	Cerebrovascular diseases	53.2	Heart diseases	55.6	Heart diseases	60.2
3	Heart diseases	38.2	Heart diseases	39.3	Heart diseases	46.9	Cerebrovascular diseases	48.0	Cerebrovascular diseases	44.4
4	Transport accidents	25.3	Intentional self-harm	24.7	Intentional self-harm	31.2	Pneumonia	28.9	Pneumonia	37.8
5	Diseases of liver	22.8	Diabetes mellitus	24.2	Diabetes mellitus	20.7	Intentional self-harm	26.5	Intentional self-harm	24.3
6	Diabetes mellitus	22.6	Diseases of liver	17.2	Pneumonia	14.9	Diabetes mellitus	20.7	Diabetes mellitus	17.9
7	Chronic lower respiratory diseases	16.7	Transport accidents	16.3	Chronic lower respiratory diseases	14.2	Chronic lower respiratory diseases	14.8	Diseases of liver	13.3
8	Intentional self-harm	13.6	Chronic lower respiratory diseases	15.5	Diseases of liver	13.8	Diseases of liver	13.4	Chronic lower respiratory diseases	13.2
9	Hypertensive diseases	8.9	Hypertensive diseases	9.3	Transport accidents	13.7	Transport accidents	10.9	Hypertensive diseases	11.3
10	Pneumonia	8.1	Pneumonia	8.5	Hypertensive diseases	9.6	Hypertensive diseases	9.9	Transport accidents	9.8

SOURCES: Statistics Korea 2011, 2016, 2018b.

TABLE 6.3 Diabetes and hypertension management trends in Korea (population aged 30 years and older, age-adjusted)

	Diabetes				Hypertension			
	2001	2005	2010	2015	2001	2005	2010	2015
Prevalence total	8.5	9.1	9.6	9.5	28.5	28.0	26.8	27.8
Male	9.5	10.5	11.0	11.0	33.2	31.5	29.3	32.6
Female	7.9	7.6	8.2	8.0	25.3	23.8	23.8	22.9
		2007–09	2010–12	2013–15		2007–09	2010–12	2013–15
Awareness rate		72.4	71.2	68.2		65.3	63.1	63.5
Male		71.7	69.3	66.2		61.6	59.5	61.9
Female		73.3	73.4	71.6		70.3	69.1	65.9
Treatment rate		57.2	62.2	60.8		59.1	57.5	59.6
Male		55.0	60.3	58.5		54.9	54.2	57.3
Female		59.7	64.6	64.7		65.2	62.9	63.1
Control rate*		29.1	28.2	26.7		41.4	40.4	43.4
Male		32.6	29.4	28.1		38.0	39.4	42.0
Female		24.1	25.9	25.4		46.2	43.2	47.3

SOURCE: KCDC 2017b.
NOTE: *Control rate among those with diabetes or hypertension.

Diabetes Epidemiology: Prevalence, Management, and Burden

As shown in table 6.3, the prevalence of diabetes in the general population (people aged 30+) was about 8.5% in 2001 and consistently increased to 9.5% in 2015 (KCDC 2017b). Hypertension is the most prevalent chronic condition in Korea and is also often a comorbid condition of diabetes. The prevalence of hypertension is much higher than diabetes in the general population (27.8% in 2015). Both diabetes and hypertension are more prevalent among men than women. A recent study projected that the prevalence of type 2 diabetes in Korea will increase to 29.3% (95% CI: 27.6–30.8) among men and 19.7% (95% CI: 18.2–21.2) among women by 2030, using risk factors identified from national statistics and a nationally representative survey, the Korea National Health and Nutrition Examination Survey (KNHANES) (Baik 2019). Among people aged 65 or older, the unadjusted prevalence of diabetes (22.2%) and hypertension (64.7%) were more than double those of the general population (10.6% for diabetes and 32.0% for hypertension) in 2015.

Along with its high prevalence, inadequate management of diabetes is another policy issue. In spite of various policy efforts, the recognition rates of diabetes and hypertension in the general population in 2015 were still about 68.2% and 63.5%, and the treatment rates were slightly lower at about 60.8% and 59.6%, respectively, based on the KNHANES data from a representative sample. Moreover, the control rate among people with each condition was much lower, at 26.7% among people with diabetes and 43.4% among those with hypertension. These statistics show there is an urgent need to improve the quality of chronic disease management (CDM) in Korea. In addition, a better understanding and more tailored approaches are necessary to reduce the gender gap in the prevalence and management of both chronic conditions.

The economic burden of diabetes management on the national health insurance system has increased over time, as shown in table 6.4 (NHIS 2001, 2006, 2011, 2016). During the last 15 years, the total number of patients of all ages receiving diabetes treatment increased about 2.6 times, from 957,690 in 2000 to 2,521,850 in 2015, while the total expenditure for diabetes management increased almost 7.5 times (from US$241.7 million in 2000 to $1,815.9 million in 2015). As for inpatient service use, the number of patients with diabetes increased about 2.5 times (from 57,327 to 91,384), and the expenditure for diabetes inpatient care almost quadrupled (from $58.9 million to $239.3 million) between 2000 and 2015. On the other hand, the number of patients and amount of expenditure on outpatient service use dramatically increased 2.6 times and 8.7 times, respectively, during the same period. In a study of people aged 15 or older with diabetes, using national health insurance sample cohort data from 2002 to 13 (Kim and Cheng 2018), the mean outpatient visits (physician consultations) per year was 26.89 (SD = 23.68) in 2002, and it increased to 31.41 (standard deviation = 31.10) in 2013. The frequency of physician consultations was much higher than that of the general population in Korea (16.0 per person per year), which was also much higher than the average number of physician consultations (6.9) in 32 OECD countries (OECD 2017).

Lastly, some of those inpatient service uses are preventable. The diabetes-related avoidable hospitalization (DRAH) rate is a widely used quality indicator of diabetes primary care across OECD countries. The age-sex standardized DRAH rate among 100,000 people in Korea was 348.1 in 2010, and the rate decreased somewhat to 281.0 in 2015; yet Korea was the county with the second highest DRAH rate, following Mexico (291.8), among 33 OECD member countries that reported the quality indicators in 2015, with the mean DRAH rate at 137.2 (OECD 2017). In a recent study of DRAH rates

TABLE 6.4 Medical care utilization of people with diabetes in Korea (all ages)

	2000	2005	2010	2015
Total				
Number of patients	957,690	1,610,575	2,016,261	2,521,850
Days	8,822,936	15,307,855	18,067,571	20,904,045
Days per patient	9.2	9.5	9.0	8.3
Total expenditure (USD, millions)	241.7	304.8	1,350.4	1,815.9
Total cost per patient (USD)	252.35	189.24	669.74	720.08
Inpatient				
Number of patients	57,327	67,536	85,984	91,384
Days	945,179	1,393,262	2,347,004	2,411,162
Days per patient	16.5	20.6	27.3	26.4
Total expenditure (USD, millions)	58.9	84.5	171.0	239.3
Total cost per patient (USD)	1,028.52	1,250.93	1,989.22	2,618.92
Outpatient				
Number of patients	948,170	1,599,643	1,999,612	2,500,933
Days	7,886,757	13,914,593	15,720,567	18,492,883
Days per patient	8.3	8.7	7.9	7.4
Total expenditure (USD, millions)	182.8	220.3	1,179.4	1,576.6
Total cost per patient (USD)	192.79	137.72	589.81	630.4

SOURCES: NHIS 2001, 2006, 2011, 2016.

NOTE: 1 USD=1,000 Korean won (1₩).

among people aged 15 or older in Korea and Taiwan, using comparable national health insurance administrative data from 2006 to 13 (Kim and Cheng 2018), the risk of DRAH in Korea was significantly higher among diabetes patients with multimorbidity, living in rural areas, and/or with fewer physician consultations.

Policy Efforts to Improve Diabetes Management

Diabetes management:
Clinical guidelines and first-line treatment

Treatment Guidelines for Diabetes (hereafter diabetes guidelines) were first released by the Korea Diabetes Association (KDA) in the 1990s, and the fifth revision of the KDA diabetes guidelines was released in October 2015 (KDA 2015). Focused on primary diabetes care, *Evidence-Based Guidelines for*

Type 2 Diabetes in Primary Care was released in January 2018 by the Korean Academy of Medical Sciences (KAMS) and Korea Centers for Disease Control and Prevention (KCDC) (KAMS and KCDC 2019). Diabetes screening is offered as a part of the National Health Screening Program administered by the National Health Insurance Services (NHIS), the single public insurer in Korea. The screening program was established under the basic health screening law in 2008 (KMHW 2019). Diabetes screening based on a fasting blood sugar test was originally included in the National Health Screening Program mainly for people aged 40 and over, and in 2019 the program was extended to all adults aged 20 or over. If an abnormal test result is found, further diagnosis tests are provided to confirm diabetes. First-line treatment of diabetes is mostly conducted in clinics in the community and/or outpatient clinics in hospitals, as well as in public health centers. Korea is known for providing good access to outpatient and inpatient care with a relatively low copayment under NHI (WHO 2015), which results in the higher number of physician consultations by diabetes patients as well as the general population (described above) in Korea compared with other OECD countries (OECD 2017); the quality and efficiency of diabetes care, however, need to be improved.

Government-initiated diabetes management programs

Several CDM programs targeting diabetes and often also hypertension in primary care settings have been implemented, and four major programs are briefly described here. First, the Hypertension-Diabetes Registration and Management Program based in community health centers (CHCs) led by the KCDC started in 2007 (Yang and Lee 2015). About 31 out of 258 CHCs in the communities (*si-gun-gu*, the smallest administrative units in Korea) partic-ipate in the program, and about 410,000 adults aged 30 and over residing in the communities have been registered since September 2017 (Kim 2018).

Second, the Clinic-Based Chronic Disease Management Program begun in 2012 aims to encourage people to manage hypertension and diabetes in community clinics rather than in the outpatient clinics of general hospitals (Kim 2018; Paik et al. 2015). As a nationwide program led by the NHIS, about 22.2 million hypertension and/or diabetes patients were enrolled in the program through 7,885 clinics in 2017. When participants designate a doctor in a local clinic as their primary doctor, they receive a discount on copayments for consultation fees starting with their second visit. Patients also receive health support services including health information sent via SMS, health counseling services, and rental services for self-monitoring devices for blood pressure and/or blood sugar.

Along with the Clinic-Based Chronic Disease Management Program, a pay-for-performance (P4P) program with quality monitoring by the Health Insurance Review and Assessment Service (HIRA) has been implemented (HIRA 2017). HIRA started an annual assessment of the appropriateness of hypertension and diabetes care at local clinics in 2011, and since 2012 has assessed the quality of care and provided a form of financial incentive to about the top 20 percent of clinics treating hypertension and diabetes patients. The quality measures have been revised over time. In 2017, a total of seven measures in the three areas of treatment consistency, prescriptions, and lab tests were used along with three monitoring (test) measures. A total of 3,194 clinics received incentives totaling ₩39 billion (US$1 = ₩1,000) for diabetes care (5,341 clinics and ₩118 billion for hypertension care) based on the performance evaluation in 2016 (HIRA 2017).

Third, in the wake of consensus on the need for more engagement and leadership by primary care physicians in the communities, another program, the Community-Based Primary Care Demonstration Program, was implemented in 2014 (Kim 2018; Kim, Hee Sun, et al. 2016, 2017). The program targets local clinics and aims to strengthen the roles of community physician associations; providers deliver care plans and education for disease management and health promotion to their patients with hypertension and diabetes who routinely visit the local clinics. If needed, the clinics refer their patients to a health support center at the CHC or the local office of the NHIS in the community, in which nurses and nutritionists provide tailored education and counseling. Participating clinics are reimbursed for their services by the NHIS through a special fee schedule for the pilot program, and the supporting centers are operated by the local government with local funding and subsidies from the central government. About 741 local clinics and approximately 101,000 patients in 16 *si-gun-gu*s have participated as of May 2018 (Kim 2018).

Fourth, the Demonstration Payment Program for Chronic Disease Management began in September 2016 (Kim 2018; Kim, Yoo, and Lee 2018) with the aim of strengthening the role of local clinics as primary care providers by examining the NHI reimbursement fee schedule and its criteria for a new CDM program, including non-face-to-face as well as face-to-face care that promote the quality of CDM in primary care settings. As part of this nationwide program, participating community clinics register patients; manage diabetes or hypertension via care-planning through face-to-face meetings with patients during visits; continue management via text messages or phone counseling between the visits, and include a follow-up visit for evaluation and re-planning. Patients send their blood pressure and/or blood sugar readings regularly through a mobile app/internet and can receive phone counseling up to twice per month. The fee schedule consists of three parts: planning-check-evaluation, continuing management, and phone counseling. Primary care physicians received on average approximately US$30 per patient per month in 2018, and the copayment was waived for participating patients during the pilot program. A relatively small number of clinics (1,173) participated in the demonstration program, and 51,000 patients had registered by July 2018.

Evidence on the economics of diabetes care and policy impacts

Evidence on the economics of diabetes care. A small number of published empirical studies have reported on the economic burden of diabetes care in Korea, showing the importance of prevention and management. Cho (2016) examined healthcare expenditure using national health insurance sample data from 2015 and reported that the healthcare expenditure per person per year for patients with both macro- and micro-vascular complications was about 32.1 times higher than for diabetes patients with no complications. The additional expenditure mostly occurred due to inpatient care and lab tests. In a nine-year prospective cohort study using detailed clinical records from six hospitals, Kim et al. (2012) also reported a significantly higher economic burden for patients with type 2 diabetes and vascular complications than for their counterparts without such complications. Another study estimated the economic burden of hypoglycemia among patients with type 2 diabetes in Korea (Kim, Gyuri, et al. 2016).

Sohn, Kwon, and Park (2012) conducted a study on the financial burden of out-of-pocket expenditure for prescription drugs (OOP-PD) among outpatients with one or more of four major chronic conditions including hypertension, diabetes, osteoarthritis, and asthma under the national health insurance system in Korea; diabetes was the chronic condition that contributed the most to OOP-PD (using Korea Health Panel Survey data from 2008–09). Suh, Kim, and Lee (2018) examined the effects of the price-cut reform introduced in April 2012 on the cost and utilization of anti-diabetic drugs using multi-year (2009–13) data from about 1 million outpatient claims. Using interrupted time series analyses, the study showed that the reform had immediate cost-containment effects by decreasing the cost per patient overall for anti-diabetics, while the volume (incidents) of medical and surgical procedures related to diabetes complications did not much change; the authors concluded that this implied there were no serious negative impacts on the clinical outcomes of patients during the study period.

Evidence on policy impacts. In an earlier study, Jeong et al. (2008) examined the cost-effectiveness of diabetes screening in the National Health Screening Program of the NHIS. A Markov model was constructed using 10-year cohort data from the people screened in 1996. The results showed an increase of 0.76 life-years gained (LYG) for diabetes patients without symptoms and 0.23 quality-adjusted life-years (QALY), and at the same time, a cost-per-person decrease of US$370 from the insurer's perspective and $729 from the societal perspective (US$1 = ₩1,000). In conclusion, the incremental cost-effective ratio was $−3,132/QALY and $−943/LYG. The study results support the social benefit of the National Health Screening Program.

There are a relatively small number of studies on the major CDM programs in Korea explained above. As for the Hypertension-Diabetes Registration and Management Program, Lee (2010) examined the satisfaction with the program in Gwangmyeong-si, Gyeonggi-do, among 1,014 patients, 65 doctors, and 93 pharmacists. The satisfaction rates of the three groups were 76.1%, 79.7%, and 83.9%, respectively. About 95% of participating patients reported they would recommend the program to other patients. In an evaluation of clinical outcomes among older participants in Gwangmyeong-si in 2009, KCDC (Yang and Lee 2015) also found an improvement in medication compliance and an increase in the proportion of patients receiving consistent diabetes treatment, from 42.8% one year before participation in the program to 57.6% and 60.8% in the first and second years of participation, respectively. Lee, Lee, and Park (2014) compared the quality of life among 68 patients registered in the Hypertension-Diabetes Registration and Management Program in Daegu City and who had completed an eight-session comprehensive education program. The education program had positive impacts on their quality of life, measured using EQ-5D.[1] The small sample size is a major limitation of the study. Yoon (2013) also conducted an evaluation study of pilot programs in Daegu-si and reported some positive improvements in healthcare utilization patterns.

Subsequently, Yim (2012) and Cheong et al. (2013) evaluated the effects of a clinic-based chronic disease registration program in the collaboration with CHCs in Incheon-si for patients with hypertension or type 2 diabetes. Using a retrospective cohort design with a one-year follow-up, the authors found no significant difference in blood glycemic control between the experimental and control groups. They also discussed the limitations of lecture-based education programs for diabetes patients. As for the Clinic-Based Chronic Disease Management program, the NHIS (Paik et al. 2015) found that participants with

---

1   EQ-5D is a standarized instrument for measuring health-related quality of life.

hypertension and/or diabetes were significantly more likely to visit the same clinics consistently and had better medication adherence than did people not participating in the program. Among the participants, those who used a health support service, including education and tailored counseling, also had significantly better outcomes in both measures than their counterparts.

In a recent evaluation of the P4P program for diabetes using one-year (2015–16) claims data, HIRA (2017) reported that only about 41.3 percent of diabetes patients received diabetes treatment in a single medical institution while others used multiple institutions (providers). Among the single-institution users, about 63.4 percent used clinics and public health centers, and the others received diabetes management at hospital-level institutions. Three variables were considered: consistency of diabetes treatment, appropriateness of medication prescription, and lab tests to prevent complications. Overall, the P4P program was reported to have increased the number of patients who manage hypertension and/or diabetes in local clinics and improved the quality of care in the participating clinics. Clinic users had better consistency in treatment measured by the rate of physician visits per three months (93.2% vs. 85.9% in total), but the rates of prescription and lab tests including HbA1c (clinic users: 72.7% vs. total: 76.7%) were lower among clinic users compared to total participants. The low rates of lipid tests (78.1%) and fundus examinations (43.0%) in the total imply an urgent need for the improvement of complication management.

Kim, Hee Sun, et al. (2016, 2017) evaluated the Community-Based Primary Care Demonstration Project at three, six, and twelve months. Compared to control groups, project participants had a significantly higher blood-sugar control rate at the six-month follow-up and better healthcare utilization patterns (medication compliance, number and days of clinic visits) at both the six-month and one-year follow-ups. In a qualitative study of the patient experience and effects of the program (Joo et al. 2017), participants reported a strengthening of trust in the patient-physician relationship and increases in the meeting of socio-psychological needs through one-to-one tailored education; they also reported better motivation for self-care and lifestyle changes. Limited access to the community support center due to geographic distance and a lack of other community resources were indicated as barriers to the success of the program. These results are consistent with and complementary to another, quantitative, evaluation of the same project (Cho, Kwon, and Jung 2015).

Conclusion

Despite the various policy efforts described above, diabetes management in Korea is still sub-optimal. Facing rapid population aging, the prevalence of diabetes and the economic burden of diabetes care are expected to increase. There are several limitations in the existing diabetes management programs (Kim 2018; Kim, Yoo, and Lee 2018; Park 2018). Low rates of registration overall and of the completion of educational components are partly due to a lack of tailored programs and a low rate of participation among physicians and local clinics. For example, both patients and physicians had little incentive to participate in the CDC Management Program, and this ended up being a key barrier to the scaling-up of the program.

To overcome the redundancy and limitations of existing CDM programs and build a comprehensive service delivery system for chronic care, the government began a new CDM pilot program at community primary care clinics in January 2019 (Park 2018). This pilot, the Primary Care-Chronic Disease Management (PC-CDM) Demonstration Program, has several new features and targets citizens 40 or older who have diabetes or hypertension. The PC-CDM Demonstration Program was developed by integrating the existing Community-Based Primary Care Demonstration Program and the Demonstration Payment Program for Chronic Care Management; the Ministry of Health and Welfare also plan to integrate the two other existing CDM programs—the Hypertension-Diabetes Registration and Management Program and the Clinic-Based Chronic Disease Management Program.

The program introduces comprehensive patient management through both face-to-face and online monitoring. Care coordination services conducted by registered nurses or nutritionists trained for the role are also being tested. The NHIS is paying for a set of three services: comprehensive assessment and care planning, patient management, and counseling. To facilitate patient participation, the total amount of out-of-pocket costs per patient per year would be limited to about US$10–20, and a tailored voucher for lab tests would be provided during the demonstration period. Community medical associations, meanwhile, hold a key role in organizing and implementing the program, and networking with CHCs and the local office of the NHIS in designated communities.

Several future research and policy priorities for diabetes management in a rapidly aging Korea can be drawn from this review. It is critical to develop and implement effective diabetes care delivery and payment models across the country. To this end, the success of the new demonstration program, which aims to integrate and surpass the previous such programs, is important. The clinical and economic impacts of the new program and its implementation process should be carefully evaluated with methodological rigor, which was not done well in the earlier policy efforts.

Although the roles of the government, insurer, and providers are widely regarded as important, patient engagement and empowerment in diabetes care is lacking, or at least, not likely the emphasis of current policy discussions on diabetes care in Korea. In the meanwhile, evidence from other countries that support self-care is critical for successful diabetes management (Eva et al. 2018). A more patient-centered approach in Korea's own context is needed. In addition, better governance and collaboration among various stakeholders, including patients, in diabetes care delivery is the key to establishing an integrated care-delivery system.

Besides the evaluation of the new demonstration program itself, a wider range of research is needed to support evidence-based policymaking to improve the quality of care and also the health and well-being of patients with diabetes. Risk models for the mortality and major complications of Koreans with diabetes need to be developed; several Asian countries have developed their own risk models (Yang et al. 2008; Tanaka et al. 2013), and such models perform better to predict the health outcomes of their own citizens. The economics of diabetes care is an important field of research to be explored in Korea. Net-value studies on diabetes care at the national level and also in cross-national contexts would be useful (Eggleston et al. 2009), and require longitudinal cohort data and high-quality clinical information. Comparative research on chronic care policies and system performance using health big data among Asian counties and beyond is another key area for future investigation; Kim and Cheng's study (2018) is an example. Innovation in diabetes-care-related medication, devices, and technology in aging Asia is an emerging topic with increasing research needs.

References

Baik, Inkyung. 2019. "Projection of Diabetes Prevalence in Korean Adults for the Year 2030 Using Risk Factors Identified from National Data." *Diabetes and Metabolism Journal* 43 (1): 90–96.

Cheong, Won, Jun Yim, Dae-kyu Oh, Jung-soo Im, Kwangpil Ko, and Kim Yunmi Kim. 2013. "Effects of Chronic Disease Management Based on Clinics for Blood Pressure or Glycemic Control in Patients with Hypertension or Type 2 Diabetes Mellitus." *Journal of Agricultural Medicine and Community Health* 38 (2): 108–15.

Cho, Dongsoon. 2016. "Research on the Medical Expenses of the NHIS about Diabetes Complications by Using HIRA's Patient Sample Data." Master's dissertation, Yonsei University.

Cho, Jung-Jin, Yong-Jin Kwon, and Sung-Hoon Jung. 2015. "Community Based Health Care Service Design on Chronic Disease for Enhancing Primary Care and the Status of Community Based Primary Care Project." *Korean Journal of Family Practice* 5 (3): 173–78.

Eggleston, Karen N., Nilay D. Shah, Steven A. Smith, Amy E. Wagie, Arthur R. Williams, Jerome H. Grossman, Ernst R. Berndt, Kirsten Hall Long, et al. 2009. "The Net Value of Health Care for Patients with Type 2 Diabetes, 1997 to 2005." *Annals of Internal Medicine* 151 (6): 386–93.

Eva, Jafrin Jahan, Yaman Walid Kassab, Chin Fen Neoh, Long Chiau Ming, Yuet Yen Wong, Mohammed Abdul Hameed, Yet Hoi Hong, and Md Moklesur Rahman Sarker. 2018. "Self-Care and Self-Management among Adolescent T2DM Patients: A Review." *Frontiers in Endocrinology* 9: 489.

HIRA (Health Insurance Review & Assessment Service). 2017. *The Assessment of the Appropriateness of Diabetes Management: 2015 Report.* Wonju: HIRA.

Jeong, Hyunjin, Hyeyoung Kwon, Juntae Han, Yoojoeng Kim, and Aekyung Lee. 2008. "Cost-Effectiveness Analysis of Type 2 DM Screening Program of National Health Insurance Corporation." *Korean Journal of Health Economics and Policy* 14 (1): 20–50.

Joo Jungmin, Jung-Jin Cho, Yong-Jin Kwon, Yulim Lee, and Dong-wook Shin. 2017. "A Qualitative Study of Satisfaction with the Community-Based Primary Care Project among Primary Care Patients and its Efficacy." *Journal of the Korean Medical Association* 60 (2): 173–82.

Kim, Gyuri, Yong-ho Lee, Mi Hye Han, Eui-Kyung Lee, Chong Hwa Kim, Hyuk Sang Kwon, In Kyung Jeong, Eun Seok Kang, and Dae

Jung Kim. 2016. "Economic Burden of Hypoglycemia in Patients with Type 2 Diabetes Mellitus from Korea." *PloS One* 11 (3): e0151282.

Kim, Hee Sun, Bit-Na Yoo, and Eun Whan Lee. 2018. "Evaluation of the National Chronic Diseases Management Policy: Performance and Future Directions." *Public Health Affairs* 2 (1): 105–20.

Kim, Hee Sun, et al. 2016. *The Community-based Primary Care Demonstration Project: The First Evaluation Study*. [In Korean.] Seoul: Korean Ministry of Health and Welfare (KMHW) and National Evidence-based Healthcare Collaborating Agency (NECA).

Kim, Hee Sun, et al. 2017. *The Community-based Primary Care Demonstration Project: The Second Evaluation Study* [In Korean.] Seoul: KMHW and NECA.

Kim, Hongsoo, and Shou-Hsia Cheng. 2018. "Assessing Quality of Primary Diabetes Care in South Korea and Taiwan Using Avoidable Hospitalizations." *Health Policy* 122 (11): 1222–31.

Kim, Namhee. 2018. "Chronic Disease Management Program for Strengthening Community-Centered Primary Medicine: An Overview and Future Agenda." *HIRA Policy Trends* 12 (5): 18–27.

Kim, Tae Ho, Ki-Hong Chun, Hae-Jin Kim, Seung-Jin Han, Dae-Jung Kim, Jiyeong Kwak, Young-Seol Kim, Jeong Taek Woo, Yongsoo Park, Moonsuk Nam, Sei Hyun Baik, Kyu Jeung Ahn, and Kwan Woo Lee. 2012. "Direct Medical Costs for Patients with Type 2 Diabetes and Related Complications: A Prospective Cohort Study Based on the Korean National Diabetes Program." *Journal of Korean Medical Science* 27 (8): 876–82.

KAMS (Korean Academy of Medical Sciences) and KCDC. 2019. *The Evidence-based Guideline for Type 2 Diabetes in Primary Care*. [In Korean.] Seoul: KAMS & KCDC.

KCDC (Korea Centers for Disease Control and Prevention). 2017a. *2017 Chronic Diseases: Current Status and Issues*. [In Korean.] Sejong: KCDC.

KCDC. 2017b. *2016 Trends of National Health Statistics*. Sejong: KCDC.

KDA (Korean Diabetes Association). 2015. *2015 Treatment Guideline for Diabetes (fifth edition)*. Seoul: KDA.

KMHW (Korean Ministry of Health and Welfare). 2019. *2019 National Health Screening Program: A Guide*. [In Korean.] Sejong: KMHW.

Korea National Cancer Center. n.d. "The National Cancer Screening Program: Overview." [In Korean.] http://www.ncc.re.kr/main.ncc?uri=manage01_4, accessed May 3, 2019.

Kwon, Tai-Hwan. n.d. "Population Change and Development in Korea." *Center for Global Education*. https://asiasociety.org/education/population-change-and-development-korea, accessed May 3, 2019.

Lee, Jung Jeung, Hye Jin Lee, and Eun Jin Park. 2014. "Effect of Staged Education Program for Hypertension, Diabetes Patients in a Community (Assessment of Quality of Life Using EQ-5D)." *Journal of Agricultural Medicine and Community Health* 39 (1): 37–45.

Lee, Wonyoung. 2010. *The Second Year Effectiveness Evaluation of the Gwangmyeong-si CVD Patient Registry Project*. Seoul: Korea Centers for Disease Control and Prevention.

National Archives of Korea. 2014. "Plan to Expand the Coverage of Four Major Serious Diseases." [In Korean.] National Archives of Korea. http://www.archives.go.kr/next/search/listSubjectDescription.do?id=009197&pageFlag=, accessed May 3, 2019.

NHIS (National Health Insurance Services). 2001. *2000 National Health Insurance Statistics*. [In Korean.] Wonju: NHIS.

NHIS. 2006. *2005 National Health Insurance Statistics*. [In Korean.] Wonju: NHIS.

NHIS. 2011. *2010 National Health Insurance Statistics*. [In Korean.] Wonju: NHIS.

NHIS. 2016. *2015 National Health Insurance Statistics*. [In Korean.] Wonju: NHIS.

OECD (Organization for Economic Cooperation and Development). 2015. *Cardiovascular and Diabetes: Policies for Better Health and Quality of Care*. Paris: OECD Publishing.

OECD. 2017. *Health at a Glance 2017*. Paris: OECD Publishing.

OECD. 2019. *OECD Health Statistics 2018*. Paris: OECD Publishing.

Paik, J. H., S. M. Lee, D. S. Kwak, H. R. Kang, and Y. D. Yoon. 2015. *An Impact Analysis of the Health Support Services through Chronic Disease Management Program on Healthcare Utilization*. [In Korean.] Wonju: NHIS.

Park, H. G. 2018. *Primary Care-Chronic Disease Management Demonstration Program: An Introduction*. [In Korean.] Seoul: Korea Health Promotion Institute.

Sohn, Hyun Soon, Jin-Won Kwon, and Eun-Ja Park. 2012. "Out-of-Pocket (OOP) Expenditure for Prescription Drugs among South Korean Outpatients under the National Health Insurance System: Focus on Chronic Diseases including Diabetes." *Journal of Diabetes and Metabolism* 3 (5): 197.

Statistics Korea. 2011. *Causes of Death Statistics: 2010 Report.* [In Korean.] Seoul: Korea Statistics.

Statistics Korea. 2016. *Causes of Death Statistics: 2015 Report.* [In Korean.] Sejong: Korea Statistics.

Statistics Korea. 2018a. *2018 Statistics on the Aged.* [In Korean.] Sejong: Korea Statistics.

Statistics Korea. 2018b. *Causes of Death Statistics: 2017 Report.* [In Korean.] Sejong: Korea Statistics.

Statistics Korea. 2019a. *Special Projection of Future Population: 2017-2067.* [In Korean.] Sejong: Korea Statistics.

Statistics Korea. 2019b. "Country Major Indicators: Number of House-hold Members, 1970-2017." [In Korean.] http://www.index.go.kr/unify/idx-info.do?idxCd=4030, accessed May 3, 2019.

Suh, Hae Sun, Jee-Ae Kim, and Iyn-Hyang Lee. 2018. "Effects of a Price Cut Reform on the Cost and Utilization of Antidiabetic Drugs in Korea: A National Health Insurance Database Study." *BMC Health Services Research* 18 (1): 429.

Tanaka, Shiro, Sachiko Tanaka, Satoshi Iimuro, Hidetoshi Yamashita, Shigehiro Katayama, Yasuo Akanuma, Nobuhiro Yamada, Atsushi Araki, Hideki Ito, Hirohito Sone, and Yasuo Ohashi. 2013. "Predicting Macro-and Microvascular Complications in Type 2 Diabetes: The Japan Diabetes Complications Study/the Japanese Elderly Diabetes Intervention Trial Risk Engine." *Diabetes Care* 36 (5):1193–199.

WHO (World Health Organization), Regional Office for the Western Pacific. 2015. *Republic of Korea Health System Review.* Manila: WHO Regional Office for the Western Pacific.

World Bank. "Data Bank Microdata Data Catalog." https://databank.worldbank.org/data/home.aspx, accessed May 3, 2019.

Yang, H., and D. Lee. 2015. "Achievements and Challenges in a Community Based Registration and Management Programme for Hypertension and Diabetes." [In Korean.] *Public Health Weekly Report, KCDC* 8 (35): 827–34.

Yang, Xilin,, Wing Yee So, Peter C. Y. Tong, Ronald C. W. Ma, Alice P. S. Kong, Christopher W. K. Lam, Chung Shun Ho, Clive S. Cockram, Gary T.C. Ko, Chun-Chung Chow, Vivian C. W. Wong, and Juliana C. N. Chan. 2008. "Development and Validation of an All-Cause Mortality Risk Score in Type 2 Diabetes: The Hong Kong Diabetes Registry." *Archives of Internal Medicine* 168 (5): 451–57.

Yim, Jun. 2012. *The Effects Assessment of Chronic Care Management Based on Primary Clinics for Hypertension, Diabetes Patients*. [In Korean.] Seoul: Korean Health Promotion Foundation.

Yoon, SeokJun. 2013. *The Development of Model for Efficient Management of Hypertensive Patients and Diabetics*. [In Korean.] Osong: Korea Centers for Disease Control and Prevention.

7 Noncommunicable Disease Management in Hong Kong

Current Policies and the Potential Role of Economics Research

Janet Tin Kei Lam, Sabrina Ching Tung Wong, and Jianchao Quan

S imilar to other developed regions in East Asia, Hong Kong faces the challenge of an aging population stemming from rising longevity and low fertility rates. The proportion of elderly persons in Hong Kong rose from 13% in 2011 to 18% in 2019, and is projected to further increase to 26% in 2030 (FHB and Department of Health 2018). Such rapid aging within a few decades poses major health, social, and financial challenges for the Hong Kong population.

Like many developed economies, Hong Kong's epidemiological profile has transitioned from predominately infectious diseases to noncommunicable diseases (NCDs). Major NCDs, such as cardiovascular disease, cancer, diabetes mellitus, and chronic respiratory diseases accounted for 55 percent of all registered deaths in Hong Kong in 2016, and contributed to an estimated 104,600 potential years of life lost before the age of 70 (FHB and Department of Health 2018). As the prevalence of NCDs increases with age, population aging will only intensify their impact. In terms of financial support, many people with NCDs will develop disabilities or other comorbidities and require institutional care. The population aged over 65 consume more healthcare resources—six times more inpatient bed-days and nine times more general specialty bed utilization—than those aged below 65 years.

Hong Kong has a mixed public-private healthcare system with spending roughly equally split between public and private financing (FHB 2018). The public healthcare system offers universal coverage and is heavily subsidized by general government revenue with only small user charges. Unusually for a high-income economy, household out-of-pocket payments account for over 30 percent of total healthcare financing. The public system bears the burden of treating the complications of chronic disease as it provides 90 percent of inpatient bed-days and around half of outpatient specialist care. Population aging is expected to both increase health needs and shrink the labor force. The public health expenditure is projected to increase from the current 5.9 percent of gross domestic product (GDP) to 8.7 percent in 2030 (FHB 2008). Given the narrow tax base in Hong Kong, this raises serious concerns about the sustainability of the healthcare financing system.

The process of aging leads to increasing frailty, resulting in more complex health and social needs. Although chronic disease management in the form of community care has long been on the agenda of the Hong Kong government, there is still a mismatch between the care currently provided and the care which meets citizens' health needs. For example, outreach services like community nursing are inadequate, and primary care initiatives typically offer a very limited scope of services (Poon, So, and Loong 2014, 47). While the Hong Kong government has made healthy aging one of its important and resounding themes, critics argue that the government adopts a narrow interpretation, with programs mainly limited to continuous education and neighborhood-based mutual help networks (Leung 2014, 108). The problem of pivoting away from the current emphasis on acute episodic hospital-based care toward continuous holistic care in the community, focusing on individual needs, remains largely unaddressed.

This chapter will elucidate the health and economic burden brought by NCDs and summarize current government policies to achieve healthy aging in Hong Kong. We outline the demography of aging and epidemiological trends of various NCDs in Hong Kong, followed by a brief overview of Hong Kong's healthcare system and its current healthy aging policies, including economic initiatives on NCDs in the local setting. Lastly, we review the existing health economics research and present early findings on the net value of chronic disease management using a population cohort of diabetes as an illustrative approach to evaluate the cost-effectiveness of the healthcare system.

Trends of Aging and Noncommunicable Diseases in Hong Kong

The demography of aging in Hong Kong

Based on current forecasts, the population of Hong Kong will grow by 9 percent from 7.34 million in 2016 to 8 million in 2031, whereas its labor force is estimated to decline by 3.04 percent from 3.62 million to 3.51 million (CSD 2017a, 2017b). We discuss the impact of migration, and changes in birth and mortality rates below.

Historically, Hong Kong is a city of migrants. During the period 1969–73, migration contributed to 21.7 percent of the total population increase as Chinese inhabitants were allowed free entry into Hong Kong (Fan 1974). In recent years, migration has become the most important driver of net population growth, contributing 90 percent. Much of this is due to the One-way Permit Holders (OWPHS) scheme and the majority of new entrants are of working age (Research Office 2018). However, future government adjustments to the scheme are expected to reduce the number of permits from 54,750 to 36,500 each year, leading to fewer workers joining the labor force (CSD 2017b).

In terms of local population demographics, Hong Kong is experiencing one of the fastest rates of population aging in the world, with rapid declines in both its mortality and fertility rates in recent years. The proportion of people aged 65 years and over is the second highest in Asia, at 19 percent in 2019 (World Bank n.d.). With post-war baby boomers entering old age by 2030, more than one in every four people (26.4 percent) will be 65 years or older. The major contributor to population aging is the rapidly declining fertility rate. The total fertility rate has been consistently below replacement levels (1.205 in 2016). These demographic shifts have led to a top-heavy population pyramid and a shrinking dependency ratio. By 2030, each person aged 65 years or over will be supported by just 2.1 working-age persons, compared to 6.6 in 2000 and 4.3 in 2016 (CSD 2017a).

The large declines in mortality rates in recent decades have translated into sizeable increases in life expectancy. Improvements in longevity are expected to push average life expectancy to 83.8 years for males and 89.8 years for females by 2030, among the highest in the world.

Trends in the incidence and prevalence of noncommunicable diseases

In Hong Kong, information on NCDs is gathered from various sources to enable surveillance and international comparison. Notably, some government data may not fully meet the formal World Health Organization (WHO) specifications. Many surveys depend on self-reporting, and are conducted too infrequently for detailed analysis of trends. For example, the Department of Health Population Health Survey is only conducted in 10-year cycles. Nevertheless, the prevalence of NCDs has clearly increased. The prevalence of diabetes increased from 3.8% in 2004 to 5.5% in 2015, while cardiovascular disease also increased, from 2.7% to 3.5%. The only notable exception has been the prevalence of chronic respiratory diseases, which fell from 3.3% in 2004 to 2.3% in 2015.

Specific research data can be used to supplement gaps in official health data. An analysis of electronic health record data held by the public health-care system showed that the overall prevalence of diabetes mellitus in Hong Kong increased from 7.2 percent in 2006 to 10.3 percent in 2014 (Quan et al. 2017a). This trend is consistent with local Population Health Survey estimates that rely solely on self-reported diagnoses (Department of Health and Department of Community Medicine 2004; Department of Health 2017). Notably, a small decline in incidence was observed from 10.01 per 1,000 person-years in 2006 to 9.46 per 1,000 person-years in 2014. Subsequent analysis showed divergent incidence trends among age groups, with significant increases among the 40 to 59-year-olds, but significant decreases among the 60–79 and over-80 age groups, suggesting earlier detection or earlier onset of disease.

There have also been major shifts in the causes of death in the population, from infectious diseases to NCDs, which now account for the majority of deaths in Hong Kong (55% in 2016) (FHB 2018, 15). Cancer has been the leading cause of death, accounting for about one-third of deaths (30.5% in 2016), but other top 10 causes of mortality include heart diseases (13.3%), cerebrovascular diseases (6.8%), and diabetes (0.9%) (Department of Health 2018a).

Government Policy on Healthy Aging and NCD Management

Elderly services are coordinated by a multitude of government agencies in Hong Kong. The Hospital Authority collectively manages all public hospitals and outpatient clinics, providing acute care and specialist services. The Department of Health administers 18 Elderly Health Centres that provide health assessment, counselling, education, and curative treatment for enrolled older persons, and oversees visiting health teams that train people caring for the elderly. The Department of Health also coordinates disease prevention policies in Hong Kong. Community-based long-term care services are administered by the Social Welfare Department.

In 2018, the Hong Kong government launched Towards 2025, a strategic framework to incorporate WHO-recommended interventions for the prevention of NCDs into local policies. This action plan tackled four NCDs (cardiovascular diseases, cancers, chronic respiratory diseases, and diabetes) and four shared behavioral risk factors (unhealthy diet, physical inactivity, tobacco use, and use of alcohol).

The government has also attempted to improve the management of chronic diseases, especially preventative care for elderly patients and more patient-centered case management. These initiatives include the Multi-disciplinary Risk Factor Assessment and Management Programme (RAMP), Patient Empowerment Programme (PEP), and Nurse and Allied Health Clinics (NAHCS) (FHB 2010, 39).

Healthcare provision for the elderly: A system overview

Hong Kong maintains a dual-track healthcare system run by both the public and private sectors and that has been in place since colonial times. The Hospital Authority was established in 1990 to manage all public hospitals; the private sector's involvement remains fragmented. While healthcare financing is roughly equally split between the public and private sectors, there is a significant imbalance in utilization. Among patients with at least one chronic illness, 81.6% seek care in the outpatient public sector (Yeoh 2018, 16). The public sector shoulders 87% of total hospital beds and 90% of inpatient bed-days (FHB 2013). In a self-reported population survey, 70% of all respondents who were admitted in the past 12 months, regardless of their condition, received care from public hospitals (CSD 2017c). The macro-organization of healthcare in Hong Kong is also imbalanced at different levels of care. Primary healthcare in Hong Kong is mainly provided by private general practitioners, as public primary care services have limited daily quotas. For example, applicants for membership in the Elderly Health Centres, established solely for providing primary care to older persons, might find themselves on wait-lists for up to 37 months (Department of Health 2018b). Specialist care is evenly split between public and private sectors, with long waiting times for public appointments. Hong Kong's health system is still weighted toward the provision of inpatient care for acute episodic illness, with tertiary care dominating healthcare funding (Our Hong Kong Foundation 2018, 45). Although strengthening primary care is associated with better health and lower overall costs, only 10 percent of government expenditure on health goes toward primary and preventative care service, a fraction compared to spending on specialized care.

Patients in Hong Kong, particularly the elderly with multiple comorbidities, are usually managed through multiple specialty or sub-specialty clinics (run by both the public and private sectors), when their needs could be better coordinated at lower levels of care. In a study of 11 developed countries, Hong Kong ranked last as a consistent source of care for elderly people suffering from multiple comorbidities (Wong et al. 2017). Hong Kong's current fragmented health system and the limited sharing of data between private providers struggles to meet the population's need for continuous and coordinated care to manage chronic conditions. Policies to establish a primary source of care are needed to reduce the heavy burden on public secondary and tertiary care services.

In Hong Kong, most funding for public healthcare services comes from government revenue. The government subsidizes 97 percent of all medical service costs in the public sector (Poon and Ng 2018). Residents are charged nominal out-of-pocket user fees per day for services that include consultation, investigations, and formulary medications (see table 7.1). These charges are largely affordable, though median monthly household income for elderly households stands at US$768 (HK$6,020), inclusive of the government's cash social benefits like the Old Age Living Allowance (CSD 2018). Of concern is the high level of household out-of-pocket spending, which is above the levels recommended by WHO (31 percent of total health expenditure), and the limited contributions from pooling by insurance. A new government-regulated voluntary insurance scheme was launched on April 1, 2019.

TABLE 7.1 Public sector charges for various medical services, by eligibility for subsidization

	Eligible persons*		Ineligible persons[†]	
	USD	HKD	USD	HKD
Inpatient (acute general beds) admission per day	—	—	650	5,100
First day	15	120	—	—
Second day onwards	10	75	—	—
Accident and emergency visit	23	180	157	1,230
Specialist outpatient visit	—	—	152	1,190
First attendance	23	180	—	—
Second attendance onwards	17	135	—	—
Per drug item	2	15	—	—
Primary care visit	6	50	57	445
General community nursing visit	10	80	68	535

SOURCE: Hospital Authority 2017.
NOTE: *Charges for eligible persons at subsidized cost; [†]charges for ineligible persons set on a cost-recovery basis; charges at cost-recovery basis reflect actual costs of the services as of 2018 (last price adjustment as of June 2017, Hospital Authority).

The availability of prescription medications in the public sector is set out in the Hospital Authority Drug Formulary. Drugs are classified into four categories: general drugs, special drugs, self-financed items with safety net coverage, and self-financed items without safety net coverage. General drugs with well-established indications and cost-effectiveness are provided to patients at standard charges, but special drugs can only be offered to patients at standard charges under more stringent indications. More expensive medications are self-financed by patients. There are no published cost-effectiveness assessment criteria or funding threshold for inclusion in the formulary. As a result, the formulary has a limited range of medications, forcing patients toward private provision if they can afford it. For both hospital and drug charges, there are safety nets for low-income patients who cannot afford the drug or visit charges; examples include the Samaritan Fund and the Community Care Fund Medical Assistance Programme (Hospital Authority 2018a).

Despite the growth in government expenditure on healthcare services, patients for public hospital services still suffer from long waiting times at specialist outpatient clinics and insufficient hospital beds. For example, the waiting time for non-urgent specialist care can reach three years. The Hong Kong government has launched multiple healthcare reform consultations in attempts to shift the public-private balance. In 2019, the Voluntary Health Insurance Scheme was launched to try to steer 1.5 million people toward the private health sector. Given the limited pooling, it is likely that most elderly patients will continue to rely on public healthcare provision.

Primary care for the elderly

In Hong Kong, primary care outpatient visits are found to contribute positively to NCD care. In particular, one population-based study of diabetes patients in Hong Kong found a negative correlation between public primary care outpatient visits and the probability of a diabetes-related avoidable admission; on the contrary, specialist outpatient visits were associated with more avoidable admissions (Quan et al. 2017b).

However, primary care in Hong Kong has underperformed as a gatekeeper for secondary and tertiary care. Much focus is on treatment for acute episodic diseases with a lack of emphasis on disease prevention and chronic disease follow-up (FHB 2010, 12). A local study finds that only 4 percent and 12 percent of primary care consultations were done for the purposes of disease prevention and long-term disease follow-up, respectively (Lee et al. 2007). Most people are not familiar with principles of family medicine or attributes of good primary care. For example, chronic disease patients would prefer to receive follow-up services in a hospital than in primary care settings, due to perceived quality differences. Meanwhile, emergency care is a popular alternative for self-limiting conditions, such as upper respiratory tract infections and gastroenteritis, that can be managed in primary care.

Efforts to set standards has led to the publication of evidence-based clinical guidelines from the Primary Care Office under the Department of Health, such as the Hong Kong Reference Frameworks for Preventive Care for Older Adults in Primary Care Settings, Hypertension, and Diabetes. These frameworks set out preventive and screening strategies, including vaccination, healthy lifestyle, and social support, in addition to specifying clinical pathways for identifying high-risk groups for screening, diagnosis, and life-course management. However, best practice recommendations are constrained by the drug formulary. For example, sulphonylurea, an older, relatively affordable drug, is recommended as a second-line treatment for diabetes over other newer but more expensive agents that are classified as special drugs (Hospital Authority 2018b).

Since 2010, the Hospital Authority has attempted to enhance care for the elderly with chronic NCDs in the primary care setting through several pilot programs, highlighted below together with a brief evaluation of their effectiveness.

The **Chronic Disease Self-Management Programme** was developed from the patient perspective to shift the focus from clinical outcomes (e.g., HbA1c levels in patients with diabetes) to daily help with chronic conditions (e.g., choosing healthy food, managing pain and fatigue). Under this initiative, a territory-wide Patient Empowerment Programme (PEP) commenced in 2010 to strengthen patient involvement and partnership with community service providers. PEP was effective in lowering the cumulative incidence of all-cause mortality, diabetes complications, and cardiovascular events (Lian et al. 2017). Despite the positive feedback, low participant retention (a dropout rate of 52 percent) and difficulty engaging community service providers (only 11 percent of invited non-governmental organizations submitted tenders) hinder coverage (Audit Commission 2012).

The **Risk Factor Assessment and Management Programme** (RAMP) initiative was launched in 2009 to set up multidisciplinary teams at primary care clinics for diabetes (RAMP-DM) and hypertension (RAMP-HT). Both RAMP programs have proven to be effective in delaying disease progression and preventing complications: RAMP-DM reduced diabetes-related complications by 13.3 percent, saving US$7,185 (HK$56,043) per person over a five-year period (Fung et al. 2012; Jiao et al. 2018; Wan et al. 2018; Yu et al. 2015, 2017).

The Hong Kong government established **Public-Private Partnerships** (PPPs) **for elderly services** in 2008, allowing private sector delivery of public services to increase efficiency (Efficiency Unit 2008). The Hospital Authority has launched several PPP projects to encourage patients to choose private providers and reduce reliance on public healthcare services, including the General Outpatient Clinic (GOPC) PPP program for primary care services, the Shared Care program to enhance support for patients with chronic diseases, and the Haemodialysis PPP program (Audit Commission 2012).

All the PPP initiatives were launched as pilots, with a narrow group of eligible participants selected. For example, only three geographical districts out of 18 are included in the GOPC-PPP program, and only 6 percent of the invited participants took up the Shared Care program. Moreover, providers (private medical practitioners, community medical organizations, and NGOs) had a muted response to PPP programs as the financial rewards were unattractive, leading to low take-up rates (Audit Commission 2012). Furthermore, Hong Kong's PPP approach in healthcare differed from that of other countries: in Hong Kong individual PPP programs attempted to re-balance the utilization of existing public-private healthcare services, whereas in the United Kingdom and Singapore, PPPs were typically used to build, fund, and manage hospitals and increase capacity (Fong and Ho 2017).

Elderly care in the community: An enabling environment

An enabling environment supports older people's aging processes in their local communities and is a crucial component of aging-friendly policies. Here we briefly touch on the physical and social environment; for a more detailed discussion, readers are encouraged to review the Institute of Ageing reports (CUHK Jockey Club Institute of Ageing 2017).

Physical environments. A high poverty rate among older age groups in Hong Kong—34.4 percent in 2016 (CUHK Jockey Club Institute of Ageing 2018)—and a lack of family support means many older people resort to residential care home for the elderly (RCHE). For those who have the financial resources, several housing schemes offered by the Hong Kong Housing Society provide integrated accommodation and related support facilities for elders under one roof. Currently, Hong Kong has one of the highest ratios of residential care beds to elderly people in the world, with around 8.5 percent of those aged 65 years and above living in an RCHE (Luk et al. 2009). However, applicants to government-subsidized RCHEs faced substantial waiting times of up to 37 months in 2015 (Research Office 2015), whereas private RCHEs have shorter waiting times but variable service quality—the average net per-resident floor area is 7.5 m², just one-third of the space in government-subsidized ones (Audit Commission 2014). With no statutory accreditation requirement, only 8 percent of RCHEs in Hong Kong are accredited, which raises concerns about their quality.

The poor standard of care in RCHEs negatively impacts residents' health. A lack of continuity between treatment in hospitals and care in RCHEs leads to a "revolving door" between the two. Common examples include severely disabled elderly patients who are admitted for conditions such as pneumonia or pressure sores, improve after a lengthy period of hospital stay and are discharged back to a nursing home, only to be rapidly re-admitted for the same problems (Sim and Leung 2000). An audit at a tertiary hospital showed that 26.8 percent of unplanned re-admissions to medical inpatient wards were from private RCHEs (Mok 2018).

The Hospital Authority Strategic Service Framework for Elderly Patients established a blueprint for enhancing the well-being of elderly people and to reduce unplanned re-admissions (Hospital Authority 2012). A Community Health Call Centre (CHCC) service established to follow up with targeted patients within two days post-discharge has reduced emergency admissions by 25 percent (Mok 2018). Outreach services provided by Community Geriatric Assessment Teams (CGATs), which covered over 90 percent of RCHEs in Hong Kong in 2016, have also been effective in reducing emergency hospitalizations and visits (Mok 2018).

Medico-social environments. In recent years, there has been an increasing trend toward older people living alone and a decrease in perceived social support (CUHK Jockey Club Institute of Ageing 2018). The Global AgeWatch Index 2016, which ranks jurisdictions according to their elderly residents' social and economic well-being, places Hong Kong at 70 out of 97 jurisdictions in the domain of social connections (CUHK Jockey Club Institute of Ageing 2018). Although the Social Welfare Department has launched the Opportunities for the Elderly Project and Neighbourhood Active Ageing Project to promote social inclusion among older people, most activities are conducted by subsidizing or outsourcing to social service and district organizations, with no territory-wide coverage (CUHK Jockey Club Institute of Ageing 2017).

Resources are similarly scarce for rehabilitative care in the community. In Hong Kong, the overall prevalence of people with disabilities increased from 5.2% in 2007 to 8.1% in 2013, with the largest increase among the older age groups (CSD 2014). As rehabilitative care is provided separately by various non–Hospital Authority parties (NGOs and voluntary groups), medical social workers are needed to coordinate the myriad rehabilitation services in out-of-hospital settings. However, with only 438 medical social workers in 2016 (Government of Hong Kong 2016), 36.7% of persons with functional disabilities and 33.1% of patients with chronic diseases expressed difficulty in seeking rehabilitative care (CSD 1999).

The current development of rehabilitation services still prioritizes hospital settings over community care. For instance, 85% of stroke patients received inpatient rehabilitation, yet only 20% received day and outpatient rehabilitation (Hospital Authority 2016). This impedes the re-integration of patients into the community and creates unnecessary pressure on public hospitals, a problem that will further increase as the population ages.

Economic incentives

The government has initiated economic incentives for elderly care in Hong Kong, mostly on the demand side in the form of vouchers. Adopting the "money-following-the-user' approach, the Elderly Health Care Voucher (EHCV) scheme was introduced in 2009 to divert elderly healthcare users from public services to private providers for disease prevention and management. As of 2018, all persons above 65 years old will receive an annual voucher amount of US$255 (HK$2,000) with a maximum accumulation limit of US$638 (HK$5,000) for use at a wide range of private healthcare providers, including Chinese and Western medical practitioners, dentists, and other allied health disciplines (Government of Hong Kong SAR 2018a). There is also a pilot scheme for the elderly to use services in the University of Hong Kong–Shenzhen Hospital in mainland China (Government of Hong Kong SAR 2018b).

An interim report of the pilot EHCV scheme in 2011 concluded that the scheme encouraged only one-third of eligible participants to use the vouchers and seek private medical services, despite 70 percent awareness of the scheme. The elderly's willingness-to-pay threshold for chronic conditions is much lower than that for acute illnesses, and the EHCV could potentially facilitate management of currently neglected NCDs (FHB 2011). The EHCV did not change the health-seeking behaviors of two-third of respondents, particularly those not accustomed to using private medical services (Yam et al. 2011). A qualitative study conducted in 2018 suggests that the low usage rate of EHCV for NCD prevention and management stems from the public's inadequate knowledge about the aims of the scheme, and the non-specific areas in which EHCV can be used. The majority of the EHCV subsidy has been used for optometry services, prompting the government to introduce a cap on these services. The subsidy is likely to be too low given the high quality of public services, and the expense of private services (Lai et al. 2018).

Similar voucher schemes were also piloted for community care services and residential care services by the Social Welfare Department in 2013 and 2017, respectively. In the second phase of the Community Care Service Voucher

(CCSV) scheme, launched in 2016, those on the waiting list for subsidized long-term care services are eligible to choose one of five service packages according to need, and redeem the voucher at non-governmental providers of home-based or day-center-based care. The value of the service packages ranged from US$501 to $1,197 (HK$3,930 to $9,390) in 2018–19. Elderly users are required to copay in a rate proportional to their financial conditions (Social Welfare Department 2019). Mid-term evaluation of the first phase of the CCSV scheme showed some benefits for current users, including better general health, better quality of life, and lower caregiver burden. However, many eligible people chose not to participate, citing the poor flexibility of service packages and perceived high copayment amounts (Lum et al. 2015).

Given the long waiting time for residential care homes, a feasibility study for the Residential Care Service Voucher (RCSV) was commissioned in 2016, which showed that one-third of those on the waiting list for elderly homes would be willing to copay for private residential care homes. About half of the respondents currently on the means-tested Comprehensive Social Security Assistance (CSSA) would choose RCSV and withdraw from the CSSA if given the option (Chui et al. 2016).

The current RCSV Pilot Scheme offers a redemption of US$1,694 (HK$13,287) for a standard service package in recognized elderly homes (Social Welfare Department 2018a). Only moderately impaired elderly on the central waiting list for government-subsidized RCHEs are eligible. There is also an attempt by the Hong Kong government to shift demand for elderly care homes to mainland China through a pilot Residential Care Services Scheme in Guangdong (Social Welfare Department 2018b). The success of these two pilot schemes has yet to be evaluated.

Existing Health Economics Studies on NCDs

There is relatively scant health economics or cost-effectiveness research on healthy aging and NCD control policies in Hong Kong. Studies of the economic burden of NCDs among the elderly estimate that direct medical costs will increase more than threefold from 2006 to 2036 (table 7.2) (McGhee et al. 2009; Yu et al. 2010, 2012; Chau et al. 2012). These direct medical costs were estimated based on the attributable risk for public sector utilization; costs incurred in the private sector were not included.

TABLE 7.2 Current and projected medical costs attributable to some NCDs in the public healthcare sector in Hong Kong

Disease	Base year	Attributable medical costs in the public sector		Projected total attributable medical costs in the public sector in 2036	
		USD	HKD	USD	HKD
Diabetes mellitus	2006	172M	1,350M	446M	3,500M
Per patient		1,519	11,915	—	—
Chronic obstructive pulmonary disease	2006	108M	844M	995M	7,800M
Per patient		8,452	66,287	—	—
Stroke	2006	170M	1,332M	507M	3,979M
Per patient		3,118	24,452	—	—
Dementia	2010	207M	1,624M	537M	4,212M
Per patient		1,971	15,456	—	—

SOURCES: Chau et al. 2012; McGee et al. 2009; Yu et al. 2010, 2012.

There have been some cost-effectiveness studies examining the direct healthcare costs saved by various NCD interventions in the local setting. The Risk Factor Assessment and Management Programme, a multidisciplinary tertiary prevention program in the public primary care setting, has already been previously discussed (Jiao et al. 2018). A Patient Empowerment Programme (PEP) for diabetes patients, which provided follow-up care in public primary care clinics, cost US$14,465 (HK$113,445) for each death avoided, which the authors concluded to be cost-effective (Lian et al. 2017). Lastly, a short message service intervention targeting patients with impaired glucose tolerance was found to be cost-effective, with a net cost of US$42 (HK$329) per subject resulting in a 5 percent reduction in diabetes onset, saving US$118 (HK$926) per subject over two years (Wong et al. 2016). However, these are mostly small-scale cost-effectiveness studies of pilot interventions, and do not address the bigger question of whether increased investment in health has improved the quality of elderly care in Hong Kong.

Most policy initiatives have focused on the demand side. To address the acute shortages in supply, the Hong Kong government has commissioned local researchers to review current and future healthcare human resource needs (FHB 2017). A full evaluation of voucher schemes for the elderly has also been commissioned (Lum et al. 2015); however, further economic analyses are still sorely needed in Hong Kong.

Net Value of NCD Care

Given the lack of economic studies on the current performance of NCD management in Hong Kong, it is imperative to assess the net value of healthcare spending: that is, whether the health system is achieving its potential "value for money" in terms of increased survival and health benefits over the past decade, given the increased healthcare spending over the same period. This net value approach is being applied to diabetes care, which will be one of the first studies to evaluate the performance of Hong Kong's public health system in managing a noncommunicable disease. The results will have crucial implications for future healthcare policy, given the increasing burden of NCDs and public pressure for increased investment. The research methodology can be readily applied to other healthcare systems and other diseases for comparative studies of Hong Kong's efforts in managing aging and NCDs.

Conclusion

Hong Kong faces the problems of rapid population aging, a rising burden of noncommunicable diseases, and increasing health and social care needs. The Hong Kong government has launched several policy initiatives aimed at improving the quality of life of older people, especially those with chronic diseases. However, most of these projects focus solely on the demand side, and remain in pilot phases with capacity constraints unable to benefit all eligible residents. Economic evaluation of these initiatives remains patchy, though future studies will help to assess their net value and cost-effectiveness. Such studies are urgently needed to establish a base for future evidence-based policymaking, and hopefully strengthen the political will to appropriately invest resources to manage the current demographic transition.

References

Audit Commission. 2012. *Hospital Authority: Public-private Partnership (PPP) Programmes*. Hong Kong Special Administrative Region (SAR).

Audit Commission. 2014. *Provision of Long-Term Care Services for the Elderly*. Report No. 63. Hong Kong SAR. https://www.aud.gov.hk/pdf_e/e63cho1.pdf.

CSD (Census and Statistics Department). 1999. *Social Data Collected via the General Household Survey: Special Topics Report—Report No.23*. Hong Kong SAR.

CSD. 2014. *Persons with Disabilities and Chronic Diseases (No. 62)*. Special Topics Report. Hong Kong SAR.

CSD. 2017a. "Hong Kong Population Projections 2017–2066." Hong Kong SAR.

CSD. 2017b. "Hong Kong Labour Force Projections for 2017 to 2066, Hong Kong Monthly Digest of Statistics." Hong Kong SAR.

CSD. 2017c. *Thematic Household Survey Report No. 63*. Hong Kong SAR.

CSD. 2018. *Thematic Report: Older Persons, 2016 Population By-census*. Hong Kong SAR.

Chau, Pui Hing, J. Chen, J. Woo, W. L. Cheung, Kwun Chuen Gary Chan, S. H. Cheung, C. H. Lee, and Sarah McGhee. 2012. *Trends of Disease Burden Consequent to Chronic Lung Disease in Older Persons in Hong Kong: Implications of Population Ageing*. Hong Kong SAR: Hong Kong Jockey Club.

Chui, Ernest, C. K. Law, Xue Bai, David Dai, Daniel Lai, Carol Ma, and Teresa Tsien. 2016. *Feasibility Study on Introducing a Voucher Scheme on Residential Care Services for the Elderly: Final Report*. Elderly Commission, Hong Kong SAR.

CUHK Jockey Club Institute of Ageing. 2017. *Topical Report on Enabling Environment, AgeWatch Index for Hong Kong*. Hong Kong SAR: Hong Kong Jockey Club.

CUHK Jockey Club Institute of Ageing. 2018. *Report on AgeWatch Index for Hong Kong 2016 and Hong Kong Elder Quality of Life Index*. Hong Kong SAR: Hong Kong Jockey Club.

Department of Health and Department of Community Medicine. 2004. *Population Health Survey 2003/2004*. Hong Kong SAR: University of Hong Kong.

Department of Health. 2017. *Report of Population Health Survey 2014/2015*. Hong Kong SAR: Surveillance and Epidemiology Branch,

Centre for Health Protection.

Department of Health. 2018a. "Health Facts of Hong Kong: 2018 Edition." Hong Kong SAR: Department of Health.

Department of Health. 2018b. "Waiting Time of Enrolment for Elderly Health Centres." Elderly Health Service. http://www.elderly.gov.hk/english/about_us/waiting_time.html, accessed January 17, 2019.

Efficiency Unit. 2008. "Serving the Community by Using the Private Sector: An Introductory Guide to Public Private Partnerships (PPPs)." Hong Kong SAR.

Fan, Shuh Ching. 1974. *The Population of Hong Kong*. Paris: Committee for International Coordination of National Research in Demography.

Fong, Ben Yuk Fai, and Wing Tung Ho. 2017. "Public-Private Partnership in Health and Long-Term Care: The Hong Kong Experience." In *Sustainable Health and Long-Term Care Solutions for an Aging Population*, edited by Ben Fong, Artie Ng, and Peter Yuen. Hershey, PA: IGI Global.

FHB (Food and Health Bureau). 2008. "Synopsis of Healthcare Financing Studies: Projection of Hong Kong's Healthcare Expenditure." Food and Health Bureau, Hong Kong SAR.

FHB. 2010. "Our Partner for Better Health: Primary Care Development in Hong Kong: Strategy Document." Food and Health Bureau, Hong Kong SAR.

FHB. 2011. "Interim Review of Elderly Health Care Voucher Pilot Scheme." Food and Health Bureau, Hong Kong SAR.

FHB. 2013. "Role and Development of Public and Private Healthcare Services, Legislative Council on Health Services Subcommittee on Health Protection Scheme." Legislative Council, Hong Kong SAR.

FHB. 2017. "Strategic Review on Healthcare Manpower Planning and Professional Development." Food and Health Bureau, Hong Kong SAR.

FHB. 2018. "Hong Kong's Domestic Health Accounts (DHA)." Food and Health Bureau, Hong Kong SAR.

FHB and Department of Health. 2018. *TOWARDS 2025: Strategy and Action Plan to Prevent and Control Non-communicable Diseases in Hong Kong: Summary Report*. Hong Kong SAR.

Fung, Colman S. C., Weng Yee Chin, Daisy S. K. Dai, Ruby L. P. Kwok, Eva L. H. Tsui, Yuk Fai Wan, Wendy Wong, Carlos K. H. Wong, Daniel Y. T. Fong, and Cindy L. K. Lam. 2012. "Evaluation of the Quality of Care of a Multi-Disciplinary Risk Factor Assessment and Management Programme (RAMP) for Diabetic Patients." *BMC Family Practice*

13 (1): 116.

Government of Hong Kong SAR. 2016. "Hong Kong: The Facts: Rehabilitation." Hong Kong SAR.

Government of Hong Kong SAR. 2018a. "Background of Elderly Health Care Voucher Scheme." Health Care Voucher. https://www.hcv.gov.hk/eng/pub_background.htm.

Government of Hong Kong SAR. 2018b. "The Elderly Health Care Voucher Scheme of the Government of the Hong Kong Special Administrative Region ("HKSARG")—Pilot Scheme at the University of Hong Kong—Shenzhen Hospital (HKU-SZ Hospital)." Health Care Voucher. https://www.hcv.gov.hk/eng/pub_sz_bg.htm.

Hospital Authority. 2012. "Strategic Service Framework for Elderly Patients." Hospital Authority, Hong Kong SAR.

Hospital Authority. 2016. "Strategic Service Framework for Rehabilitation Services." Hospital Authority, Hong Kong SAR.

Hospital Authority. 2017. "Fees and Charges." June 18, 2017. http://www.ha.org.hk/visitor/ha_visitor_index.asp?Content_ID=10045&Lang=ENG, accessed November 11, 2019.

Hospital Authority. 2018a. "Drug Formulary Management." HA Drug Formulary. http://www.ha.org.hk/hadf/en-us/Frequently-Asked-Questions, accessed December 18, 2018.

Hospital Authority. 2018b. "Hospital Authority Drug Formulary (v14.2)." Hospital Authority, Hong Kong SAR.

Jiao, Fang Fang, Colman Siu Cheung Fung, Eric Yuk Fai Wan, Anca Ka Chun Chan, Sarah Morag McGhee, Ruby Lao Ping Kowk, and Cindy Lo Kuen Lam. 2018. "Five-Year Cost-effectiveness of the Multidisciplinary Risk Assessment and Management Programme–Diabetes Mellitus (RAMP-DM)." *Diabetes Care* 41 (2): 250–57.

Lai, Angel Hor-Yan, Zoey Kuang, Carrie Ho-Kwan Yam, Shereen Ayub, and Eng-Kiong Yeoh. 2018. "Vouchers for Primary Healthcare Services in an Ageing World? The Perspectives of Elderly Voucher Recipients in Hong Kong." *Health & Social Care in the Community* 26 (3): 374–82.

Lee, A., F. L. Lau, C. B. Hazlett, C. W. Kam, P. Wong, T. W. Wong, and S. Chow. 2007. "Utilisation of Accident and Emergency Services by Patients Who Could Be Managed by General Practitioners." *Hong Kong Medical Journal* 13 (Suppl 4): S28–31.

Leung, J. C. B. 2014. "Active Ageing in Hong Kong." In *Active Aging in Asia*, Routledge Studies in Social Welfare in Asia, edited by Alan Walker and Christian Aspalter. London: Routledge.

Lian, Jinxiao, Sarah M. McGhee, Ching So June Chau, Carlos K. H. Wong, William C. W. Wong, and Cindy L. K. Lam. 2017. "Five-Year Cost-Effectiveness of the Patient Empowerment Programme (PEP) for Type 2 Diabetes Mellitus in Primary Care." *Diabetes, Obesity and Metabolism* 19 (9): 1312–16.

Luk, James Ka Hay, Patrick Ka Chun Chiu, and Leung Wing Chu. 2009. "Factors Affecting Institutionalization in Older Hong Kong Chinese Patients after Recovery from Acute Medical Illnesses." *Archives of Gerontology and Geriatrics* 49 (2): e110–14.

Lum, Terry, Vivian Lou, Andy H. Y. Ho, Gloria H. Y. Wong, Jennifer Y. N. Tang, Hao Luo, Mandy Lau, Wing W. S. Kan, and Olive P. L. Yek. 2015. *Evaluation Study of the First Phase of the Pilot Scheme on Community Care Service Voucher (CCSV) for the Elderly: Mid-term Evaluation Report.* Hong Kong SAR: Sau Po Centre on Ageing.

McGhee, Sarah M., W. L. Cheung, Jean Woo, Pui Hing Chau, J. Chen, K. C. Chan, Sai Hei Cheung, and Peter Chan. 2009. *Trends of Disease Burden Consequent to Diabetes in Older Persons in Hong Kong: Implications of Population Ageing.* Hong Kong: Hong Kong Jockey Club.

Mok, C. K. Francis. 2018. "Achievements and Challenges in Elderly Service Development in Hong Kong." Presented at the Hospital Authority Convention 2018. Hospital Authority, Hong Kong SAR.

Our Hong Kong Foundation. 2018. *Fit for Purpose: A Health System for the 21st Century: Research Report.* Hong Kong SAR: Our Hong Kong Foundation.

Poon, Lai Fong, and Shirley Ng, eds. 2018. "Health." In *Hong Kong Yearbook 2017.* Hong Kong: Information Services Department, Hong Kong SAR.

Poon, Peter King-Kong, Angelina So, and Eve Lai-Ching Loong. 2014. "Self-Management in Community-Based Rehabilitation Programme for Persons with Chronic Diseases." In *Community Care in Hong Kong: Current Practices, Practice-Research Studies and Future Directions,* edited by Kar-wai Tong and Kenneth Nai-kuen Fong. Hong Kong: City University of HK Press.

Quan, Jianchao, T. K. Li, H. Pang, C. H. Choi, S. C. Siu, S. Y. Tang, N. M. S. Wat, J. Woo, J. M. Johnston, and G. M. Leung. 2017a. "Diabetes Incidence and Prevalence in Hong Kong, China During 2006–2014." *Diabetic Medicine* 34 (7): 902–08.

Quan, Jianchao, Huyang Zhang, Deanette Pang, Brian K. Chen, Janice M. Johnston, Weiyan Jian, Zheng Yi Lau, Toshiaki Iizuka, Gabriel M. Leung, Hai Fang, Kelvin B. Tan, and Karen Eggleston. 2017b.

"Avoidable Hospital Admissions from Diabetes Complications in Japan, Singapore, Hong Kong, and Communities outside Beijing." *Health Affairs* 36 (11): 1896–903.

Research Office. 2015. "Challenges of Population Ageing." Research Brief no. 1. Hong Kong SAR: Information Services Division, Legislative Council Secretariat.

Research Office. 2018. "Livelihood of New Arrivals from the Mainland." (ISSH18/17-18). Statistical Highlights. Information Services Division, Legislative Council Secretariat, Hong Kong SAR.

Sim, T. C. and E. M. F. Leung. 2000. "Geriatric Care for Residents of Private Nursing Homes." *Journal of the Hong Kong Geriatrics Society* 10 (2): 84–89.

Social Welfare Department. 2018a. "The Pilot Scheme on Residential Care Service Voucher for the Elderly." Government of Hong Kong SAR. https://www.swd.gov.hk/en/index/site_pubsvc/page_elderly/sub_residentia/id_psrcsv, accessed December 18, 2018.

Social Welfare Department. 2018b. "Pilot Residential Care Services Scheme in Guangdong." Government of Hong Kong SAR. https://www.swd.gov.hk/en/index/site_pubsvc/page_elderly/sub_residentia/id_guangdong, accessed December 18, 2018.

Social Welfare Department. 2019. "Pilot Scheme on Community Care Service Voucher for the Elderly (CCSV)." Government of Hong Kong SAR. https://www.swd.gov.hk/en/index/site_pubsvc/page_elderly/sub_csselderly/id_psccsv/, accessed January 17, 2019.

Wan, Eric Yuk Fai, Colman Siu Cheng Fung, Fang Fang Jiao, Esther Yee Tak, Yu, Weng Yee Chin, Daniel Yee Tak Fong, Carlos King Ho Wong, Anca Ka Chun Chan, Karina Hiu Yen Chan, Ruby Lai Ping Kwok, and Cindy Lo Kuen Lam. 2018. "Five-Year Effectiveness of the Multi-disciplinary Risk Assessment and Management Programme-Diabetes Mellitus (RAMP-DM) on Diabetes-Related Complications and Health Service Uses—A Population-Based and Propensity-Matched Cohort Study." *Diabetes Care* 41 (1): 49–59.

Wong, Carlos K. H., Fang-Fang Jiao, Shing-Chung Siu, Colman S. C. Fung, Daniel Y. T. Fong, Ka-Wai Wong, Esther Y. T. Yu, Yvonne Y. C. Lo, and Cindy L. K. Lam. 2016. "Cost-Effectiveness of a Short Message Service Intervention to Prevent Type 2 Diabetes from Impaired Glucose Tolerance." *Journal of Diabetes Research* 2016 (1219581).

Wong, Samuel Yeung-Shan, Dan Zou, Roger Y. Chung, Regina W. Sit. Dexing Zhang, Dicken Chan, Eng Kiong Yeoh, and Jean W. Woo. 2017. "Regular Source of Care for the Elderly: A Cross-National

Comparative Study of Hong Kong with 11 Developed Countries." *Journal of the American Medical Directors Association* 18 (9): 807. e1–807.e8.

World Bank. N.d. "DataBank | World Development Indicators." http://databank.worldbank.org/data/reports.aspx?source=world-development-indicators, accessed December 9, 2018.

Yam, Carrie H. K., Su Liu, Olivia H. Y. Huang, E. K. Yeoh, and Sian M. Griffiths. 2011. "Can Vouchers Make a Difference to the Use of Private Primary Care Services by Older People? Experience from the Healthcare Reform Programme in Hong Kong." *BMC Health Services Research* 11 (1): 255.

Yeoh, Eng Kiong. 2018. "What are the Disruptions Necessary and Sufficient for Integrating Health Systems?" Presented at the Towards an Integrated Person-Centred Health System for Hong Kong, Hong Kong.

Yu, Esther Yee Tak, Eric Yuk Fai Wan, Karina Hiu Yen Chan, Carlos King Ho Wong, Ruby Lai Ping Kwok, Daniel Yee Tak Fong, and Cindy Lo Kuen Lam. 2015. "Evaluation of the Quality of Care of a Multi-Disciplinary Risk Factor Assessment and Management Programme for Hypertension (RAMP-HT)." *BMC Family Practice* 16 (1): 7.

Yu, Esther Y. T., Eric Y. F. Fan, Carlos K. H. Wong, Anca K. C. Chan, Karina H. Y. Chan, Sin-yi Ho, Ruby L. P. Kwok, and Cindy L. K. Lam. 2017. "Effects of Risk Assessment and Management Programme for Hypertension on Clinical Outcomes and Cardiovascular Disease Risks after 12 Months: A Population-Based Matched Cohort Study." *Journal of Hypertension* 35 (3): 627–36.

Yu, Ruby, Pui Hing Chau, Sarah M. McGhee, June Chau, Che Hei Lee, Man Yee Chan, Sai Hei Cheung, and Jean Woo. 2012. *Trends of Disease Burden Consequent to Stroke in Older Persons in Hong Kong: Implications of Population Ageing.* Hong Kong: Hong Kong Jockey Club.

Yu, Ruby, Pui Hing Chau, Sarah M. McGhee, Wai Ling, Cheung, Kam Che Chan, Sai Hei Cheung, and Jean Woo. 2010. *Dementia Trends: Impact of the Ageing Population and Societal Implications for Hong Kong.* Hong Kong: Hong Kong Jockey Club.

8 Creating National Demonstration Areas for the Integrated Prevention and Control of Noncommunicable Diseases in China

Jianqun Dong, Fan Mao, Wenlan Dong, Yingying Jiang, Shiwei Liu, and Maigeng Zhou

Chronic and noncommunicable diseases (NCDs) are estimated to kill around 38 million people every year, accounting for 68 percent of all deaths worldwide. The main NCDs (cardiovascular disease, cancer, chronic respiratory diseases, and diabetes) are among the top 10 causes of death. Nearly 80 percent of NCD deaths—30 million—occur in low-, middle-, and high-income countries that are not part of the Organisation for Economic Co-operation and Development (OECD), where NCDs are fast replacing infectious diseases and malnutrition as the leading causes of disability and premature death (WHO 2015). Notably, the economic burden of NCDs, particularly as an impediment to social development, is even greater than that brought about by the 2007–08 global financial crisis (Kong 2012). NCDs have become a conspicuous global public health issue that threatens socioeconomic development.

In 2011, the role of governments in preventing and mitigating NCDs was first officially put forward based on a political declaration on NCDs adopted at the United Nations General Assembly. It was emphasized again in an outcome document on NCDs adopted at the UN General Assembly in 2014, which included a road map of government commitments. The World Health Organization's Global Action Plan for the Prevention and Control of NCDs 2013–2020, which was endorsed by the World Health Assembly in May 2013, set priorities and provided strategic guidance on how countries could implement the road map of commitments. It also included a series of voluntary targets that focus on risk factors such as tobacco use, high blood pressure, high salt intake, obesity, and physical inactivity, as well as targets for access to essential medicines and technologies, and drug therapy and counseling for NCDs (WHO 2013).

China has experienced an epidemiological transition from infectious to chronic diseases in a shorter period than other countries, along with rapid industrialization, urbanization, population aging, and lifestyle changes. According to a 2015 report on chronic disease and nutrition in China, 30.1 percent of Chinese adults were overweight and 11.9 percent were obese. The prevalence rates of hypertension and diabetes were 25.2 percent and 9.7 percent, respectively (NHFPC 2016). In response to the severe and urgent need for NCD prevention and control, the National Health and Family Planning Commission[1] (NHFPC) launched a pilot program in 2010 establishing national demonstration areas (*shifan qu*) for the integrated prevention and control of NCDs, for the purpose of demonstrating and then scaling up measures to prevent and control NCDs nationwide.

At the beginning of 2009, the NHFPC's Bureau of Disease Prevention and Control began to prepare for the establishment of national demonstration areas. The bureau set up the Office of the National Demonstration Area for Comprehensive Prevention and Control of Chronic Disease[2] (hereafter the National Demonstration Area Office), which was put in charge of the areas' day-to-day management. In November 2010, the "Guidelines for Construction of National Demonstration Areas for Integrated Prevention and Control of NCDS" (NHFPC 2010) were published, based on several rounds of expert discussions and a systematic review of the relevant literature. These guidelines were followed by the "Regulation of National Demonstration Areas for Integrated Prevention and Control of NCDS" (NHFPC 2011) and the "National Demonstration Area for the Comprehensive Prevention and Control of Chronic Diseases: Assessment and Evaluation Workbook (revised)" (National Demonstration Area Office for Comprehensive Prevention and Control of Chronic Disease 2012).

Purpose and Goals

The general objective of national demonstration areas is to demonstrate integrated approaches to and mechanisms of NCD prevention and control at the district and county levels. Such a goal requires cooperation among multiple sectors, with the government taking the lead (NCNCD 2014). Those strategies that are proven to be effective will then be summarized and promoted on a larger scale. The expectation is that through health education and

1   The NHFPC was integrated into the National Health Commission as of 2018.

2   The office is situated in the National Center for Chronic and Noncommunicable Disease Control and Prevention, within the Chinese Center for Disease Control and Prevention.

promotion, early diagnosis and treatment, and standardized management, the burden of NCDs can be reduced.

According to the "China National Plan for NCD Prevention and Treatment (2012–2015)," a 2015 target was set for 300 national demonstration areas, expected to cover more than 10 percent of China's counties/districts (NHFPC 2012). All provinces, autonomous regions, and municipalities, and more than 50 percent of prefecture-level cities of the eastern provinces, were also expected to have at least one national demonstration area by 2015.

Based on the latest plans released by the State Council of China, namely, "Health Plan for the Thirteenth Five-Year Period" (State Council 2016) and "Medium- to Long-Term Plan (2017–2025) on the Prevention and Treatment of Chronic Diseases" (General Office of the State Council 2017), national demonstration areas' coverage is planned to reach 15 percent by 2020 and 20 percent by 2025. Setting these long-term goals guarantees the sustainability of national demonstration areas and is expected to help foster a healthier China (Central Committee and State Council 2016).

Guidelines for National Demonstration Areas

Strong safeguard measures regarding leadership, policy, funding, and human resources are fundamental to the construction of national demonstration areas. In each jurisdiction, a group will be set up to spearhead the effort, led by a senior leader from the local government. A multi-sectoral cooperative mechanism that involves all related departments is also to be established, and directors from these departments are to serve as group members in order to gain enough support for NCD prevention and control. Under the leadership of the group, a specific office is set to regulate and coordinate work related to the construction of national demonstration areas. Policies supporting NCD prevention and control, such as media communications and public welfare campaigns, promotion of a healthy diet and physical activities, stricter tobacco control, and referral and two-way referral for high-risk groups, are to be introduced by the government and related departments. In addition to financial support from the NHFPC, funds for NCD prevention and control will be included in local financial budgets and be used as special funds. Meanwhile, a fund guarantee mechanism supported by government leadership and social forces, such as private charitable foundations and non-state corporations, is expected to be established to ensure long-term and sustainable investments in NCD prevention and control. A professional department for NCD prevention and control will be set up at local centers for disease control and prevention and a technical guidance panel will be founded by experts in relevant fields to provide technical guidance and policymaking consultation. Guidance and training systems should be established, and district-/county-level medical institutions and centers for disease control should provide standard training and technical guidance on a regular basis to local medical and health personnel, improving their capacity to prevent and control NCDs.

Collect basic information on NCDs at the county/district level. A database was set up for collecting, sorting out, and analyzing basic information on county/district characteristics, the main NCDs observed, and common risk factors to determine target populations, priority areas, as well as appropriate strategies and measures.

Establish and improve the NCD monitoring system. This should encompass the total population and include data on causes of death, a cancer registry, reports on cardiovascular and cerebrovascular events, risk factor surveillance, and information on basic public health service projects related to NCDs. The quality and quantity of data should be upgraded continuously. In addition, an information management platform relating to NCD prevention and control should be built and updated on a regular basis.

Carry out extensive health education and promotion. Several recommendations are pertinent here: give full play to the role of mass media in NCD prevention and control, highlight local characteristics, carry out health education and promotion activities (around controlling tobacco consumption, advocating a balanced diet, and promoting fitness activities), and establish a long-term operating mechanism for such efforts.

Encourage a healthy lifestyle for all. A comprehensive program to promote healthy lifestyles should involve tools appropriate to the targeted populations. Mass physical exercise programs could be founded under the government's leadership and in cooperation with multiple sectors, encouraging extensive participation. Private enterprises and public institutions could create a supportive environment for physical exercise, implement a work-break exercise fitness program for employees, and carry out a nationwide exercise program aimed at students. Some restaurants and other communal spaces should be designated as smoking-free under the government's leadership to provide examples that others might replicate.

Pay attention to NCD detection among high-risk populations and conduct appropriate interventions. Regular physical examinations of employees will be arranged and medical institutions at all levels will ensure that the blood pressure of adults aged 35 and above is measured at their initial clinical visit. Health indicator self-check stations will be established to provide measures of height, weight, waistline, blood pressure, and blood glucose for all people to find high-risk groups vulnerable to NCDs. Dental examinations of children will be conducted, and dental cavity filling and pit and fissure sealing will be provided for children in need.

Regulate patient management. The National Essential Public Health Service will implement norms for NCD management, integrated with an information management system. Patients with hypertension, diabetes, and a history of strokes are encouraged to participate in chronic disease self-management groups organized by community health service centers to learn the relevant information on NCD prevention and control, and exchange experience on disease control, so as to improve their self-management capacity.

Evaluation System

In order to guarantee the accuracy and completeness of data, the National Demonstration Area Office (2012) developed a handbook for how areas should be created and evaluated. The handbook quantifies the elements laid out in the earlier guidelines in order to aid implementation and monitoring. Specifically, an evaluation index system including 7 categories, 24 items, and 71 specific indicators was constructed based on several rounds of expert consultation to aid in the comprehensive evaluation of interventions in certain districts or counties (see table 8.1). Among the 71 indicators, 11 are considered core indicators and 14 are considered additional. Each indicator was assigned a score, for a total of 1,280 points. This includes a basic score of 1,000 points (including a core 240 points) and an additional score of 280 points.

Taking into account regional differences in the incidence of NCDs and in stages of economic development, the standards for determining qualifying scores is slightly different among eastern, midland, and western regions, mainly focusing on the additional score (see table 8.2).

At the end of 2016, a revised evaluation system was released by the NHFPC to guide national demonstration areas. Some indicators in the old evaluation system were retained while higher standards were put forward. In addition, some new indicators consistent with current policies or strategies on NCD prevention and control were added into the revised version. The newly revised evaluation system includes seven categories: namely, supportive policy; an enabling environment; system integration; health education and health promotion; NCDs' management, monitoring, and evaluation; innovation; and guidance, with a full score of 300 points (National Health Commission 2016). Although the number of indicators has decreased overall, several more specific requirements were added.

TABLE 8.1 Evaluation index system for national demonstration areas

Category	Item	Notes
Political commitment	Institutional structure	Mobilization of local government leaders to participate in and lead the prevention and control of chronic diseases
	Financial support	Availability of necessary funds for the prevention and control of chronic diseases
	Policy/strategy support	
	Manpower	Appropriate numbers of chronic disease prevention and control personnel
Community diagnosis	Community diagnosis	
Surveillance	Mortality surveillance	
	NCD risk factor surveillance	
	Cancer registry	
	Cardiovascular/cerebrovascular incident reports	
Health education/ promotion	Mass media	
	Information materials development	
	Enabling environment	
	Health promotion among children and teenagers	Health education courses and in-school physical activity
	NCD Special Day	Large-scale health education and health promotion activities, e.g., World No Tobacco Day, UN Day for Diabetes
"Healthy lifestyle for all" campaign	Workplace interventions	Implementation of work-break exercises
	Community fitness campaign	
	Healthy diet	E.g., promoting nutritional labeling on foods and reducing salt intake
	Tobacco control	E.g., making all medical/health institutions smoke-free and decreasing the adult male smoking rate
	Models for community/ office/canteen/restaurant	
High-risk population management	Identification of high-risk groups	
	Interventions targeting high-risk groups	
	Dental hygiene	E.g., filling cavities and groove sealing for children of appropriate age
NCD patient management	Equalization of essential public health services	Registering and management of patients with hypertension and/or diabetes
	Patient self-management	Implementation and coverage of Chronic Disease Self-management Program

SOURCE: NHFPC 2010.

NOTE: NCD = noncommunicable disease.

TABLE 8.2 Qualification standards for national demonstration areas, by region (points)

Region	Total score	Basic score	Additional score	Core score
Eastern	≥850	≥650	≥200	≥180
Midland	≥800	≥650	≥150	≥180
Western	≥750	≥650	≥100	≥180

SOURCE: National Demonstration Area Office for Comprehensive Prevention and Control of Chronic Disease 2012.
NOTES: The eastern region includes 9 provinces, autonomous regions, and municipalities: Beijing, Tianjin, Liaoning, Shanghai, Jiangsu, Zhejiang, Fujian, Shandong, and Guangdong. The midland includes 10: Hebei, Shanxi, Jilin, Heilongjiang, Anhui, Jiangxi, Henan, Hubei, Hunan, and Hainan. The western region includes 12: Mongolia, Guangxi, Chongqing, Sichuan, Guizhou, Yunnan, Tibet, Shaanxi, Gansu, Qinghai, Ningxia, Xinjiang, and Xinjiang Production and Construction Corps.

Application and Review

To provide research-based guidance for the creation of national demonstration areas in different places, the National Demonstration Area Office developed regulations that contain specific provisions for implementation, regular management, and assessment, these were issued by NHFPC in March 2011.

The national demonstration area application and review process is illustrated in figure 8.1. From 2011 to 2015, all counties and districts willing to host a national demonstration area were invited to submit an application in the name of the local government to the municipal administrative department of health, which then submitted all the applications within its jurisdiction to the provincial administrative department of health. After being considered using the evaluation system outlined above, qualified applications were recommended to the National Center for Chronic and Non-communicable Disease Control and Prevention. Under the leadership of the NHFPC, the National Demonstration Area Office organized related experts on NCD prevention and control to evaluate the applications received. Qualified counties and districts were then recommended to receive an on-site review. A list of the counties/districts entitled to host a national demonstration area is released publicly on the NHFPC's website at the end of each year. The counties/districts that do not pass the review process are allowed to reapply in the next round, after improving their situation and application materials.

Since the end of 2016, the application form has been adjusted based on the revised regulations of national demonstration areas. Only those counties/districts designated as having a provincial demonstration area for one year are permitted to participate. In addition, considering the regional leading role of national demonstration areas, the NHFPC has begun to allocate the

FIGURE 8.1 National demonstration area application and review process

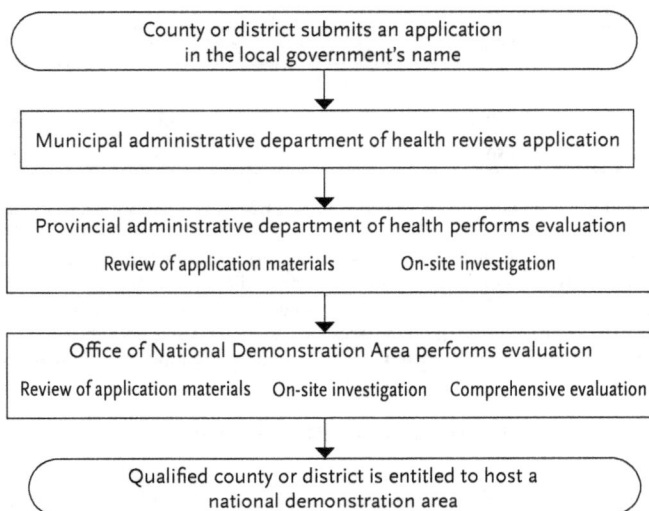

```
┌─────────────────────────────────────────────────────┐
│         County or district submits an application     │
│              in the local government's name           │
└─────────────────────────────────────────────────────┘
                          ↓
┌─────────────────────────────────────────────────────┐
│  Municipal administrative department of health reviews application │
└─────────────────────────────────────────────────────┘
                          ↓
┌─────────────────────────────────────────────────────┐
│  Provincial administrative department of health performs evaluation │
│                                                       │
│   Review of application materials      On-site investigation │
└─────────────────────────────────────────────────────┘
                          ↓
┌─────────────────────────────────────────────────────┐
│   Office of National Demonstration Area performs evaluation │
│                                                       │
│ Review of application materials   On-site investigation   Comprehensive evaluation │
└─────────────────────────────────────────────────────┘
                          ↓
┌─────────────────────────────────────────────────────┐
│         Qualified county or district is entitled to host a │
│                  national demonstration area          │
└─────────────────────────────────────────────────────┘
```

SOURCE: NHFPC 2011.

corresponding quotas for each province based on its current number, replacing the previous voluntary and open-ended process. The concrete review process is the same as before.

Progress and Achievements

From the beginning of the program to 2015, a total of 365 counties/districts from 30 provinces and the Xinjiang Production and Construction Corps submitted application materials to the National Demonstration Area Office, and 265 were named as national demonstration areas. From 2016 to the end of 2017, based on the quotas allocated by the NHFPC, another 103 counties/districts were named as national demonstration areas. After an adjustment to administrative divisions, two counties/districts were merged with other nearby demonstration areas. That brings the latest total of national demonstration areas to 366, covering all of China's provinces. Table 8.3 shows that national demonstration areas are found in 49.7 percent of prefecture-level cities; the coverage rate for counties/districts, 12.8 percent, is shown in table 8.4. In general, eastern provinces have achieved more than midland and western provinces. Among all provinces, Shanghai hosts the highest percentage of national demonstration areas, covering 100 percent of the counties/districts in its jurisdiction.

TABLE 8.3 Coverage rates of national demonstration areas in prefecture-level cities

Region	Prefecture-level cities containing at least one national demonstration area	Prefecture-level cities	Coverage rate (%)
Eastern	51	88	58.0
Midland	61	119	51.3
Western	56	131	42.7
Total	168	338	49.7

SOURCE: Authors.

TABLE 8.4 Coverage rates of national demonstration areas at county/district level

Region	National demonstration areas	Counties/districts	Coverage rate (%)
Eastern	148	676	21.9
Midland	108	1,086	10.0
Western	110	1,089	10.1
Total	366	2,851	12.8

SOURCE: Authors.

The creation of national demonstration areas has enabled NCD prevention and control to gain increased attention from governments at all levels. Where the national demonstration areas are located, governments have established high-ranking leading groups to guide NCD prevention and control within their jurisdictions. Plans for NCD prevention and treatment at the county/district level were drawn up to promote the implementation of related work. All the required policies, funds, and human resources are fully guaranteed at the local levels. Most counties/districts have taken this opportunity to establish special departments responsible for NCD prevention and control.

In several counties/districts, the responsibilities of various departments are outlined in detail, and department leaders have been asked to sign a responsibility declaration before the local government to ensure the implementation of corresponding NCD prevention and control work. For example, an industrial and commercial department might be in charge of the nutrition labeling of prepackaged food. The construction sector could be asked to prepare public venues and facilities for health-related events, the education department to ensure that information on NCD prevention and control and dental health be provided to students in primary and middle schools, and the sports department to train a certain number of fitness instructors to guide mass sporting activities.

Simply put, the creation of national demonstration areas has strengthened supportive environments for NCD prevention and control. The creation of these areas has further enhanced the key responsibilities of local governments in the prevention and control of NCDs and has allowed the wide recognition of the importance of mobilizing social resources and involving all citizens in this effort. Among the positive results are many valuable, practical experiences in promoting multi-department cooperation in the prevention and control of NCDs. Since 2015, the presence of a national demonstration area is one of the public health and medical criteria that need to be met before a municipality can apply to be designated as a National Health City.

Next Steps

In recent years, the creation of national demonstration areas has provided a platform for governments at all levels to improve resource integration and NCD prevention and control. This is due to great attention from local governments and support from related departments. Several issues need to be further emphasized in the future to promote the sustainable development of related efforts.

First, an evaluation system of multi-sector cooperation needs further development to gradually perfect such cooperation and help each department to fulfill its corresponding duties in NCD prevention and control. Second, dynamic management of national demonstration areas should be further strengthened through such mechanisms as annual reports and monitoring systems to guarantee the quality and effect of local NCD prevention and control. Finally, replicable experiences in NCD prevention and control should be summarized and exchanged to better support NCD prevention and control on a larger scale.

References

Central Committee of the Communist Party of China and the State Council. 2016. "'Jiankang Zhongguo 2030' guihua gangyao" ['Healthy China 2030' plan outline]. http://www.gov.cn/zhengce/2016-10/25/content_5124174.htm.

General Office of the State Council of the People's Republic of China. 2017. "Guowuyuan Bangong Ting guanyu yinfa Zhongguo fangzhi manxingbing zhong changqi guihua (2017–2025 nian) de tongzhi" [Circular of the General Office of the State Council on the issuance of China's medium- to long-term plan (2017–2025) on the prevention and treatment of chronic diseases]. http://www.gov.cn/zhengce/content/2017-02/14/content_5167886.htm.

Kong, Ling-Zhi. 2012. "Zhongguo manxingbing fangzhi guihua jiedu" [Interpretation of national plan for NCDs prevention and treatment] *Zhongguo manxingbing yufang yu kongzhi* [Chinese journal of prevention and control of chronic disease] 20 (5): 502–03.

National Demonstration Area Office for Comprehensive Prevention and Control of Chronic Disease. 2012. *Guojia manxing fei chuanran xing jibing zonghe fangkong shifan qu: kaohe pingjia gongzuo shouce (shixing)* [National Demonstration Area for comprehensive prevention and control of chronic diseases: Assessment and evaluation workbook (revised)]. National Center for Chronic and Noncommunicable Disease Control and Prevention, Chinese Center for Disease Control and Prevention. http://www.gxcdc.com/uploadfile/ywdh/uploadfile/201401/20140109090959327.pdf.

National Health Commission. 2016. "Guojia manxingbing zonghe fang kong shifan qu jianshe guanli banfa" [Measures for the construction and management of National Demonstration Areas for the comprehensive prevention and control of chronic diseases]. National Health Commission notice no. 44, issued October 16. Available at "Weijiwei yinfa guojia manxingbing zonghe fang kong shifan qu jianshe guanli banfa" [Health and Family Planning Commission issues management measures for the construction of a national chronic disease prevention and control demonstration zone], Zhongguo xinwen wang [China news], November 1, 2016, http://www.chinanews.com/sh/2016/11-01/8050083.shtml.

NCNCD (National Center for Chronic and Non-communicable Disease Control and Prevention, Chinese Center for Disease Control and Prevention). 2014. "Manxingbing zonghe fang kong shifan qu xiangmu jieshao" [Introduction to the National Demonstration Area for the comprehensive prevention and control of chronic disease]. http://ncncd.chinacdc.cn/xmgz/manxingbzhfksf/xmjs/201406/t20140618_98308.htm.

NHFPC (National Health and Family Planning Commission of the People's Republic of China). 2010. "Manxing fei chuanran xing jibing zonghe fangkong shifanqu gongzuo zhidao fang'an" [Guidelines for construction of National Demonstration Areas for integrated prevention and control of NCDs]. Department of Health, Disease Control, and Prevention notice no. 172. http://www.gov.cn/gzdt/2010-11/16/content_1746847.htm.

NHFPC. 2011. "Manxing fei chuanran xing jibing zonghe fangkong shifanqu guanli banfa" [Regulation of National Demonstration Areas for integrated prevention and control of NCDs]. Department of Health, Disease Control, and Prevention notice no. 35. http://www.gov.cn/zwgk/2011-03/24/content_1830841.htm.

NHFPC. 2012. "Zhongguo fangzhi manxingbing guihua (2012–2015)" [China national plan for NCD prevention and treatment (2012–2015)]. http://politics.people.com.cn/GB/70731/17948200.html.

NHFPC. 2016. Report on Situation of Chronic Disease and Nutrition among Residents in China. Beijing: People's Medical Publishing House.

State Council of the People's Republic of China. 2016. "'Shisanwu' weisheng yu jiankang guihua" [Health plan for the thirteenth five-year period]. http://www.gov.cn/zhengce/content/2017-01/10/content_5158488.htm.

WHO (World Health Organization). 2013. Global Action Plan for the Prevention and Control of NCDs 2013–2020. Geneva: WHO.

WHO. 2015. Health in 2015: From MDGs to SDGs. Geneva: WHO.

9 Avoidable Hospital Admissions of Diabetes Patients and Associated Medical Spending in Rural China

Evidence from Zhejiang Province

Min Yu, Yiwei Chen, Hui Ding, Jieming Zhong, Ruying Hu, Chunmei Wang, Kaixu Xie, Xiangyu Chen, Pedro Gallardo, and Karen Eggleston

Diabetes mellitus poses a critical public health issue in many countries around the globe, including low- and middle-income countries with health systems ill-prepared to manage chronic disease within primary care. China, especially in rural areas, represents an interesting and important case of strengthening population health and primary care management for diabetes. Such prevention and control may not only improve patients' health and quality of life, but also potentially save resources by reducing avoidable hospital admissions. We propose age- and sex-standardized medical expenditures of avoidable admissions, alongside the more standard metric of number of avoidable admissions, as a new way of measuring primary care management of diabetes and comparing progress over time and across regions.

In China, rapid economic development and urbanization have contributed to alarming increases in the incidence of diabetes. In 2013, an estimated 10.9 percent of adults had type 2 diabetes (Xu et al. 2013). Although there is greater prevalence of type 2 diabetes in urban areas, diabetes is associated with greater excess mortality in rural China (Bragg et al. 2017). As the morbidity and mortality burden of diabetes rises in both urban and rural China, so, too, will the costs associated with medical care. From 2002 to 2008, the direct medical cost of type 2 diabetes in China rose from US$2.27 billion to $8.65 billion (Hu et al. 2015).

The authors thank Mr. Haibin Wu and others at the Zhejiang CDC and Tongxiang CDC who assisted with the collection of the data and early phase of the analyses. This research was reviewed for ethical approval by both the Zhejiang provincial and Stanford University institutional review boards.

Avoidable admissions for ambulatory care-sensitive conditions (ACSCS) such as diabetes are used by the Organisation for Economic Cooperation and Development (OECD) and others as a Health Care Quality Indicator. Avoidable admissions for ACSCS are useful for signaling resource use that could be diverted elsewhere with improved ACSC control. To date, literature regarding avoidable admissions and diabetes-related health expenditures in China, especially rural China, remains limited, despite nationwide efforts to strengthen chronic disease management and adopt a family doctor system. We contribute to the literature by estimating avoidable admissions and associated medical expenditures for one ACSC, diabetes, with data from a county in rural southeast China that, based on its socioeconomic development, may presage the future of rural and peri-urban China.

Tongxiang County in Zhejiang Province is one of southeast China's richest counties; in 2015, per capita disposable incomes of urban and rural residents were ¥44,725 and ¥27,357, respectively (Wu et al. 2018). In that same year, Tongxiang had a registered population of 689,000, among whom 20,699 (3 percent) were type 2 diabetes patients over the age of 15; this is considerably lower than the 10.9 percent national prevalence of type 2 diabetes reported in 2013. However, expenditures on the complications of diabetes absorb a substantial amount of resources, burdening patients with out-of-pocket spending and adding to pressures on social insurance coverage. After adjusting for confounders, Wu et. al (2018) found patients in Tongxiang with at least one type 2 diabetes complication had, respectively, 83.55% and 38.46% higher total inpatient and outpatient costs. Our study expands on these findings by reporting age- and sex-standardized avoidable admission rates of type 2 diabetes patients in Tongxiang and associated medical expenditures, and comparing these to other regions and countries.

We assembled and linked hospital admissions data from Tongxiang's diabetes management system and rural resident health insurance claims data. To code an admission as diabetes-related, we counted any admission with at least one ICD10 code for diabetes-related procedures or services (E10, E11, E13, E14). Using these data, we calculated the avoidable admissions, standardizing for age and sex according to the criteria set by OECD Health Care Quality Indicators 2014–15.

In 2015, 19.9 percent (4,120) of Tongxiang's registered diabetic patients had at least one hospital admission. Of the 6,709 total hospitalizations, 1,038 admissions (15.47 percent) were coded as diabetes-related. After standardizing for age and sex to the OECD standard population, there were 1,108.76 hospitalizations of diabetes patients per 100,000 people. Using the same age- and sex-standardization, there were 163.64 avoidable admissions

FIGURE 9.1 Hospitalization expenditures per managed diabetes patient for diabetes-related hospitalizations (top panel) and for all hospitalizations (bottom panel), by patient's sex and age (2015 USD)

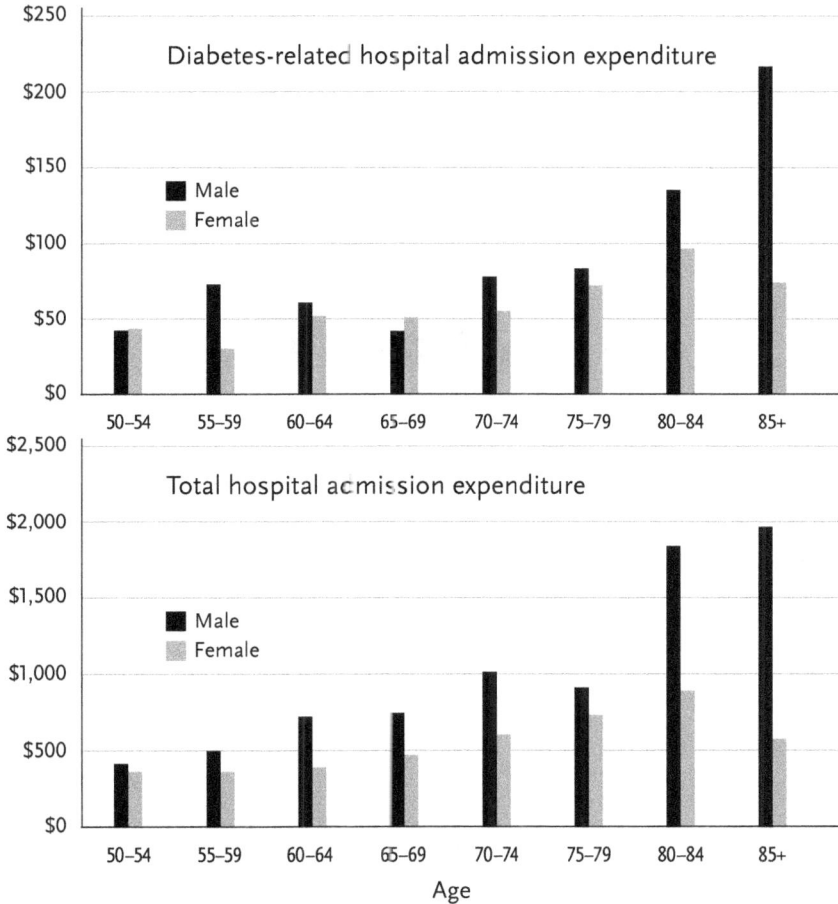

SOURCE: Authors' analysis of Tongxiang County data.
NOTE: The expenditures are per individual with diabetes in that age-sex group, not per individual who was hospitalized. Therefore, the higher average spending for those above 70 reflects both more hospitalizations as well as greater spending per hospitalization. For example, based on the top panel and as noted in the text, hospitalizations directly related to diabetes in 2015 cost approximately ¥384 (US$59) per managed diabetes patient, which is similar to the columns shown for those aged 70–74.

FIGURE 9.2 Diabetes patients' hospitalizations and related healthcare expenditures, by sex, 2015

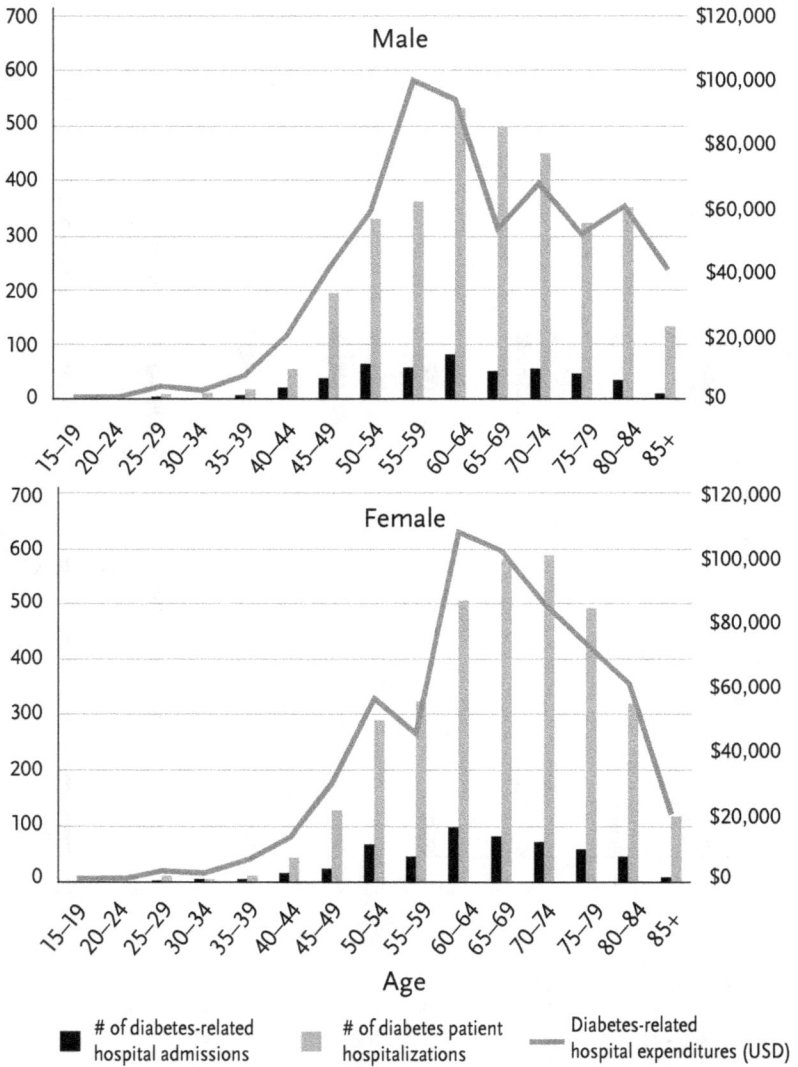

SOURCE: Authors' analysis of Tongxiang County data.

(diabetes-related hospital admissions) per 100,000 people.

We can compare this rate to age- and sex-standardized admissions in other populations. In 2011, avoidable admissions for diabetes per 100,000 people, using the same standardization, were 162.3 for Japan and 248.1 for Singapore, above the OECD average of 149.8 (Quan et al. 2017). The same study reported peri-urban Beijing and Hong Kong to have rates of 271.6 and 147.9 avoidable diabetes admissions per 100,000 people, respectively. Our estimate of 163.64 for Tongxiang is quite close to that of Japan, and in between those estimated for peri-urban Beijing and Hong Kong. Importantly, the aforementioned study also found a negative correlation between the number of outpatient visits made by diabetes patients in one year and the probability of an avoidable admission the following year. This finding underscores the promising potential for improved primary care management of chronic disease to offset costlier avoidable diabetes patient admissions.

Hospitalizations of patients with diabetes were costlier for older age groups (see figures 9.1 and 9.2). Diabetes-related hospitalizations of male patients generally cost more per capita compared to their female counterparts, especially for those over the age of 80 (among whom hospitalizations may no longer be avoidable).

Overall, Tongxiang diabetic patients' 2015 health expenditures on hospitalizations totaled approximately ¥75.8 million (US$11.6 million), 37.9 percent of which was out-of-pocket expenditure. Hospitalizations directly related to diabetes in 2015 cost approximately ¥7.9 million (US$1.21 million), or ¥384 (US$59) per managed diabetes patient. After standardizing for age and sex, diabetes-related hospitalizations cost ¥12.9 per capita, equivalent to 28 percent of per capita spending on essential population health services.

The external validity of our findings merits investigation. Data limitations precluded strict adherence to the inclusion and exclusion criteria of the OECD guidelines. Therefore, our rate of diabetes-related admissions may be an underestimate; we also report the rate based on any hospitalization for individuals with diagnosed diabetes, as an upper bound on the true avoidable admissions rate.

Limitations notwithstanding, our results highlight the resources that society and households absorb for unnecessary hospitalizations. Importantly, our findings could be compared across countries and regions to illustrate the per capita resources that might be re-directed to strengthen ambulatory management and control the diabetes epidemic in China and globally.

References

Bragg, Fiona, Michael V. Holmes, Andri Iona, Yu Guo, Huaidong Du, Yiping Chen, Zheng Bian, Ling Yang, William Herrington, Derrick Bennett, Iain Turnbull, Yongmei Liu, Shixian Feng, Junshi Chen, Robert Clarke, Rory Collins, Richard Peto, Liming Li, and Zhengming Chen. 2017. "Association between Diabetes and Cause-Specific Mortality in Rural and Urban Areas of China." *JAMA* 317 (3): 280–89.

Hu Huimei, Monika Sawhney, Lizheng Shi, Shengnan Duan, Yunxian Yu, Zhihong Wu, Guixing Qiu, and Hengjin Dong. 2015. "A Systematic Review of the Direct Economic Burden of Type 2 Diabetes in China." *Diabetes Therapy* 6 (1): 7–16.

Quan, Jianchao, Huyang Zhang, Deanette Pang, Brian K. Chen, Janice M. Johnston, Weiyan Jian, Zheng Yi Lau, Toshiaki Iizuka, Gabriel M. Leung, Hai Fang, Kelvin B. Tan, and Karen Eggleston. 2017. "Avoidable Hospital Admissions from Diabetes Complications in Japan, Singapore, Hong Kong, and Communities outside Beijing." *Health Affairs* 36 (11): 1896–903.

Wu, Haibin, Karen N. Eggleston, Jieming Zhong, Ruying Hu, Chunmei Wang, Kaixu Xie, Yiwei Chen, Xiangyu Chen, and Min Yu. 2018. "How Do Type 2 Diabetes Mellitus-Related Complications and Socioeconomic Factors Impact Direct Medical Costs in Rural Southeast China?" *BMJ Open* 8 (11): e020647.

Xu, Yu, Limin Wang, Jiang He, Yufang Bi, Mian Li, Tiange Wang, Linhong Wang, Yong Jiang, Meng Dai, Jieli Lu, Min Xu, Yichong Li, Nan Hu, Jianhong Li, Shengquan Mi, Chung-Shiuan Chen, Guangwei Li, Yiming Mu, Jiajun Zhao, Lingzhi Kong, Jialun Chen, Shenghan Lai, Weiqing Wang, Wenhua Zhao, and Guang Ning. 2013. "Prevalence and Control of Diabetes in Chinese Adults." *JAMA* 310 (9): 948–59.

10 Exploring and Promoting the Family Doctor System in an Aging China

Rize Jing and Hai Fang

According to the National Bureau of Statistics, China had a population of 1.39 billion in 2017, among which 158.47 million were aged 65 and over, accounting for 11.4% of the total population, and its elderly dependency ratio had reached 15.9%. Furthermore, the newly born population in 2017 was 17.23 million, down by 0.62 million year-on-year. The aging trend in China has been accompanied by an increasingly higher incidence of various chronic diseases among the elderly. Taking hypertension as an example, the two-week consultation rate and hospitalization rate for hypertension rose from 8.0% and 1.2% in 2003 to 21.4% and 4.9% in 2013, respectively (National Health Commission 2018). In addition, health expenses in China have continued to rise; after new medical reform in 2009, they had nearly doubled by 2017 (National Health Commission 2018). As China faces an aging population, a changing disease spectrum, intertwined health factors, and an enhanced public concept of health, diversified and individualized demands for health products and services continue to grow in the nation. Urgent problems in this aging society vary from the skyrocketing incidence of chronic diseases and rapid growth of medical expenses, to deteriorating doctor-patient relationships and a lack of effective health management. Many non-Chinese studies have proved that the family doctor system can effectively control chronic diseases such as hypertension and diabetes (Bass, McWhinney, and Donner 1986; Fang, Ayala, and Loustalot 2015; LeBlanc et al. 2017), highlighting the potential importance of this system in promoting healthy aging. As a "gatekeeper" of health, the family doctor system can provide continuous, personalized, and comprehensive health services via contractual partnerships, thereby achieving a combination of the source control and prevention/treatment combination of chronic diseases. The family doctor system is essentially a set regulations of family doctors' behaviors. In China, family doctors work mainly in the primary healthcare sector and play an important role in China's primary healthcare system. Currently, primary healthcare services are provided in China by urban community health centers, rural township health centers, and village clinics. Some community health stations are affiliated with local health centers, while others are comparatively independent, only receiving technical support from local health centers. Most village clinics are not government owned and receive technical guidance from township health centers; some are affiliated with local township health centers (Meng et al. 2015). This chapter gives an overview of the family doctor system in China, including its development, how doctors are cultivated, service patterns, incentive mechanisms, and supporting conditions.

The Development of China's Family Doctor System

In China, the family doctor system has undergone a long-term conceptual evolution. The system plays an important role in strengthening community health services and building up healthcare networks in primary healthcare institutions.

Concept

China's demand-oriented system of community health service institutions, led by higher-level health authorities, aims to meet the basic health needs of families in each community, especially the needs of women, children, the elderly, patients with chronic diseases, the disabled, and other vulnerable groups. It integrates prevention, healthcare, rehabilitation, and technical guidance on family planning and health education, aiming to provide effective, economic, convenient, comprehensive, and continuous primary healthcare services for each family. The family doctor system implements a community health coordinating strategy, builds a two-way referral mechanism, and provides network information services. The ultimate goal is to protect the health of residents, improve their quality of life, and reduce total medical expenditures (Bao et al. 2011).

According to a guidance report jointly issued by the National Health Commission and National Administration of Traditional Chinese Medicine of the People's Republic of China (2018), family doctors in contemporary China can be divided into three groups: (1) registered general practitioners (GPs) in primary healthcare institutions, qualified doctors in township health hospitals, qualified village doctors, and qualified doctors of traditional Chinese medicine; (2) clinicians in general medicine or those who undergo professional GP training, and are conducting multi-site practices in primary healthcare institutions; (3) retired clinicians holding a medium- or higher-grade professional title who have received GP training.

Reform history

In China, the concept of "general practitioner" predated that of "family doctor," which derives from it. An overview of the history of the family doctor system is shown in table 10.1. In 2011, the State Council unveiled *Guidelines on Establishing a General Practitioner System*, which set the requirements for being a GP. According to these guidelines, GPs serve as health "coordinators" who provide integrated primary services to the general population, including preventive services, primary healthcare (treatment and referral of patients with common diseases), rehabilitation, and management of chronic diseases (State Council 2011). Primary healthcare services are provided by urban community health centers, rural township health centers, and village clinics in which GPs or family doctors work. Establishing a hierarchical medical system, implementing family doctor service contracts, and clarifying individual doctors' responsibility are the major development directions of China's healthcare reform, according to the State Council, which holds that these same development directions are common to and have succeeded in other countries (State Council 2011). A GP system that is suitable for China's particular conditions could optimize the allocation of medical resources, facilitate rational functional divisions between primary healthcare institutions and city hospitals, and make basic medical services more continuous, coordinated, and convenient so as to solve the existing problem of "high medical expenses and difficult-to-access medical treatments" (State Council 2011). The guidelines suggest at least

TABLE 10.1 Establishment of the family doctor system in China

Year	
2009	New healthcare reforms call for the establishment of a community health service model
2011	General practitioner system is established
2015	Hierarchical medical system is established; proposal is made for the contracting of doctors
2016	Family doctor service contracts begin
2018	Content of family doctor contract services is standardized

SOURCE: Authors.

one qualified GP in each urban community healthcare institution and rural township health center in 2012, and two to three GPs per 10,000 residents by 2020 (State Council 2011). The 2015 State Council–issued "National Health Service System Planning Outline (2015–2020)" re-emphasized that by 2020 there would be two GPs per 10,000 residents and specified a goal of 1.07 per 10,000 by 2013 (General Office of the State Council 2015a). In 2018 the General Office of the State Council issued another document indicating that by 2030 there should be five qualified GPs per 10,000 residents nation-wide, and GP teams would be able to meet the basic needs of the Healthy China 2030 campaign. By that time, a standardized GP training model and a service model of seeking care first in primary healthcare institutions would be formed, providing residents with easier and more continuous access to primary health services (State Council 2011).

In 2015, the government proposed to establish a hierarchical medical system and gradually improve supporting policies to promote the coordination and functional division among healthcare institutions (General Office of the State Council 2015a). The hierarchical medical system promotes the downward flow of high-quality health sources to primary healthcare institutions and reinforces the development of human resources in primary healthcare, especially GPs, so as to further improve the utilization efficiency and overall benefits of medical resources. The hierarchical medical system emphasizes promoting the service capability of primary healthcare and strives for breakthroughs in the hierarchical diagnosis and treatment of common, frequently occurring, and chronic diseases. Supporting policies were also designed to promote the voluntary signing of service contracts between households and contracting doctor teams. A contracting doctor team consists of doctors from secondary hospitals or above and qualified primary healthcare professionals. Private clinics were also encouraged to sign service contracts. Contracting doctor services should be first provided to priority groups including the elderly, patients with chronic diseases, patients with severe mental disorders, pregnant women, children, and the disabled, and then should gradually be extended to the entire population (General Office of the State Council 2015b). The establishment of a hierarchical medical system helps primary healthcare institutions to clarify their duty to provide treatment, rehabilitation, and nursing services for patients who have been clearly diagnosed and are in stable condition, such as senile patients, patients with chronic diseases, and patients with advanced cancer. GPs play an important role in performing this duty (General Office of the State Council 2015b).

In 2016, 200 Chinese cities that were piloting public hospital reforms introduced family doctor service contracts (*jiating yisheng qianyue fuwu*). Other regions were also encouraged to actively conduct similar pilot programs. This was the first time that the concept of family doctors had been formally recorded on a national document, according to which registered GPs (assistant GPs and traditional Chinese medicine GPs), competent township hospital doctors, and village doctors were qualified to be family doctors (Medical Reform Office of the State Council 2016). Priority groups include seniors, pregnant women, children, the handicapped, patients with chronic diseases like hypertension, diabetes and tuberculosis, as well as those with severe mental disorders. It was expected that by 2017 contractual services from family doctors would cover more than 30 percent of the entire population, including over 60 percent of the priority population; by 2020, contractual services would gradually be extended to the entire population via a stable long-term contractual relationship, so that the family doctor system would have essentially achieved full coverage.

In 2018, the National Health Commission and National Administration of Traditional Chinese Medicine of the People's Republic of China jointly issued a document to further standardize the contract services provided by family doctors. It clarified the concept of family doctors (teams) and focused on enriching the content of family doctors' contract services and making appropriate arrangements for contract service fees (National Health Commission and National Administration of Traditional Chinese Medicine 2018).

Family doctor services in Shanghai's Changning District

The family doctor system was explored and promoted comparatively earlier in Shanghai; there, in 2006, "promoting the service model of a community GP team" was first explicitly proposed (Shanghai Municipal Health Commission 2006). Implementation of the family doctor system gradually began in 2010 and by 2013 covered all of Shanghai. In 2015, a series of documents[1] were issued that marked the beginning of a new round of comprehensive reform of community health services (Shanghai Municipal Health Commission 2015; Huang and Gao 2017). Changning District in Shanghai was the pilot district for community health service reform and the application of the family doctor system. The implementation path of the family doctor system in Changning District was based on residents' compliance and their

---

1   These were the "1+8" documents, a main document entitled *Guidelines on Further Deepening the Comprehensive Reform and Development of Community Health Services in Shanghai* and eight supporting documents.

health demands, following a five-layer concentric structure (Ge et al. 2012). In that structure, the primary beneficiary group of the family doctor system is the poor. Family doctor services are next extended to patients with chronic diseases and the disabled. Services are gradually provided to the elderly, and then finally all households. The community healthcare centers in Changning District actively carried out pilot projects based on local conditions, achieving a qualitative transformation of the family doctor system.

The Changning District family doctor system adopted what was called a "1-3-5-3-3" work pattern:

1. The system centers on the health management of community residents (*one center*).
2. It relies on *three collaborations*—between the family doctor team and the healthcare center, between the healthcare center and the technical services of other health institutions, and between the healthcare center and community resources.
3. It provides *five types of services*: contractual, interactive, follow-up, caring, and monitoring.
4. The system maintains *three relationships*: a long-term stable one with community residents, a partnership for health promotion, and a targeted service relationship with key populations.
5. It aims to embody *three effects*: promoting health, harmonious doctor-patient relationships, and government's service awareness.

The practice of the family doctor system in Changning District resulted in an increase in the management rate of hypertension and diabetes by 10 percent and 30 percent, respectively, within three years (2013–15). Over the same three-year period the management rate of residents with chronic diseases increased; the management rate of residents with a family doctor was always higher than that of non-contracted residents (Huang and Gao 2017).

The Cultivation and Development of Family Doctors in China

It is not easy to strictly distinguish between family doctors (*jiating yisheng*) and general practitioners (*quanke yisheng*) in China, because almost all family doctors are registered GPs, clinicians who major in general medicine or undergo professional GP training, and who work in primary healthcare institutions. Below we discuss the development and cultivation of GPs, which reflect the current situation of Chinese family doctors.

In some community health centers, there is little deliberate distinction made between a family doctor and a GP, whether by the general public or medical staff. Nonetheless, the idea of GPs pre-dated that of family doctors in most places and family doctors were developed on the basis of GPs (Zhao, Ge, and Jiang 2016). At present, family doctors mainly include registered GPs in primary healthcare institutions (including assistant GPs and traditional Chinese medicine GPs), qualified doctors at township health centers, and village doctors. Retired physicians are also encouraged to work in urban community health centers as family doctors, especially those who were health professionals in internal medicine, gynecology, pediatrics, and traditional Chinese medicine.

The growth in the number of China's GPs from 2012 to 2017 is shown in table 10.2. There were only 1.82 GPs per 10,000 people in 2017, a long way from the target of five GPs per 10,000 people by 2030 (General Office of the State Council 2018). In addition, although some studies have argued that the age structure of family doctors in both community health centers and town/township health centers is reasonable, family doctors in rural areas are more likely to be elderly, to be male, and to have lower educational levels and position titles; doctor-nurse ratios are also more imbalanced (Wu, Zhao, and Cao 2017). Therefore, the foundation for establishing a sound family doctor system in China is the cultivation of family doctors and the improvement of primary healthcare human resources.

TABLE 10.2 General practitioners in China, 2012–17

Year	Total	Type of healthcare institution			Type of GP		GPs per 10,000 population
		Hospitals	Community health centers (stations)	Town/township health centers	Registered GPs	Individuals with GP certificate	
2012	109,794	21,074	47,363	38,557	37,173	72,621	0.81
2013	145,511	25,758	60,181	56,825	47,402	98,109	1.07
2014	172,597	30,428	68,914	70,296	64,156	108,441	1.26
2015	188,649	31,382	73,288	80,975	68,364	120,235	1.37
2016	209,083	34,634	78,337	92,791	77,631	131,452	1.51
2017	252,717	49,400	83,933	110,900	96,235	156,482	1.82

SOURCE: *Zhongguo weisheng tongji nianlan* [China health statistical yearbook] 2013–18.

Chinese family doctor training and cultivation

In China, GPs have been trained based on a "5+3" training model since 2011, meaning five years of undergraduate education in clinical medicine (including traditional Chinese medicine) and three years of GP standardized training. The three-year GP standardized training can be carried out in two ways: through standardized training after graduation or by postgraduate education in clinical medicine. The specific content of training programs is determined by the province, the autonomous region, or the municipality. Most of those who participate in standardized training after graduation are graduates of clinical medicine with a bachelor's degree or above and are managed by the GP standardized training bases under the joint guidance of the health department (including the traditional Chinese medicine management department) and the education department. Those who fulfill their three-year training through postgraduate education in clinical medicine are trained according to the unified requirements of GP standardized training and are managed mainly by the education department. If these individuals pass the examination after their postgraduate education, they will be awarded the GP standardized training certificate.

GP standardized training, which aims to improve the clinical and public health practice abilities of GPs, is carried out at nationally granted GP standardized training bases. The standardized training involves a tutor management system (trainees are assigned tutors) and credit management system (which ensures trainees receive an adequate amount of training). Participants in GP standardized training are required to take part in, at the minimum, two-year rotations in different clinical departments, public health departments, and community practice platforms. They also must, for a specified period of time, undergo service training in primary healthcare practice bases and professional public health institutions. During GP standardized training, participants can perform clinical work such as medical examinations, disease investigations, and medical treatments, or take hospital duties under the guidance of their instructors. As part of their training they also need to take the National Medical Licensing Examination. Those who meet the requirements, earn the required number of credits in the types of diseases and number of cases, show basic competence in clinical and public health practice abilities, and are of professional quality will be granted a GP standardized training certificate. Registered GPs must go through three years of GP standardized training and obtain qualifications through the National Medical Licensing Examination. Individuals possessing five-year bachelor's degrees or above in clinical medicine who pass the GP standardized training will be awarded corresponding professional degrees in clinical medicine (GP direction, or *quanke yixue fangxiang*).

While the cultivation of GPs has always been an important task for China's healthcare system, since 2005 there has been an urgent need for a large number of GPs (Wang et al 2007). In order to solve the current conflict between the urgent need for family doctors in primary healthcare institutions and the long cultivation cycle of GP standardized training, the Chinese government has proposed adjusting the GP training model. One such solution is to provide qualified primary healthcare physicians or assistant physicians with 1–2 years of transfer training, as needed, to improve their basic medical and public health service capabilities. Transfer training is carried out in nationally granted GP standardized training bases. After passing unified examinations organized by provincial health administrative departments, they can obtain the GP transfer training certificate to be a registered GP or assistant GP. For five-year GP-oriented clinical medicine graduates, the internship can be extended as appropriate to improve their clinical skills and public health practices. In addition, three-year program graduates who work in underdeveloped rural areas can be registered as an assistant GP after receiving two years of training in clinical and public health skills and obtaining qualification as assistant doctors.

Since 2012, China has seen good results in the training of GPs. The total number of GPs has quadrupled from 2012 to 2017, and the number of GPs per 10,000 people has increased yearly, going from 0.81 in 2012 to 1.82 in 2017.

Corresponding GP training programs have been developed in different regions in China and are constantly updated. Provinces and municipalities adopt similar training programs to cultivate GP talents by promoting college education in general medicine, training in general medicine after graduation, and continuing education in general medicine (see table 10.3).

Family Doctor Service Contracts

In the Chinese family doctor system, a family doctor team provides contract services for residents. Below we discuss the provider of family doctor contract services, how services are provided in the contract, what is actually provided, and how contract fees are paid.

A contractual service model is widely used in China's family doctor system. Primary healthcare institutions furnish service sites and ancillary services for residents who sign agreements. Qualified non-government medical institutions (including private clinics) are encouraged to provide contractual services and allowed to enjoy the same payment policy. As China cultivates

TABLE 10.3 GP cultivation goals in various provinces or municipalities

Province/ Municipality	GPs/10,000 people	College education in general medicine	Training in general medicine after graduation	Continuing education in general medicine
			Cultivation Goals	
Beijing	2020: ≥3 2030: 5	1,000 undergraduates and 800 junior college graduates majoring in clinical medicine for community health centers and village clinics within 8–10 years (2018–26). 400 students in traditional Chinese medicine within 5–8 years.	Adjust the enrollment preference of the standardized residency program by giving GPs priority. By 2020, 20% of all trainees in residency programs will be GPs.	By 2030, 20 municipal-level key disciplines in general medicine will be established, and 220 critical GP talents will be trained.
Shanghai	2020: 4 2030: 5 2035: 5.5	Medical colleges should strengthen the construction of teaching bases in affiliated hospitals, and build a "university-hospital-community" teaching system.	Expand the enrollment of GPs in standardized residency programs. By 2020, the number of enrolled GPs will reach 400 per year, and by 2030, there will be no less than 500.	Establish 10 continuing medical education bases for GPs in community health centers.
Zhejiang (Hangzhou)	2020: 3–4 2030: 5	The newly added post-graduate enrollment plan in clinical medicine and traditional Chinese medicine should be tilted toward general medicine.	Expand the enrollment of GPs in the standardized residency program. By 2020, the number of enrolled GPs will count for 20%.	Actively carry out primary-level GP training and education to upgrade academic qualifications.
Fujian (Xiamen)	2020: 2–3 2030: 5	Medical colleges should focus on the establishment of general medicine disciplines, and establish departments, majors, and research centers in general medicine.	Expand the enrollment of GPs in the standardized residency program. By 2020, the number of enrolled GPs will count for 20%.	Vigorously promote "internet + continuing medical education" programs.

SOURCES: General Office of the People's Government of Beijing Municipality 2018; General Office of the People's Government of Fujian Province 2018; General Office of the People's Government of Shanghai Municipality 2018; General Office of the People's Government of Zhejiang Province 2018.

GPs, contractual service teams in which GPs assume primary responsibilities are being established (Medical Reform Office of the State Council 2016).

Contract form: Provide services in teams

In 2016, the State Council made a series of recommendations on how family doctor services should promote contract services. The main points included the following:

1. In principle, contractual services should be provided in teams. The family doctor team is mainly composed of family doctors, community nurses, and public health doctors (including assistant public health doctors). Secondary hospitals or above should assign doctors (including traditional Chinese medicine doctors) to primary healthcare institutions to offer support and guidance. Traditional Chinese medicine services should gradually be made available in each family doctor team. Health centers in some qualified areas may recruit pharmacists, health managers, psychological counselors, and social workers into the family doctor teams.

2. Family doctors are responsible for task assignments and the management of team members. Primary healthcare institutions should clarify the tasks, working process, norms, and division of duties within the family doctor team, and appraise their performance in different tasks regularly. Other specialists and health technicians should cooperate closely with the family doctor team.

3. Based on the population size and service coverage, the areas of contracted service responsibility are rationally divided and family doctor teams are assigned to them. Accordingly, local residents or families will voluntarily choose a family doctor team within the region to sign service contracts, in which the content, methods, duration, responsibilities, rights, obligations, and other related terms of family doctor services are clarified. The contracts usually last for one year, and residents can renew their contracts or choose another family doctor team after the expiration. Residents are encouraged to sign contracts nearby, but they are also allowed to sign contracts across regions to establish an orderly competition mechanism.

To provide one example of how contractual services are provided by teams, in Xiamen (Fujian Province), the family doctor teams adopt a model of "joint management by three professionals" (JMTP, *san shi gong guan*): (1) specialists in large hospitals (such as endocrinologists and diabetes specialists, responsible for making diagnosis and treatment plans); (2) GPs in community health centers (responsible for implementing the plans, daily monitoring, and providing two-way referral of patients); and (3) health managers in community health centers (responsible for health education and patient behavior interventions). Since specialists and GPs are too busy to provide health education, nurses, nutritionists and other personnel in community health centers will be mobilized to become knowledgeable about daily diet, exercise, nutrition, and the professional skills of diabetes care, so as to assist the specialists and GPs in carrying out daily health education to improve patients' level of self-management (Yang 2017).

The linkage between hospitals and primary healthcare institutions can guide residents or families with service contracts to voluntarily choose a secondary hospital and a tertiary hospital to form a "1+1+1" combined contract. Within the combination, residents or families can choose the most suitable medical institution for their needs and are encouraged to receive primary treatment in community healthcare centers. Doctor visits outside the combination need referral by a family doctor. The "1+1+1" combined model has worked very well in Shanghai (Shanghai Municipal Health Commission 2017)

Family doctor teams provide residents with basic healthcare, public health services, and health management services. Basic healthcare covers the diagnosis and treatment of common diseases and frequently occurring diseases, effective administration of drugs, guidance on medical treatments, referrals, and appointments. Public health services cover national basic public health services and other public health services as required by the government. Basic contractual services, including basic healthcare and basic public health services, will be provided to all contracted residents according to local service capabilities and health demands. Health management services are personalized based on residents' health status and needs, and include services such as health assessment, rehabilitation guidance, family bed services, home care, traditional Chinese medicine preventive care, and remote health monitoring. At the current stage, policy aims to have the family doctor system first cover key populations (the elderly) for management of key diseases (hypertension and diabetes); subsequently, the range of services will gradually expand. Table 10.4 details the services provided in the family doctor system (National Health Commission and National Administration of Traditional Chinese Medicine 2018).

TABLE 10.4 Services provided by China's family doctor system

Service	Description
Basic healthcare services	Diagnosis, treatment, effective administration of drugs, and medical guidance on common and frequently occurring diseases
Public health services	National basic public health service project*
Health management services	Health assessment, a health management plan based on the assessment, and health guidance services in accordance with the plan during the management cycle
Health education and consultation services	Personalized health education and health consultation (face-to-face or via internet, telephone, etc.)
Priority in making appointments	Priority in making appointments in the contracted healthcare institution
Priority in referrals	A green referral channel for contracted residents
Home-visiting services	Access to treatment, rehabilitation, nursing, hospice care, health guidance, and home sickbeds for qualified contracted residents who require in-home services
Drug distribution and medication guidance	Drugs provided to contracted residents who require them and supporting medication guidance
Long-term prescriptions	Increased drug dosage and prolonged prescription cycle (4–8 weeks in principle) for chronic disease patients who are in stable condition and have shown good compliance in terms of medication safety
Traditional Chinese medicine services	Health education, health assessment, and health intervention using traditional Chinese medicine

SOURCE: Authors.
NOTE: *Basic public health services are provided to all residents by urban and rural basic health institutions, such as the Center for Disease Control and Prevention, urban community health service centers, and township hospitals. These are public welfare interventions that are mainly used for disease prevention and control. For more information, see Primary Health Department, National Health Commission of the People's Republic of China (2019).

Looking specifically at the elderly of Xiamen, there are ample personalized services that assist in coping with the medical problems that accompany aging. These include follow-ups, regular checkups, and full-time health management services for those over 65 years of age, and free on-site services during at least one visit per year for those over 80. Contracted seniors can also take advantage of services such as blood pressure testing, physical examinations, medication guidance, and health consultations (Xiamen Development and Reform Commission 2016).

The family doctor team provides residents who enroll with a benefit package of contractual services, which are co-paid by health insurance funds and basic public health service funds, and by contracted residents in the form of annual service contract fees. The specific payment standards and sharing ratios are jointly determined by local health departments, human resources and social security departments, and finance and price departments, in light of which contractual services are being provided, the population distribution of contracted residents, and the pressures on basic medical insurance funds and public health funds. Medical assistance is offered to those meeting the requirements for assistance. The costs of basic public health services provided in contractual services are paid by special public health service funds. For example, the service contract fee in Hangzhou (capital of Zhejiang Province) is ¥10 per month, in which only ¥1 is paid by residents; those over 60 years old, families that have lost their only child, and those living in extreme poverty do not have to pay at all. Table 10.5 shows the distribution of service contract fees in Hangzhou and Xiamen. Contracted residents can obtain all the services available in the family doctor benefit package for a small out-of-pocket price. However, in some areas there are upgraded benefit packages available that require contracting residents to pay more for some contracted services.

TABLE 10.5 Distribution of service contract fees in Hangzhou and Xiamen

	Hangzhou	Xiamen
Public finances	¥9 per person per month, paid by municipal and district public finances	¥30 per person per year, paid by basic public health service funding
Health insurance funding	—	¥70 per person per year
Out-of-pocket payments	¥1 per person per month	¥20 per person per year
Total	¥120 per person per year	¥120 per person per year

SOURCE: Hangzhou and Xiamen Municipal Health Commissions.

Incentives and Compensation Mechanisms for Family Doctors

The key indicators in the performance appraisal system for Chinese family doctor teams include the number and structure of residents, service quality, health management effects, residents' satisfaction, and control of medical expenses. Also discussed below are the comprehensive incentive and competition mechanisms and reform of payment and compensation mechanisms for family doctor teams.

Performance appraisals

The performance of family doctor teams is assessed regularly and representatives from family doctor teams and residents are encouraged to participate in the assessment. The assessment results, linked to health insurance subsidies, basic public health service funds distribution, and team or individual allowances distribution, are disclosed to the public in a timely manner. For family doctor teams whose assessment results are unsatisfactory and who receive a significant number of negative comments from their patients, a corresponding punishment mechanism is established. China's family doctor performance appraisal system has a number of characteristics. The first is that there are diverse assessment methods. For example, the Desheng health service center in Beijing's Xicheng District applies a quantitative points-based assessment system that measures the quantity of services provided, the quality of those services, and the satisfaction associated with them. This particular assessment system has shown good results (Hang et al. 2009). Changning District in Shanghai adopts a time-based assessment method by identifying quantitative workload indicators; this approach not only significantly improves the workload, service efficiency, and performance of family doctor teams, but also helps kindle their enthusiasm and develop their potential (Jiang et al. 2017). Second, assessments are based on teams, not individuals. A study by Xiao, Huang, and Chen (2015) compared individual performance appraisals with team-based ones and found that the latter created a "community of interests," allowing for better collaboration, more enthusiasm, and enhancing service capabilities. In team-based assessments, the second round of appraisal in the team focuses on team leaders, so that team leaders can better coordinate the tasks within the team.

Incentive and competition mechanisms

In many aspects of their professional lives, family doctors are provided with preferential treatment, including *bianzhi* (the offer of a permanent working position), employment opportunities, promotions, on-the-job-training, and the opportunity for awards. Outstanding personnel may be included in governmental preferential policy programs aimed at talented individuals, so they can be promoted to higher levels sooner. The goal of such preferential treatment is to attract more people to become GPs, thus accelerating the construction of GP teams and hastening the implementation of contractual services. The State Council has also made other recommendations, including:

- Efforts should be made to rationally set the proportion of high- and mid-level GP positions in primary healthcare institutions, and expand the space for professional title promotions. The assessment results of contractual services serve as an important factor for title promotion, and personnel with outstanding results are more likely to be promoted.
- Those family doctors and their teams with outstanding performance should be upheld as good examples and be awarded in accordance with state regulations.
- Family doctor teams should continue to receive medical training (i.e., continuing medical education), so training channels at home and abroad will be expanded, and doctors in secondary hospitals and above will regularly go to primary health centers to offer guidance. Family doctors and their teams should also go to clinical teaching bases for regular clinical training to improve the quality of their services.

Payment and compensation mechanisms reforms

International evidence shows that compensation policies for family doctor teams are of great significance in the provision of health services. Service fees, salaries, and capitation each have affected the performance of family doctors differently (Scott et al. 2011). In China, most areas with family doctors still adopt a fee-for-service system.

The State Council has recommended that primary healthcare institutions in some qualified areas can explore paying for contract services by capitation (a fixed amount of money per year). Primary healthcare institutions or family doctor teams will be paid part of the referral fees for the patients they refer to hospitals. Efforts can be made to explore the payment of a global budget to a cooperative medical group, such as a vertical-cooperated medical group. Thus, family doctors can play the role of a "coordinator" for health insurance payment control in order to guide two-way referrals in a rational manner.

The Jiangsu street community in Shanghai's Changning District began to reform its payment system in October 2012, gradually establishing a new capitation payment mechanism in which family doctor teams were paid based on the number of contracted residents. This payment system reform improved the incomes of Changning District family doctor teams by 25 percent on average (Wu and Shi 2013). The direction of the future payment system for family doctors is a capitation system within the global budget (Medical Reform Office of the State Council 2015). This payment method can effectively curb the unreasonable growth of medical insurance expenses and control the supplier-induced demand or supply-side moral hazard (i.e., excess utilization because it brings doctors more income), thereby saving medical resources.

Promoting the Family Doctor System

Technical support for the family doctor team needs to be strengthened. The family doctor system has different models in different provinces or municipalities, but all need the policy support of the local government. The health information system is also a very important supporting element of China's family doctor system.

Examinations and laboratory tests are important services provided by family doctor teams and provide critical support for the daily operation of the family doctor system. Therefore, in the implementation of the family doctor system, it is of critical importance how equipment used for examinations and laboratory tests is allocated. Equipment allocation is based on three principles:

1. Classification and function—the different types of urban community health centers (town/township health centers) should be equipped in line with their technical levels, the types of services they offer, and the workload levels of their family doctor teams.
2. Reasonable procedures—before purchasing expensive medical equipment, institutions should conduct sufficient research and follow strict approval procedures.
3. Resource sharing—when planning the use of the equipment, decision-makers should take social welfare and equipment efficiency into consideration to achieve practical and efficient resource sharing.

The implementation of the family doctor system depends on the support of the local government. However, because each provincial or municipal government faces different local conditions, it has established different family doctor systems where funding, management, supervision, and so on are all suitable for local conditions. Table 10.6 summarizes four representative family doctor system models in China.

TABLE 10.6 China's four representative family doctor system models

City	Model	Explanation
Shanghai	"1+1+1" combined model	Residents can choose the most suitable primary health institution plus a secondary and a tertiary hospital when they are in need of them.
Hangzhou	Integrating medical treatments, long-term care, and nursing care	Family beds are established for persons ill in bed and the elderly. Extra fees are added to the total annual medical insurance expenses, including family bed fees (¥80 per capita), family bed inspection fees (¥40 per capita), and visiting fees for medical staff with sub-senior titles or above (¥60 per capita).
Xiamen	Joint management by three professionals	The family doctor team includes specialists in large hospitals, general practitioners, and health managers in community health centers.
Yanchen	Service package	Differentiated service packages including a free service package, and primary, intermediate, and advanced service packages.

SOURCE: Wu, Zhao, and Cao 2017.

Health information systems

Information plays an important role in the implementation of the family doctor system in China, and the creation of health information platforms will also assist implementation. A one-card system—which has patient personal information, health insurance reimbursement details, and health service utilization information—can facilitate patients' medical consultations in medical institutions at all levels and their easy access to medical services, improving the efficiency and quality of medical services. eHealth innovations have helped to facilitate reforms and strengthen the gatekeeping function of community healthcare providers. For example, in Anhui Province, family doctor teams use a free messaging application to facilitate consistent communication between patients and service providers. Electronic health records are used across the province, helping to capture referrals and share patients' information across the health service delivery system (World Health Organization 2018).

Conclusion

China's family doctor system is currently playing an important role in the form of service contracts, but there are still some obstacles to further growth (Tang, Song, and Xu 2016). Several empirical studies in China have shown the positive effects of the family doctor system, especially on patients with chronic diseases, for example, hypertension (Sun, Zhai, and Zhang 2014), diabetes (Jin, Jing, and Ding 2013), and stroke (Liu et al. 2015). The elderly are at higher risk of these chronic diseases, so in the context of aging China, the implementation of the family doctor system will help this country to achieve healthy aging.

References

Bass, Martin J., Ian R Mcwhinney, and Allan Donner. 1986. "Do Family Physicians Need Medical Assistants to Detect and Manage Hypertension?" *Canadian Medical Association Journal* 134 (11): 1247–55.

Bao, Yong, Xueli Du, An Zhang, Wei Sun, Su Xu, and Junjie Ni. 2011. "Family Doctor System Study in China Based on Community Health Management." [In Chinese.] *Chinese Journal of General Practice* 9 (6): 831.

Fang, Jing, Carma Ayala, and Fleetwood Loustalot. 2015. "Primary Care Providers' Recommendations for Hypertension Prevention, DocStyles Survey, 2012." *Journal of Primary Care & Community Health* 6 (3): 170–76.

Ge, Min, Ping Jiang, Wei Lu, Hong Liang, and Xiaolin He. 2012. "Jiating yisheng zhidu de tuijin lujing, fuwu moshi he zhidu jiagou de tantao: Yi Changning wei lie" [Discussion on the promotion path, service mode and institutional framework of the family doctor system: Taking Changning City as an example]. *Zhongguo weisheng ziyuan* [Chinese health resources] 15 (5): 420–22.

General Office of the People's Government of Beijing Municipality. 2018. "Beijing shi guanyu gaige wanshan quanke yisheng peiyang yu shiyong jili jizhi de shishi fangan" [Guidelines of the General Office of the People's Government of Beijing Municipality on reforming and improving the training and incentive mechanism for general practitioners]. October 19, 2018. No. 39. http://www.beijing.gov.cn/zfxxgk/dxq354/qtwj/2018-10/29/content_9040e802ee054aea95959602a05c89dc.shtml.

General Office of the People's Government of Fujian Province. 2018. "Fujian sheng renmin zhengfu bangongting guanyu gaige wanshan quanke yisheng peiyang yu shiyong jili jizhi de shishi yijian" [Guidelines of the General Office of the People's Government of Fujian Province on reforming and improving the training and incentive mechanism for general practitioners]. October 16, 2018. No 81. http://www.fujian.gov.cn/zc/zxwj/szfbgtwj/201810/t20181017_4541704.htm.

General Office of the People's Government of Shanghai Municipality. 2018. "Guanyu benshi gaige wanshan quanke yisheng peiyang yu shiyong jili jizhi de shishi fangan" [Guidelines of the General Office of the People's Government of Shanghai Municipality on reforming and improving the training and incentive mechanism for general practitioners]. December 25, 2018. No. 34. http://www.shanghai.gov.cn/nw2/nw2314/nw2319/nw12344/u26aw58014.html.

General Office of the People's Government of Zhejiang Province. 2018. "Zhejiang sheng renmin zhengfu bangongting guanyu yinfa zhejiang-sheng gaige wanshan quanke yisheng peiyang yu shiyong jili jizhi shishi fangan de tongzhi' [Guidelines of the General Office of the People's Government of Zhejiang Province on reforming and improving the training and incentive mechanism for general practitioners]. July 12, 2018. No 65. http://www.zj.gov.cn/art/2018/7/24/art_1582412_25818. html.

General Office of the State Council. 2015a. "Guowuyuan bangong ting guanyu tuijin fenji zhenliao zhidu jianshe de zhidao yijian" [Guidelines of the General Office of the State Council on promoting the construction of hierarchical medical system]. Office of the State Council, no. 70, September 8, 2015. http://www.gov.cn/zhengce/content/2015-09/11/content_10158.htm.

General Office of the State Council. 2015b. "Guowuyuan bangong ting guanyu yinfa quanguo yiliao weisheng fuwu tixi guihua gangyao (2015–2020 nian) de tongzhi" [Notice of the General Office of the State Council on Issuing the Outline for the Planning of the National Medical and Health Service System (2015-2020)]. Office of the State Council, no. 14, March 16, 2015. http://www.gov.cn/zhengce/content/2015-03/30/content_9560.htm.

General Office of the State Council. 2018. "Guowuyuan bangong ting guanyu gaige wanshan quanke yisheng peiyang yu shiyong jili jizhi de yijian" [Guidelines of the General Office of the State Council on reforming and improving the training and incentive mechanism for general practitioners]. Office of the State Council, no. 3, January 14, 2018. http://www.gov.cn/zhengce/content/2018-01/24/content_5260073. htm.

Hang, Chengcheng, Yi Feng, Xiaonghong Liu, Yuehong Zhang, Chunhong Ma, Yanfang Zhang, Qi Lu, Juhong Liu, Lei Zhang, Aisheng Zhou, and Jiangong Zhao. 2009. "Effect of Practice of Performance Appraisal and Distribution System to Motivation in Desheng Community Health Service Center." [In Chinese.] *Chinese General Practice* 12 (1): 71–74.

Huang, Jiaoling, and Zhenyao Gao. 2017. "Health Management and Effect Analysis of Family Doctor System: A Case Study from Changning District of Shanghai." [In Chinese.] *China Health Insurance* 2: 33–36.

Jiang, Ping, Jie Wang, Qi Zhao, and Yuchao Sheng. 2017. "Research on Performance Management Based on Standardized Workload of Family

Doctor Studio." [In Chinese.] *Chinese Journal of Health Policy* 10 (10): 16–22.

Jin, Yuan, Lin Jing, and Fujun Ding. 2013. "The Effective Evaluation on Family Doctor Group Service for Chronic Diseases Health Management." [In Chinese.] *Chinese Primary Health Care* 27 (11): 70–71.

Liu, Xiumei, Xinying Liu, Caiying Ge, Hongyan Jia, Min Kong, Hao Wu, Xiangdong Zhang, Jing Zhao, and Lina Lan. 2015. "The Effective Evaluation on Family Doctor Group Service for Chronic Diseases Health Management." [In Chinese.] *Chinese Journal of General Practice* 13 (4): 616–18.

LeBlanc, Emilie, Mathieu Bélanger, Véronique Thibault, Lise Babin, Beverly Greene, Stuart Halpine, and Michelina Mancuso. 2017. "Influence of a Pay-for-performance Program on Glycemic Control in Patients Living with Diabetes by Family Physicians in a Canadian Province." *Canadian Journal of Diabetes* 41 (2): 190–96.

Medical Reform Office of the State Council (*Guowuyuan yigaiban*). 2016. "Guanyu yinfa tuijin jiting yisheng qianyue fuwu zhidao yijian de tongzhi" [Announcement about issuing guidelines on promoting family doctor contract service]. Notice no. 1, June 6, 2016. http://www.gov.cn/xinwen/2016-06/06/content_5079984.htm.

Meng, Qingyue, Hongwei Yang, Wen Chen, and Xiaoyun Liu. 2015. *People's Republic of China Health System Review.* Switzerland: World Health Organization.

National Health Commission. 2018. *2018 Zhongguo weisheng tongji nianlan* [China health statistical yearbook 2018]. Beijing: China Union Medical University Press.

National Health Commission and National Administration of Traditional Chinese Medicine. 2018. "Guanyu guifan jiating yisheng qianyue fuwu guanli de zhidao yijian" [Guidelines on regulating the management of family doctor contract services]. No. 35, October 8, 2018. http://www.nhc.gov.cn/jws/s7874/201810/be6826d8d9d14e849e37bd1b57dd4915.shtml.

Office of the State Council. 2011. "Guowuyuan guanyu jianli quanke yisheng zhidu de zhidao yijian" [State Council guidelines on establishing a general practitioner system]. No. 23. http://www.gov.cn/zwgk/2011-07/07/content_1901099.htm.

Primary Health Department, National Health Commission of the People's Republic of China. 2019. "Guanyu zuohao 2019 nian jiben gonggong weisheng fuwu xiangmu gongzuo de tongzhi" [Notice on doing well on the 2019 Basic Public Health Service Projects]. No. 52,

September 4. http://www.nhc.gov.cn/jws/s7881/201909/83012210b4564f 26a163408599072379.shtml.

Scott, Anthony, Peter Sivey, Driss Ait Ouakrim, Lisa Willenberg, Lucio Naccarella, John Furler, and Doris Young. 2011. "The Effect of Financial Incentives on the Quality of Health Care Provided by Primary Care Physicians." The Cochrane Library. John Wiley & Sons, Ltd CD008451.

Sun, Hong, Fenfen Zhai, Yuling Zhang. 2014. "Family Doctor Contract Service on the Quality of Life of Patients with Hypertension in Shenzhen City." [In Chinese.] *Journal of Community Medicine* 12 (4): 7–9.

Shanghai Municipal Health Commission. 2006. "Shanghai shi quanmian tuijin shequ quanke yisheng tuandui fuwu moshi" [Shanghai comprehensively promotes the service model of community general practitioner team]. June 2, 2006.

Shanghai Municipal Health Commission. 2015. "Shanghaishi xinyilun shequ weisheng fuwu zonghe gaige" [Shanghai officially launched the new round of comprehensive community health care service reform]. June 10, 2015.

Shanghai Municipal Health Commission. 2017. "Guanyu jinyibu zuohao benshi jiating yisheng qianyue fuwu gongzuo de tongzhi" [Announcement on further work on the family doctor service contract in Shanghai municipality]. September 20, 2017.

Tang, Qi, Peipei Song, and Lingzhong Xu. 2016. "The Role of Family Physicians Contracted Healthcare in China: A 'Cardiotonic' or a 'Band-Aid' for Healthcare Reform?" *BioScience Trends* 10 (4): 325–26.

Wang, Jie, Kenneth Kushner, John J Frey, Pingdu Xue, and Qian Ning. 2007. "Primary Care Reform in the Peoples' Republic of China: Implications for Training Family Physicians for the World's Largest Country." *Family Medicine* 39 (9): 639–43.

Wu, Jun, and Qing Shi. 2013. "Thinking on Reform of Family Doctors Contract Service and Medical Insurance Payment Mode." [In Chinese.] *Chinese General Practice* 16 (34): 3346–50.

Wu, Shuang, Yan Zhao, and Zhihui Cao. 2017. *Jiating yisheng qianyue fuwu zhidu yanjiu* [A study of the family physician contract services system]. Beijing: China International Broadcasting Press.

World Health Organization. 2018. "China: Multidisciplinary Teams and Integrated Service Delivery Across Levels of Care." In *Country Case Studies on Primary Health Care*. Geneva: WHO.

Xiamen Development and Reform Commission. 2016. *Fujian: Xiamen shi jiating yisheng jiceng qianyue fuwu shishi fang'an (shixing)*

[Implementation plan for the primary healthcare contract services of family physicians in Xiamen (trial)]. August 17, 2016. http://dpc. xm.gov.cn/xwdt/tzgg/201608/t20160823_1356125.htm.

Xiao, Li, Rui Huang, and Bowen Chen. 2015. "Effect of Team Performance Appraisal Program for Community Health Service Centers." [In Chinese.] *Chinese General Practice* (31): 3781–86.

Yang, ShuYu. 2017. "Introduction of General Practitioner Education and Chronic Disease Management Mode in Xiamen." [In Chinese.] *Chinese General Practice* 20 (20): 2526–27.

Zhao, Deyu, Min Ge, and Ping Jiang. 2016. *The Development and Promotion of Family Doctor System: A New Exploration for the Changning Model*. [In Chinese.] Shanghai: Shanghai Jiaotong University Press.

11   Hypertension Control after Health Insurance Expansion

Empirical Evidence from China

Jason Li

Hypertension, or abnormally high blood pressure, is one of the most important risk factors for chronic, noncommunicable diseases (NCDs), especially cardiovascular disease—the leading cause of death and the largest part of the disease burden in China (Leeder et al. 2005). In the last 10 years, hypertension prevalence has doubled in China—a condition responsible for 55 percent of the global cardiovascular disease burden and 7 percent of all disability-adjusted life-years (DALYs) (Lim et al. 2012). However, almost half of all Chinese cases of hypertension are undiagnosed (Zhao et al. 2013). In response, China has launched a series of national healthcare reforms in the last two decades to respond to chronic diseases, most notably its dramatic insurance expansion to cover all Chinese citizens (Min et al. 2015). A challenging public health issue relying on a primary-care-centered, preventative healthcare system, hypertension is thus a compelling metric to assess China's ambitious efforts to transform its public health system to address new and urgent chronic disease challenges.

The current literature surrounding how these chronic disease control policies have affected hypertension management and health outcomes are limited. While epidemiological indicators on hypertension have been documented, source data are outdated—with most recent papers analyzing 2011 data (Zhao et al. 2013; Ma et al. 2013). Few studies characterize hypertension management and the continuum of care among the most vulnerable and fastest growing population: China's elderly. Further, no studies investigate

The author thanks Dr. Karen Eggleston for excellent research advising and gratefully acknowledges funding to support this study from Stanford Undergraduate Advising and Research.

and quantify insurance generosity and its direct role in steps within hypertension management.

With a focus on recent years, the main objective of this chapter is to characterize how China's policy efforts, particularly its insurance expansion, have impacted current hypertension epidemiology and management. To meet this goal, the chapter undertakes three specific tasks. First, using a recent, nationally representative dataset, it explores the largest gaps in hypertension management through a Cascade of Care model, which will decompose the sample into the four stages of hypertension management: hypertensive, diagnosed, treated, and controlled. Second, it examines China's ambitious health insurance expansion—successful in insuring almost all of China—by characterizing the depth of its coverage through outpatient reimbursement rates. Finally, by exploiting this variation, the chapter quantitatively examines whether increased insurance generosity leads to increased diagnosis, treatment, and control of hypertension.

The next section discusses China's growing hypertension burden, contextualized in its aging population. We then explore China's efforts to control hypertension, particularly through its unprecedented insurance expansion. We describe our approach, present results, and then discuss conclusions.

Population Aging and Hypertension Management in China

Since it typically becomes more severe with age, addressing hypertension is especially relevant in China because of the country's aging population. Indeed, hypertension prevalence grew from 27.2% in 2000 to 40.9% in 2010 among adults aged 35 to 74—a statistic that has been corroborated through multiple studies (Huang et al. 2016). One study predicts that this population aging alone will produce a 200% increase in deaths due to cardiovascular disease between 2000 to 2040 (Ibrahim and Damasceno 2012). Controlling blood pressure has been called the most cost-effective public health strategy that China should pursue (Tang, Ehiri, and Long 2013).

Preliminary analysis of recent hypertension surveillance data suggests that controlling hypertension is a complex issue that has not been addressed fully by China's recent efforts. In 2012, Feng, Pang, and Beard (2014) found that the overall prevalence of hypertension among those aged 45 and older— 40%—had not dropped; more than 40% were unaware and about half of those who were aware received no medication. In the most recent national survey, Lv et al. (2013) found that 44.7% of adults 35 years and older are hypertensive—44.7% of whom were aware of their hypertension, 30.1% were taking their medications, and 7.2% had achieved control. In contrast, in other developed countries more than 80% of people with hypertension were aware of their condition and receiving treatment (Feng et al. 2014).

Health Reform and Insurance Expansion for Chronic Disease Control

In response, China has prioritized chronic disease control programs as a central part of the nation's health policy agenda. The 2009 National Healthcare Reform represented an ambitious and unprecedented overhaul of China's health system to achieve universal coverage predicated on equitable and affordable basic healthcare (Langenbrunner, Marquez, and Wang 2011). Of the reform's five pillars, three are directly related to chronic disease control and, thus, hypertension management: a national primary healthcare system, a national essential medicine system, and universal health insurance (Feng, Pang, and Beard 2014).

China's ambitious insurance expansion is one of the country's most lauded healthcare achievements. In the 1990s, the vast majority of Chinese citizens were uninsured. By 2011, almost all of China's citizens were insured—a significant feat, and important for hypertension control (Li et al. 2017). To accomplish this, the country set up two sweeping programs for low-income urban and rural citizens: the New Rural Cooperative Medical System (NCMS), launched in 2003, and Urban Resident Basic Medical Insurance (URBMI), launched in 2007. In addition, Urban Employee Basic Medical Insurance (UEBMI)—established prior to NCMS and URBMI—expanded its eligibility to more working Chinese and became the most comprehensive form of coverage available (Li et al. 2017).

This insurance expansion has important ramifications for improving hypertension management. Indeed, coverage may encourage preventative care utilization in local community health clinics, resulting in higher screening and diagnosis rates of hypertension (Xiao et al. 2014). Coverage may also allow for the increased purchase of anti-hypertensive medication and growing rates of treatment, adherence, and thus control. By allowing for hypertension's earlier diagnosis and easier management, insurance coverage could help manage it and prevent costly hospital admissions (Huang et al. 2016).

The current literature has examined insurance generosity in health utilization, hypertension, and chronic disease management in China with conflicting results. Indeed, Feng et al. (2014) find that people covered by UEBMI—a comprehensive insurance scheme that typically reimburses outpatient costs more readily than its alternatives—were more likely to be aware of and successfully control their hypertension. Lei and Lin (2009), using multiple estimating strategies, found that participation in NCMS significantly decreases use of folk doctors and increases preventative care utilization, such as general physical examinations. Further, Zhong (2011) found that immediate reimbursement from insurance programs for health costs significantly increases the likelihood of patients seeking outpatient treatment in China when compared to those without immediate reimbursement. Especially in low-income communities where citizens may not readily borrow money to pay for health services up front, reimbursement mechanisms and their depth may be crucial to encouraging health utilization.

However, results have also shown how China's health insurance expansion has been ineffective in encouraging healthcare utilization and—importantly—improving chronic disease control. Dai (2015) found that elderly members of NCMS had low rates of treatment and use of preventive health services while grappling with the highest prevalence of chronic disease compared to other age groups. The few to receive health services did so at village clinics, which are often cheaper—not the township health centers that the government envisioned and funds. Thus, insurance programs and general health reforms seemingly have not reached their full potential in targeting those most vulnerable in hypertension management: the rural elderly. In the same vein, Cheng et al. (2015) found that NCMS had no significant effect on mortality and did not reduce out-of-pocket spending for elderly participants.

However, few if any of these studies analyze comprehensive, robust, and recent data to reveal trends in hypertension detection, management, and control. Indeed, the most recent studies exploring national hypertension epidemiology and management use older data, the most recent being 2011. This is especially important because China's reforms are relatively recent and capturing their effects on health behaviors and outcomes are challenging without more long-term surveillance. Moreover, research has suggested that the coverage depth of expanded insurance varies drastically depending on the type of insurance people have and where they live (Xiao et al. 2014). This may be the reason why, despite expanded health insurance, health utilization and hypertension management have not dramatically improved in the literature. However, no studies have quantified how China's diverse communities have unevenly expanded their insurance and linked this variation to hypertension management. Thus, this chapter aims to analyze more recent hypertension epidemiology through the Care Cascade model and explore whether variation in insurance generosity has improved hypertension management.

Cascade of Care:
A Model to Investigate Hypertension Management

Effective management requires not just diagnosis but an adequate and continuous care system, and this chapter seeks to investigate the prevalence, diagnosis, treatment, and control of hypertension in China through a Care Cascade model. Because each of these four epidemiological measures represent different aspects of the healthcare reform and raise different policy implications, the Care Cascade model—breaking down the hypertensive population visually—represents a particularly well-suited research framework to analyze the cascade of care required to effectively manage hypertension (Berry et al. 2017). For instance, a low and unchanging diagnosis rate and high treatment rate may suggest that detection in community health centers—the intended site for primary care in China's reforms—are the main "stumbling block" in hypertension management; a low treatment rate among those diagnosed may represent barriers in accessing anti-hypertensive drugs not addressed by the expansive healthcare reform. To date, a Care Cascade model has not been applied to examine the population-level management of hypertension in the China context. Thus, decomposing national trends in hypertension represents an opportunity to evaluate the complex, equitable, and patient-centered care that chronic diseases necessitate and of which health insurance has encouraged increased utilization.

Methodology

We use data collected in the harmonized China Health and Retirement Longitudinal Study (CHARLS), a de-identified and publicly available dataset from the U.S. Health and Retirement Study (HRS) family of surveys. A nationally representative sample of people aged 45 and over living in households in China, CHARLS data were collected by surveying individuals from 150 county-level units from 28 provinces and municipalities. The included information is from two sources: (1) a questionnaire administered through face-to-face interviews in the sampled household and (2) a physical examination carried out by trained interviewers in the household. The structured questionnaire collected information on individual attributes, socioeconomic characteristics, health behaviors, chronic disease history (including hypertension), and urban/rural settings from each respondent, as explained in detail by Zhao et al. (2014). The socioeconomic factors investigated were age, sex, ethnicity (Han vs other), agricultural *hukou* (household registration), urban residence, marital status, household income, and level of education. Education was categorized into three levels: (1) below secondary education—which includes those illiterate and with primary education only, (2) secondary education but no higher, or (3) tertiary education—which includes only those educated to at least a college level. Household income was split into four quartiles. Modifiable risk factors considered were body mass index, how often the subject drank alcohol—split into light, moderate, and heavy drinker status—and cigarettes smoked per day. Diabetes status was also assessed.

Importantly, anthropometric measurements of blood pressure, weight, and height were recorded in the physical exam portion of the survey, which can be used to determine whether a participant has hypertension even if unaware of it and undiagnosed based on the questionnaire. Blood pressure was measured three times (approximately 45 seconds apart) on a single occasion. Excluding the first blood pressure reading because of the "white coat effect," the mean of the last two blood pressure readings was used to determine each respondent's blood pressure level.

As of now, no studies of hypertension have used the most recent waves of CHARLS or taken advantage of the panel nature of these data. The analysis reported here was restricted to hypertensive participants in both waves with non-missing information from relevant hypertension survey questions—such as reports on past treatments or prior diagnosis—and anthropometric measurements from the physical exam. From 17,708 total participants in the 2011 wave, 13,688 participated in the physical exam (4,020 excluded); from 18,447 participants in the 2013 follow-up exam, 12,907 participated in the physical exam (5,540 excluded), and of those, 9,153 participants with complete survey and physical exam information from both waves (3,754 excluded for missing data) were included in the initial analysis for the Care Cascade model.

When examining the effect of health insurance on this cascade of care, the panel sample was further modified to include only hypertensives with positive total health costs in the last month. CHARLS has available numeric codes for primary sampling units, so that community fixed effects regressions could be run. A total of 1,637 individuals, along with the 446 communities in which they live, were included in the empirical analysis.

Cascade of care:
Hypertension measurement, diagnosis, treatment, and control

The hypertensive category was decomposed into four mutually exclusive and exhaustive subcategories to examine unmet gaps in hypertension management, modeled from a hypertension care cascade study in South Africa conducted by Berry et al. (2017). The four categories—hypertensive, diagnosed, treated, controlled—are summarized below.

Hypertensive: Individuals were defined as hypertensive if either they self-reported as hypertensive and/or had a blood pressure value above the diagnostic threshold, which is the mean systolic blood pressure (SBP) ≥ 140 mmHg and/or mean diastolic blood pressure (DBP) ≥ 90 mmHg.

Diagnosed: CHARLS collected information on individual self-reports of specific conditions with the general question: "Have you been diagnosed with hypertension by a doctor?" Individuals were defined as diagnosed if they answered yes to this question.

Treated: Hypertensive patients were categorized as under treatment if they were taking prescribed Western or Chinese medicine for management of hypertension.

Controlled: Control of hypertension was defined as anti-hypertensive treatment associated with mean SBP < 140 mmHg and mean DBP < 90 mmHg.

Measuring insurance generosity

To capture insurance generosity, a reimbursement rate variable was constructed from individual health spending responses reporting out-of-pocket and total healthcare costs from doctor visits over the month. Reimbursement from health insurance covers the gap between out-of-pocket and total healthcare costs, which can be written as:

$$Reimbursement = Total\ health\ costs - out\text{-}of\text{-}pocket\ costs$$

Thus, the reimbursement rate—the percentage of total costs covered by insurance—can be written as:

$$Reimbursement\ rate = 1 - \frac{out\text{-}of\text{-}pocket\ costs}{total\ health\ costs}$$

Statistical analysis

Descriptive statistics were generated using means for continuous variables and proportions for categorical variables for the hypertension care cascade analysis. To empirically examine insurance generosity, multi-variable regression models were used to investigate steps and gaps within the hypertension cascade of care (hypertension status, diagnosis, treatment, and control), focusing on the effect of the constructed reimbursement rate variable. Because community policies are so central to insurance generosity, we first run a linear regression model at the community level. Each community incorporates smaller areas than cities or counties and are likely more homogenous, including factors not captured by provincial-level dummies (Strauss et al. 2010). Examples of communities include urban neighborhoods or administrative villages. We then collapsed the individual-level data into community-level averages for the reimbursement rate and household income, which serves as a control for community wealth. The averages for diagnosis, treatment, and control (outcome variables) are then regressed on reimbursement rate, controlling for household income and incorporating one dummy variable for each community for fixed effects analysis. The model can be written as:

$$Y_c = \alpha + \beta'Rate_c + \gamma'Income_c + \phi_c + \varepsilon_i \qquad (1)$$

where the dependent variable Y_c indicates the outcome variable averages in community c, and $Rate_c$ and $Income_c$ are the average reimbursement rate and household income for community c, respectively. We also add community fixed effects, ϕ_c, to account for community-level heterogeneity.

For each step in the hypertension care cascade (diagnosis, treatment, and control), we also fit four logistic regressions models on the individual level with differing modifications adjusting for:

1. demographics only,
2. demographics and health variables,
3. demographics and community fixed effects, and
4. demographics, health variables, and community fixed effects.

Robust standard errors of the regression coefficients are computed, that also allow for clustering at the community and individual level where appropriate. All analyses were created within STATA, and odds ratios were computed and presented for logistic regression results.

Results

Characteristics of the overall sample for the hypertension care cascade as well as the hypertensive sample are summarized in table 11.1. The full sample included 9,153 total respondents. A total of 4,915 female (53.7%), and 4,238 male (46.3%) participants were included in this study. The mean age of all participants was 60.1 ± 9.5 (50.6–69.6) years. Of the respondents, 50.4% and 49.6% were interviewed in an urban and rural setting, respectively; 82.2% of participants had an agricultural *hukou*. The vast majority of participants were Han (93.4%) and had less than a secondary school education (89.9%). This hypertensive sample includes 1,637 hypertensives with positive health costs from the past month. Compared to the overall sample, this sample is—on average—older (63 versus 60.5) and less educated. The average body mass index increased by one point, and the percentage of the sample with diabetes doubled (13.1% versus 6.7%).

TABLE 11.1 Study sample characteristics

Variables	Full sample (n=9,153)	Hypertensive sample (n=1,637)
Characteristics		
Age (years)	60.1 ± 9.5	63 ± 9.3
Female	53.70	59.80
Han	93.40	94.10
Agricultural *hukou*	82.20	81.20
Urban residency	50.40	49.60
Married	82.60	77.00
Household income (quartile)		
First quartile	25.30	30.00
Second quartile	24.70	25.80
Third quartile	25.00	24.30
Fourth quartile	25.00	19.90
Education		
<Primary	89.90	93.10
Secondary	8.90	6.30
Tertiary	1.20	0.90
Insurance generosity		
Reimbursement rate	—	.14 ± .26

SOURCE: China Health and Retirement Longitudinal Survey.
NOTE: Values are mean ± standard deviation and percentage of sample.

The hypertension care cascade results are displayed in figure 11.1. The first stage in the cascade is being diagnosed for hypertension. Among those with hypertension, 59.7% reported that they had been told by a health professional that they had hypertension, resulting in 40% of hypertensives who had never been diagnosed. Among those who self-reported ever being diagnosed, 84% reported that they had taken either a Western or traditional Chinese blood pressure medication. Among those treated for hypertension, 43% had controlled their blood pressure (<140/90 mmHg).

FIGURE 11.1 China's hypertension care cascade, 2011–13

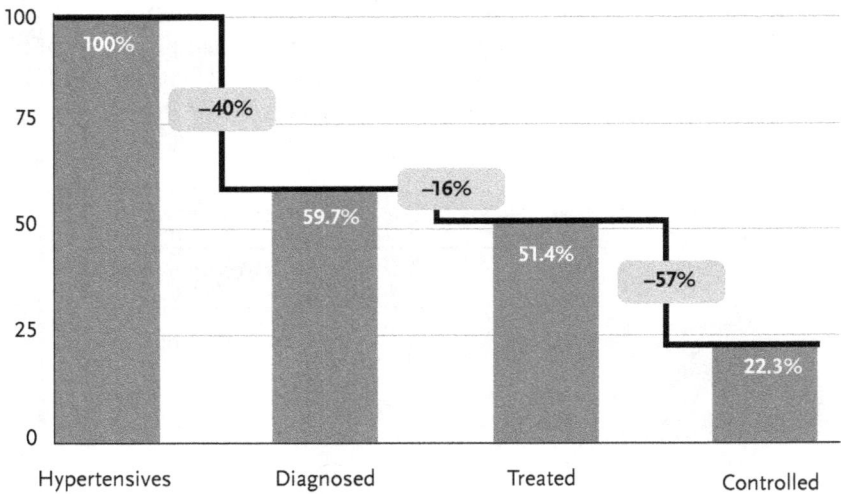

SOURCE: China Health and Retirement Longitudinal Survey.

Insurance Generosity and the Hypertension Cascade of Care

Community-level regression

A community-level regression is presented below in table 11.2. The reimbursement rate was found to be a statistically significant predictor of rates of diagnosis, treatment, and control after controlling for average community income and incorporating fixed effects.

TABLE 11.2 Community-level linear model results for diagnosis, treatment, and control

Variables	Diagnosed	Treated	Controlled
Household income average	1.37e-07	1.54e-08	1.39e-07*
	(9.07e-08)	(1.04e-07)	(7.46e-08)
Reimbursement rate	0.0646**	0.0608**	0.0386**
	(0.0283)	(0.0261)	(0.0184)
Constant	0.261***	0.202***	0.0534***
	(0.00500)	(0.00505)	(0.00327)
Communities	446	446	446
R-squared	0.028	0.020	0 020
Community FE	Yes	Yes	Yes

SOURCE: China Health and Retirement Longitudinal Survey.
NOTES: Robust standard errors in parentheses; *** p<0.01, ** p<0.05, * p<0.1. FE = fixed effects.

Individual-level results

Encouraged by the significant effect of the community reimbursement rate on all steps within the cascade, we turned to the individual-level data. The sample includes 1,657 hypertensives with positive health costs from the past month.

Diagnosis and control

Because the effect of insurance generosity on diagnosis and control are similar, they will be discussed together. Table 11.3 displays regressions predicting hypertension diagnosis and control for this hypertensive sample. In this sample, reimbursement rate had no significant effect on diagnosis or control in any model, differing with the community-level regression. Thus, hypertensive individuals, controlling for demographic characteristics and health conditions, were not more likely to be diagnosed if they had more generous reimbursement rates.

Treatment

Table 11.4 displays regressions predicting hypertension treatment for this hypertensive sample. In this sample, the reimbursement rate did significantly increase the odds of taking anti-hypertensives when not incorporating community fixed effects at the 0.05 level. When community fixed effects are incorporated, the reimbursement rate loses its significant effect on treatment, which is consistent with the fact that insurance generosity policies are set at the community level. The community drives and explains the effect of the reimbursement rate on hypertension treatment, which would thus reduce the significance of the reimbursement rate variable in models incorporating community fixed effects.

TABLE 11.3 Logistic regression results for diagnosis and control of hypertension

Variables	Diagnosed				Controlled			
	(1)	(2)	(3)	(4)	(1)	(2)	(3)	(4)
Reimbursement rate	1.293	1.349	1.219	1.542	1.318	1.3	1.19	1.348
	(0.255)	(0.306)	(0.341)	(0.509)	(0.240)	(0.264)	(0.312)	(0.415)
Demographics?	Y	Y	Y	Y	Y	Y	Y	Y
Health conditions?	N	Y	N	Y	N	Y	N	Y
Community FE?	N	N	Y	Y	N	N	Y	Y
Observations	1,637	1,637	1,270	1,270	1,637	1,646	1,270	1,270

SOURCE: China Health and Retirement Longitudinal Survey.
NOTE: Column headings are as follows: (1) adjusting only for demographics; (2) adjusting for demographics and health variables; (3) adjusting for demographics and community fixed effects; and (4) adjusting for demographics, health variables, and community fixed effects. Robust standard error in parentheses. FE = fixed effects.

TABLE 11.4 Logistic regression results for treatment of hypertension

Variables	(1)	(2)	(3)	(4)
Reimbursement rate	1.476**	1.715**	1.154	1.664
	(0.278)	(0.377)	(0.298)	(0.527)
Demographics?	Y	Y	Y	Y
Health conditions?	N	Y	N	Y
Community FE?	N	N	Y	Y
Observations	1,646	1,646	1,360	1,360

SOURCE: China Health and Retirement Longitudinal Survey.
NOTE: Column headings are as follows: (1) adjusting only for demographics; (2) adjusting for demographics and health variables; (3) adjusting for demographics and community fixed effects; and (4) adjusting for demographics, health variables, and community fixed effects. Robust standard error in parentheses. Results presented as odds ratios; ** $p<0.05$. FE = fixed effects.

Discussion and Conclusions

This chapter estimated the burden of hypertension and gaps in hypertension management in a nationally representative sample of China since the healthcare reform. This analysis suggests a high and steady hypertension prevalence of 39.5% among adults aged 45 and older—almost half of whom are undiagnosed. While this age-standardized prevalence is comparable to other countries' hypertension prevalence, the gaps in hypertension management revealed in this analysis are much wider. Importantly, of the 39.5% of the sample with hypertension, only 22.3% were treated and controlled. Thus, 77.7% of the hypertensive population are not managing their hypertension effectively.

By depicting and decomposing these losses in every step of a Care Cascade model, one sees the most substantial drops in care. Strikingly, 40% of all hypertensives in this population are undiagnosed and are thus not connected to the healthcare infrastructure and knowledge needed to manage this chronic, asymptomatic, but consequential disease. Indeed, once participants are diagnosed, they are likely to be treated: only 17% of those diagnosed were not treated, the smallest drop in this population. This confirms the hypothesis, corroborated through other hypertension studies in China, that diagnosis of hypertension is the "stumbling block" in hypertension management.

As expected, the largest losses in this cascade of care were the treated but uncontrolled hypertensives: 57% of treated hypertensives still had high blood pressure readings that met hypertension diagnosis criteria ($\geq$ 140/90 mmHg) during the physical examination. Controlling hypertension is a complex challenge that even the most developed healthcare systems struggle with; as with any often asymptomatic disease, hypertension—if only diagnosed without further surveillance—rarely motivates those affected to continue buying and taking hypertension medication (Hesketh and Zhou 2017). This is especially true in low-resource households and communities that must navigate and stretch already constrained time and financial budgets. Challenges to adherence have also been documented for other long-term treatment regimens, such as HIV anti-retroviral therapy and tuberculosis treatments, and represent significant challenges for public health systems at large (Miller et al. 2010).

In sum, China has low rates of diagnosis, treatment, and control, especially when compared to high-income countries such as the United States. Indeed, the National Health and Nutrition Examination Survey (NHANES)—a national survey in the United States—found that 87% of adults aged 40 to 75 years old were diagnosed, 73% were treated, and 61% achieved effective control (Bautista 2008). In contrast, this model found much lower rates of all three steps in the cascade: 59.7% were diagnosed, 51.4% were treated, and only 22.3% achieved effective control in the sample from China. Further, the Care Cascade model showed that diagnosis and control had the biggest losses, with a 40% and 57% loss, respectively.

Moreover, this chapter delved into China's ambitious health insurance expansion and investigated how coverage depth and generosity—uneven across communities in China—have affected steps within the hypertension cascade of care: diagnosis, treatment, and control. Results showed that reimbursement rates are low for most hypertensive individuals, which is expected given that most CHARLS individuals are elderly, unemployed, and live in rural areas. Thus, the vast majority of CHARLS respondents participate in URBMI and NCMS, the two programs with relatively shallow coverage and whose depth is dependent on community design. When individual data were collapsed, regression results found that communities with higher average reimbursement rates were associated with higher diagnosis, treatment, and control rates, though the effect is modest. Though the reimbursement rate was a significant, positive predictor in the community-level models, the variety of individual-level models showed that higher insurance generosity significantly increased the likelihood of an individual taking anti-hypertensive treatment but had no significant effect on the likelihood of diagnosis or effective control. We discuss each step in detail below.

The reimbursement rate had no effect on diagnosis, which is unsurprising given that this sample consists of hypertensives who had already visited the doctor in the past month. Those who visited the doctor in the last month are already more likely to visit the doctor regularly and are also more likely to have been diagnosed in previous visits. Thus, the proposed mechanism—increased insurance generosity encouraging more preventative care utilization—may be more pronounced in those who do not already visit the doctor regularly. However, because the reimbursement rate variable is constructed from health spending data for each individual, this sample could not include those who had zero health visits in the last month—a limitation to this study and one, if rectified, that may yield significant effects for insurance generosity on diagnosis.

The reimbursement rate had a positive, significant effect on treatment. As discussed in the proposed mechanism between insurance generosity and treatment and consistent with previous literature, patients who had more financial support for their health visits are more likely to regularly obtain and afford anti-hypertensives. Though they are more likely to get treated, sample respondents with higher insurance generosity were not more likely to control their hypertension—a surprising finding that is inconsistent with health insurance programs in other settings. Indeed, Milan et al. (2017) found that increased out-of-pocket costs in Quebec were associated with non-adherence to anti-hypertensives in older adults. In plans providing chronic disease drugs for free, participants significantly increased medication possession rates, decreased total pharmacy costs, and decreased emergency department visits (Mahoney 2005). In Mexico, expansion of healthcare coverage to uninsured people was associated with greater use of anti-hypertensive treatment and blood pressure control (Bleich et al. 2007). And while no income-related effects were found in this study, patients with low incomes were two times more likely to be non-adherent and have uncontrolled hypertension in the United States (Gu et al. 2012).

Because this chapter found that increased insurance generosity is associated with increased treatment but not increased diagnosis and control, other barriers to the cascade of care specific to China must be investigated. Though financial barriers may have decreased, an underdeveloped health and screening system limits accessibility even if cost is less of a concern. Health clinic operations and the quality and training of providers also vary enormously, and linkage to care after a positive blood pressure screening may be lacking and affect adherence. Literature has suggested that some of China's chronic disease control policies—such as expanded screening, the Essential Medicines List, and revamped hypertension clinical guidelines—have not been effectively implemented in practice (Hesketh and Zhou 2017). For instance, in a study of 3,362 primary health sites in China, high-value medications were not preferentially used or stocked; only 32.7% of them had actually stocked the high-value medications, and even fewer—11.2%—regularly prescribed them (Su et al. 2017). Therefore, while China's initiatives have rapidly expanded insurance and promoted a grassroots primary care network designed to capture undiagnosed hypertensives, some policies have wide gaps between theory and praxis—gaps which may account for the large drops in the hypertension care cascade demonstrated in this chapter.

References

Bautista, Leonelo E. 2008. "Predictors of Persistence with Antihypertensive Therapy: Results from the NHANES." *American Journal of Hypertension* 21 (2): 183–88.

Berry, Kaitlyn M., Whadi Ah Parker, Zandile J. McHiza, Ronel Sewpaul, Demetre Labadarios, Sydney Rosen, and Andrew Stokes. 2017. "Quantifying Unmet Need for Hypertension Care in South Africa through a Care Cascade: Evidence from the SANHANES, 2011-2012." *BMJ Global Health* 2(3): e000348. BMJ Publishing Group.

Bleich, Sara N., David M. Cutler, Alyce S. Adams, Rafael Lozano, and Christopher J. L. Murray. 2007. "Impact of Insurance and Supply of Health Professionals on Coverage of Treatment for Hypertension in Mexico: Population Based Study." *BMJ* 335 (7625): 875.

Cheng, Lingguo, Hong Liu, Ye Zhang, Ke Shen, and Yi Zeng. 2015. "The Impact of Health Insurance on Health Outcomes and Spending of the Elderly: Evidence from China's New Cooperative Medical Scheme." *Health Economics* 24 (6): 672–91.

Dai, Baozhen. 2015. "Does China's New Cooperative Medical Scheme Promote Rural Elders' Access to Healthcare Services in Relation to Chronic Conditions?" *International Health* 7 (1): 32–41.

Feng, Xing Lin, Mingfan Pang, and John Beard. 2014. "Health System Strengthening and Hypertension Awareness, Treatment and Control: Data from the China Health and Retirement Longitudinal Study." *Bulletin of the World Health Organization* 92 (1): 29–41.

Gu, Qiuping, Vicki L. Burt, Charles F Dillon, and Sarah Yoon. 2012. "Trends in Antihypertensive Medication Use and Blood Pressure Control among United States Adults with Hypertension: The National Health And Nutrition Examination Survey, 2001 to 2010." *Circulation* 126 (17): 2105–14.

Hesketh, Therese, and Xudong Zhou. 2017. "Hypertension in China: The Gap Between Policy and Practice." *Lancet* 390 (10112): 2529–30.

Huang, Kehui, Yu Ting Song, Yong Huan He, and Xing Lin Feng. 2016. "Health System Strengthening and Hypertension Management in China." *Global Health Research and Policy* 1 (1): 13.

Ibrahim, M. Mohsen, and Albertino Damasceno. 2012. "Hypertension in Developing Countries." *The Lancet* 380 (9841): 611–19.

Mahoney, John J. 2005. "Reducing Patient Drug Acquisition Costs Can Lower Diabetes Health Claims." *American Journal of Managed Care* 11 (5 Suppl): S170–76.

Langenbrunner, John, Patricio Marquez, and Shiyong Wang. 2011.
"Toward a Healthy and Harmonious Life in China: Stemming the Rising Tide of Non-communicable Diseases." World Bank, Washington, DC.

Leeder, Stephen, Susan Raymond, Henry Greenberg, Hui Liu, and Kathy Esson. 2005. *A Race Against Time: The Challenge of Cardiovascular Disease in Developing Economies*. New York: Columbia University.

Lei, Xiaoyan, and Wanchuan Lin. 2009. "The New Cooperative Medical Scheme in Rural China: Does More Coverage Mean More Service and Better Health?" *Health Economics* 18 Suppl 2: 25–46.

Li, Yanping, Vasanti Malik, and Frank B. Hu. 2017. "Health Insurance in China: After Declining in the 1990s, Coverage Rates Rebounded to Near-Universal Levels by 2011." *Health Affairs* 36 (8): 1452–60.

Lim, Stephen S., Theo Vos, Abraham D Flaxman, Goodarz Danaei, Kenji Shibuya, et al. 2012. "A Comparative Risk Assessment of Burden of Disease and Injury Attributable to 67 Risk Factors and Risk Factor Clusters in 21 Regions, 1990–2010: A Systematic Analysis for the Global Burden of Disease Study 2010." *The Lancet* 380 (9859): 2224–60.

Lv, Jun, Miao Liu, Yu Jiang, and Li-Ming Li. 2013. "Prevention and Control of Major Non-Communicable Diseases in China from 1990 to 2009: Results of a Two-Round Delphi Survey." *Global Health Action* 6 (February): 20004.

Ma, Yu-Quan, Wen-Hua Mei, Ping Yin, Xiao-Hui Yang, Sana Kiani Rastegar, and Jian-Dong Yan. 2013. "Prevalence of Hypertension in Chinese Cities: A Meta-Analysis of Published Studies." *PLoS One* 8 (3): e58302.

Milan, Raymond, Helen-Maria Vasiliadis, Samantha Gontijo Guerra, and Djamal Berbiche. 2017. "Out-of-Pocket Costs and Adherence to Antihypertensive Agents among Older Adults Covered by the Public Drug Insurance Plan in Quebec." *Patient Preference and Adherence* 11 (September): 1513–22.

Miller, Candace M., Mpefe Ketlhapile, Heather Rybasack-Smith, and Sydney Rosen. 2010. "Why Are Antiretroviral Treatment Patients Lost to Follow-Up? A Qualitative Study from South Africa." *Tropical Medicine & International Health* 15 (Suppl 1): 48–54.

Min, Yan, Li-Xin Jiang, Li-Jing L. Yan, Lin-Hong Wang, Sanjay Basu, Yang-Feng Wu, and Randall S. Stafford. 2015. "Tackling China's Noncommunicable Diseases: Shared Origins, Costly Consequences and the Need for Action." *Chinese Medical Journal* 128 (6): 839–43.

Strauss, John, Xiaoyan Lei, Albert Park, Yan Shen, James P. Smith, Zhe Yang, and Yaohui Zhao. 2010. "Health Outcomes and Socio-Economic Status among the Elderly in Gansu and Zhejiang Provinces, China: Evidence from the CHARLS Pilot." *Journal of Population Ageing* 3 (3–4): 111–42.

Su, Meng, Qiuli Zhang, Xueke Bai, Chaoqun Wu, Yetong Li, Elias Mossialos, George A. Mensah, Frederick A. Masoudi, Jiapeng Lu, Xi Li, Sebastian Salas-Vega, Anwen Zhang, Yuan Lu, Khurram Masir, Harlan M. Krumholz, and Lixin Jiang. 2017. "Availability, Cost, and Prescription Patterns of Antihypertensive Medications in Primary Health Care in China: A Nationwide Cross-Sectional Survey." *The Lancet* 390 (10112): 2559–68.

Tang, Shenglan, John Ehiri, and Qian Long. 2013. "China's Biggest, Most Neglected Health Challenge: Non-Communicable Diseases." *Infectious Diseases of Poverty* 2 (1): 7.

Xiao, Nanzi, Qian Long, Xiaojun Tang, and Shenglan Tang. 2014. "A Community-Based Approach to Non-Communicable Chronic Disease Management within a Context of Advancing Universal Health Coverage in China: Progress and Challenges." *BMC Public Health* 14 (2): S2.

Zhao, Yaohui, Yisong Hu, James P. Smith, John Strauss, and Gonghuan Yang. 2014. "Cohort Profile: The China Health and Retirement Longitudinal Study (CHARLS)." *International Journal of Epidemiology* 43 (1): 61–68.

Zhao, Yaling, Hong Yan, Roger J. Marshall. Shaonong Dang, Ruihai Yang, Qiang Li, and Xueying Qin. 2013. "Trends in Population Blood Pressure and Prevalence, Awareness, Treatment, and Control of Hypertension among Middle-Aged and Older Adults in a Rural Area of Northwest China from 1982 to 2010." *PLoS ONE* 8 (4): e61779.

Zhong, Hai. 2011. "Effect of Patient Reimbursement Method on Health-Care Utilization: Evidence from China." *Health Economics* 20 (11): 1312–29.

12 Private Roles for Public Goals in China's Social Services

Jack Donahue, Karen Eggleston, Yijia Jing, and Richard J. Zeckhauser

China, like other countries, has public needs that far outstrip the abilities of the government alone to deliver, including the broad array of social services that support healthy aging. In this chapter, drawing on a survey of 17 medium-sized cities, we discuss how China's local governments are seeking ways to create public value through contracting with the private sector and collaborative arrangements with some shared *discretion*, what we label "collaborative governance" (Donahue and Zeckhauser 2011; Donahue, Eggleston, and Zeckhauser 2018).[1]

China's determination to rapidly replicate—even leapfrog—the social service networks constructed over decades or centuries in the West poses a historic challenge of capacity-building. Audacious plans for "equalization of access" to eight major service areas—education, employment services, social insurance (pensions, maternity and unemployment insurance, etc.), social support services, healthcare and public health, family planning, housing security, and cultural, sports, and recreational activities—were announced in mid-2012 by the central government. The 12th (2011–15) and 13th (2016–20) five-year plans call for an expanded role for competition and outsourcing in basic public services ranging from health and education to

The authors gratefully acknowledge the work of the Fudan University students involved with the 17-city survey in early 2013, as well as the excellent research assistance of Yingtian He and Sen Zhou.

1   Collaborative governance is defined as government sharing with the private sector a real measure of *discretion* as to the means and, to some extent, the ends of collective action (see Donahue, Eggleston, and Zeckhauser 2018). The private sector includes both for-profit and non-profit entities.

affordable housing.[2]

Yet local governments bear primary responsibility for social services, and these commitments threaten to over-match their capabilities. Local governments face the dual burden of unfunded mandates from above and insufficient revenues.[3] Efficiency-promoting innovation is the only possible way out when commitments exceed capabilities.

In many Western countries, budget shortfalls are the major drivers of service-delivery innovation. In China, the good news is that central-level public-sector revenues have been on the rise. The bad news is that local governments, which provide virtually all social services, have large and growing debts, debts that are a macro-economic concern.[4] Yet ambitions remain high, and those ambitions will be a driving force fostering the innovations that reshape social service delivery. Policymakers appear to aspire to a social service system reflecting the broader ideal of a lean, efficient, and effective government within a market-based economy. The prospect of forging a hybrid social service system featuring significant private-sector engagement inspires considerable enthusiasm. In short, Chinese policymakers are in the process of embracing—or perhaps more precisely re-inventing—the underlying principles of what is sometimes called the "new public management" movement in America.[5]

Any major shift toward collaborative delivery of social services will inevitably transform China's governmental institutions as well as their relationships with private organizations and the public at large (Jing and Savas 2009; Brown, Gong, and Jing 2012; Jing 2015). The vast majority of projects highlighted in the national public-private partnership (PPP) demonstration projects, for example, fall within the more traditional categories of municipal engineering, transportation, area development, and tourism. Nevertheless,

---

2   The two plans are "The Outline of the Twelfth Five-Year Plan for National Economic and Social Development of the People's Republic of China" (Chinese version available at https://www.cmab.gov.hk/doc/12th_5yrsplan_outline_full_text.pdf) and "The 13th Five-Year Plan for Economic and Social Development of the People's Republic of China" (http://en.ndrc.gov.cn/newsrelease/201612/P020161207645765233498.pdf).

3   See, for example, Wong (1991); Oi (1995); Croll (1999); Adams and Hannum (2005); Cook (2011); Duckett (2011); Eggleston, Oi, and Wang (2017).

4   Fiscal revenues of Chinese governments grew from ¥1339.5 billion in 2000 to ¥10387.4 billion in 2011, an increase of 675 percent (National Bureau of Statistics of China 2012). But more recently, local governments have struggled to finance many services and have expanded debt considerably (Guess and Ma 2015; Wong 2016; Eggleston, Oi, and Wang 2017).

5   For a classic popular book in this tradition, see Osborne and Gaebler (1993); a more recent sample is Eggers and Macmillan (2013).

a few cases do focus on affordable housing, education, healthcare, and elder care (see CPCCC 2019, 2016a). While private involvement in social services remains embryonic, other domains have already seen significant change, including some arenas of actual or incipient collaboration (as addressed in Donahue, Eggleston, and Zeckhauser 2018).

As the United States and other Western countries have already discovered, however, private roles in social services summon special sorts of complexity. Local governments have experimented with different forms of social service provision, and the diversity of the contemporary landscape reveals the deep impacts of path dependence, serendipity, and inertia. As we show in our survey at the cusp of the most recent wave of "PPP demonstration projects" in China, originally few cases involved true collaboration. Indeed, in many cases even among the nationally recognized PPPs, the private sector is a state-owned enterprise (Bloomberg 2017). Government directives reiterate the call for leveling the playing field for the private sector, thus revealing that old practices and prejudices continue to inhibit collaborative governance between public- and private-sector actors in China.[6]

This chapter surveys the status quo of China's social service sector prior to the most recent wave of demonstration projects, presenting results from a 2013 survey we conducted of 17 medium-sized cities spanning 10 provinces. We supplement our customized survey data with relevant information from standard statistical sources. As the chapter concludes, we reflect on the potential for, and the hazards of, public-private collaboration in this uniquely important and distinctly complex policy arena for a rising and aging China.

A Tale of Seventeen Cities

Capitalizing on the good offices of co-author Yijia Jing of Fudan University, in 2013 we deployed a contingent of Fudan students to gather evidence about public service delivery models in 17 medium-sized cities or districts within larger cities. We do not claim an ideal sample of systematically

---

6   For example, the "Circular on Further Advancing the Public-Private Partnership in Public Services" (CPCCC 2016b) exhorts "finance departments at all levels shall work with relevant agencies to create a level playing field, and. . . prevent differential or discriminatory treatment on potential partners under unreasonable terms (including too high or irrelevant eligibility requirements, and excessive deposit), so as to boost private investments." Also see discussion and examples of "government NGOs" in Jing (2015): "Grassroots groups often regard government-initiated non-profit organizations as bureaucratic, rigid, less innovative and unprofessional. They often make no effort to hide their antipathy towards the monopoly status and strong political connections these groups enjoy" (601).

representative locales; indeed, the cities are a "convenience sample" of the Fudan students' hometowns. Nevertheless, our sites capture a broad range of geographic diversity and economic development, as summarized in table 12.1. They ranged in population at the time from 150,000 in Yichun to 9.9 million in Harbin, capital of Heilongjiang Province; the average population was 2.7 million. Productivity and prosperity diverged widely across the sites, from ¥11,594 (about US$1,800 on a per capita gross domestic product [GDP] basis) in Jianshi, Hubei Province, to ¥105,978 (about $17,000) at that time in Shanghai's Pudong district.

TABLE 12.1 Population and per capita GDP of the 17 cities in the sample, 2011

City	Province	Administrative level	Population (millions)	Per capita GDP (yuan)
Jianshi	Hubei	County-level	0.41	11,594
Xishui (Qingquan Town)	Hubei	County-level	0.87	14,267
Yichun (Yichun District)	Heilongjiang	County-level	0.15	20,548
Cangnan	Zhejiang	County-level	1.18	24,993
Mianyang	Sichuan	Prefecture-level	4.61	25,794
Lianyungang	Jiangsu	Prefecture-level	4.39	32,159
Cangzhou (Xinhua District)	Hebei	Prefecture-level	7.13	36,445
Tai'an	Shandong	Prefecture-level	5.51	41,791
Ningguo	Anhui	County-level	0.39	41,981
Harbin (Nangang and Xiangfang Districts)	Heilongjiang	Municipality	9.94	42,682
Changyi	Shandong	County-level	0.58	45,318
Yan'an (Baota District)	Shaanxi	Prefecture-level	2.15	51,724
Ninghai	Zhejiang	County-level	0.61	52,581
Jiading District	Shanghai	Prefecture-level	1.51	60,738
Yidu	Hubei	County-level	0.40	69,216
Cixi	Zhejiang	County-level	1.04	84,223
Pudong District	Shanghai	Prefecture-level	5.18	105,978
Average			2.71	44,825

SOURCE: Statistical yearbooks, People's Republic of China.

The data were gathered through structured (but flexible) Mandarin-language interviews of local officials about arrangements for delivering nine public services: emergency medical transport (ambulance services), medical insurance and healthcare delivery, care for the elderly, care for the disabled, compulsory education (grades 1–9), affordable housing construction and management, park management (gardening and landscaping), job training, and public transportation.[7] Some of these functions—notably park management, public transportation, and affordable housing—fall outside of most definitions of "social services," but are included here for the perspective they offer on both the bundle of duties and the opportunity to learn and improvise that local officials encounter.

Only two of the cities we examined have no significant private role in the delivery of any of the nine services—a remarkable finding all on its own for a nation so recently viewed as classically communist, and which still self-identifies as socialist while embracing a market-based economy. Private roles in social service delivery were discovered in poorer as well as richer Chinese cities, though there is a perceptible tendency for wealthier cities (as measured by average per-capita GDP) to experiment more aggressively with private roles. (Later we speculate as to why this might be the case.) Our survey examines the delegation to the private sector across a spectrum of arrangements, not just collaborative governance. The collaborative governance form would neither be expected nor recommended for the entirety or even the majority of private-sector roles.

As found by an earlier survey of American cities (Donahue and Zeckhauser 2011, ch. 9), "contracting out"—that is, delegating to private providers *without* the shared discretion that defines collaborative governance—is very common for park management. All but two cities in our sample contracted out gardening and landscaping for city parks. One of the sample sites in Zhejiang, however, actually shares discretion for elements of park management in an arrangement that bears the hallmarks of collaborative governance. In addition to this one example of park management, only long-term care for the disabled displayed examples of true public-private collaboration. (Several interviewed officials revealed that caution about more extensive sharing of discretion with private parties is driven by the concern that private parties might grab excessive profits—a classic illustration of what we term payoff discretion; see Donahue and Zeckhauser [2011]; and Donahue, Eggleston, and Zeckhauser [2018].)

Construction of affordable housing units also overwhelmingly involved contracting with private providers. It should not be surprising that private engagement has been less common for social services, which tend to be multi-dimensional, difficult to define, and politically delicate, all qualities that push appropriately toward more public control. Primary and secondary education, as well as long-term care services for the elderly and disabled,

---

7   All interview quotes have been translated by the two Chinese-speaking authors, sometimes with slight re-casting for clarity in English.

featured some private involvement; health services less; and emergency medical services none at all. (This last is hardly surprising, since at the time it was technically illegal for private organizations to deliver emergency medical services.) The finding that direct government provision completely dominates public transportation services was more unexpected, both because such services seem reasonably amenable to delegation, and because they frequently feature major private roles in other countries.[8]

The following sections report on the survey results for each social service in greater depth and situate those results within the broader context of national policy.

Health services

In our 17-community survey, we find results that are broadly consistent with both the status quo and the recent trajectory of China nationwide (e.g., see Eggleston, forthcoming). Despite signs of openness to a greater private role, in all of the surveyed cities the public sector continues to be the dominant insurer and provider. Few cities systematically contract with private providers, and no cities adopt an explicitly collaborative approach in the health sector. Existing private delivery mostly served a small bifurcated clientele: the burgeoning upper middle class, and those left out of standard public provision, such as migrant workers and new peri-urban communities with fewer public facilities. Interview subjects endorsed a larger role for private hospitals, but subject to the stipulation that they proved able to match or exceed the service quality of public hospitals. "Private hospitals certainly deliver worse services than public ones, due to their limited resources," according to a government official of Jiading County, Shanghai. A Harbin official similarly argued that:

> Private hospitals need to fight for their life and actively compete for patients. If we can have proper management, private hospitals could be truly beneficial, helping to share the burden on public hospitals and the government. Appropriate management and regulation are the most crucial factors.

Officials thus seem open to an expanded private role, and some localities have moved aggressively in that direction recently; at the national level, meanwhile, such changes have been limited.

---

8   There was one case of contracting out to a single corporation, a state-owned enterprise.

Emergency medical services

Emergency medical services—or, more prosaically, ambulances—are provided through a wide range of delivery and financing options in many countries. Private-sector roles are extensive, and in some cases dominant. China is a stark exception. Private provision of ambulance services was technically prohibited by law at the time of our survey. Nevertheless, private ambulances had been under consideration, notably in rural areas, with the motive of increasing supply. This suggests that the illegality of private involvement may not reflect a principled and durable objection, given pragmatic concerns about needed provision. Interviewed officials in our sample sites gave mixed signals about whether private ambulance services should be rejected on principle or whether a more mixed-ownership approach might deliver greater public value. One ambulance driver in Jianshi County, Hubei Province, expressed deep skepticism about private involvement—though on pragmatic rather than ideological grounds. "I think it is almost impossible for private parties to contract to provide ambulance services because of specialization and high cost. . . . Moreover, local people hardly understand the concept of private contracting." Specialization and high cost do not preclude contracting if there is a well-developed private sector for that service, which many localities in China of course lack for ambulance services or other services where private involvement is proscribed or discouraged. Thus, this quote and similar ones by local officials in other sites we surveyed reveal an instinct to preserve public-sector dominancy, and lack of understanding of the potential benefits and risks of private contracting, or else legitimate concerns about private parties extorting seriously ill or injured patients for money, which cloud judgments about other features of contracting that could be readily addressed with appropriate contractual structures and effective monitoring arrangements.

Primary and secondary education

Collaborative governance has characterized some specific types of social service provision in China for decades. Non-governmental *minban* (people-run) schools are a salient example. Far from being a twenty-first-century innovation, they date back to the Mao era. As Hannum et al. (2008) note,

> much of school finance in China during the Cultural Revolution [1966–76] relied on local community support for *minban*, or people-managed, teachers and schools. . . . Education authorities ceded authority over state-managed

elementary schools to local production teams or brigades, communes, facto-
ries, business enterprises, neighborhood revolutionary committees, etc. . . .
Minban teachers were paid in grain rations and supplementary cash wages. . .
(Hannum et al. 2008, 4).

Presumably pragmatism—serving a population that would otherwise lack
a school—trumped any ideological objections to private-sector involvement.
Minban schools, in different manifestations, survive to the present day.
The private-sector role in education has evolved over time to fit new niches
neglected by mainstream public schools, and to supplement public schools
with learning technologies and other services (for a more detailed discussion
see the chapter on education in Donahue, Eggleston, and Zeckhauser [2018]).

Results from our 17-city survey help to illustrate the important though still
circumscribed domain of the private sector—including but extending beyond
minban schools—in contemporary Chinese education. In Mianyang, Sichuan
Province, private education plays a significant role in compulsory education,
and officials consider its quality to be relatively high. Private schools even
attract students from outside Mianyang. The local government gave extensive
support to private education, assigning some teachers hired and paid by the
government to private schools and subsidizing private kindergartens. One
of the county governments within Mianyang provides funding to a private
middle school on the same terms as it offers public middle schools. Shanghai's Jiading District hosts two very different types of *minban* schools. The
first category serves migrant workers' children. While these schools are of
mediocre quality, they charge no fees to parents and comprise a vital part
of the Jiading school system, since 56 percent of residents are from other
provinces and thereby legally excluded from mainstream public schools. The
second category—more comparable to conventional private schools in the
United States—charge high tuition to supplement governmental funding.
They are run by private corporate sponsors and are perceived to be of much
higher quality. These examples from our survey confirm that, while there is
certainly room for expansion and differentiation relative to the United States
and other nations, the private sector has already carved out a meaningful
set of niches within Chinese education.

Affordable housing

Extraordinary returns to migration have fueled a massive and unprecedented
surge of urbanization that has been a great enabling force in China's rise.
Managing this tsunami of population inflow, and especially providing
appropriate housing, is one of the present day's most imposing governance

challenges. The scale is difficult for non-Chinese to appreciate, with the "floating population" of temporary migrants totaling more than 200 million—equivalent to the population of Brazil, and larger on its own than the entire population of every country but Indonesia, the United States, India, and China itself. Over the coming decades, China's cities are projected to absorb an astounding 300 million new residents (Peng 2011; Eggleston et al. 2013). For both the construction and management of affordable housing, delegation in general, and collaborative governance in particular, offer much-needed options.

How can China gain more of the benefits from private involvement in this area while controlling the costs, risks, and adverse effects? Increasing the supply of affordable housing requires that local governments cooperate with private developers—a challenging requirement, since both sides might have preferable alternatives. Local governments can harvest much higher revenues by allocating land to commercial rather than residential use (or affordable housing in particular). Developers' profits are often capped for affordable housing construction.

China's localities employ three primary methods for promoting the private provision of affordable housing, only the last of which can be considered collaborative governance (see the chapter on real estate in Donahue, Eggleston, and Zeckhauser [2018]). First, municipalities purchase existing, privately constructed housing to offer to local residents. Second—assuming that the discouraging incentives noted above can be overcome—the government contracts with private companies to build new units with specified characteristics at a specified price. Third, the local government can require commercial developers to designate a share of new units as affordable housing.

In our 17-city survey, affordable housing emerged as an active arena of private involvement in public missions. Most housing officials interviewed reported engaging private actors in the construction of affordable housing, with some turning to the private sector for housing management as well. But while more than three-fourths of the cities featured private construction or management or both, none of them reported engaging the private sector on terms where discretion was considerably shared. This may hint that there are hidden impediments to truly collaborative approaches to affordable housing in China—or alternatively, and we think more probably, may suggest the untapped potential for new approaches. The international evidence offers both good news and bad news in this regard. On the positive side is the vast number of examples of private involvement, on terms of shared discretion, in publicly supported housing. In just the United States alone, "Section 8" rental assistance, a range of tax preferences for affordable housing, and conditional permitting that requires a specified share of affordable units for mixed housing developments—among other arrangements—engage fully private entities that are influenced but not controlled by the government in the provision of housing. On the negative side, there is abundant evidence that these arrangements are prone to risks that must be monitored, such as the private parties being able to extract benefits for themselves dispropor- tionate to the public value they create.

Long-term care for the elderly and disabled

As noted elsewhere in this volume, China's low fertility, increases in longevity, and changes in living arrangements and employment (e.g., migrating for work) combine to limit the number of adult children directly providing care for elderly parents—the traditional model—thus making it imperative to develop capacity for elder care beyond the family. China's local jurisdictions have experimented with a range of options for coaxing private investment into long-term care.

Several interviewees in the cities we studied confirmed that long-term care was as yet not well developed; few private, for-profit providers found it attractive. "The biggest obstacle is attracting private firms, for it is almost impossible for a private company to run a profitable nursing home according to the national standard," said a government official of Cangnan County, Zhejiang Province. A government official from Yinchun, Heilongjiang Prov- ince, lamented, "Private nursing homes have ameliorated the shortage of supply and alleviated some of the pressure on the public sector. However, due to their limited budgets, low-quality facilities, and other problems, overall effectiveness is limited." Some officials in higher per capita income areas shared these concerns, such as one government officer from Shanghai's Jiading County: "We do not encourage the private sector to be involved in the elder-care industry. . . . Elder care should be undertaken by the government, since it is a costly activity, not a profitable business." Yet affluent cities in practice encourage private elderly homes by offering subsidies. For example, Shanghai announced it has achieved the "90-7-3 scheme" goal set in its 11th five-year plan: 90 percent of the elderly remaining in their homes, 7 percent of the elderly remaining at home but accessing community-based elderly support services, and 3 percent of Shanghai's elderly population receiving institutionalized care. Since the existing infrastructure was insufficient to meet the 3 percent target of accessible nursing home beds, both the Shanghai municipal government and district governments subsidize every new bed in nursing homes (regardless of ownership) and provide an annual subsidy if the bed is occupied. Despite official approval and support, however, expensive land and lack of urban planning for specialized homes for the elderly often have discouraged private investment in the long-term-care industry.

Approaches toward care for the disabled varied considerably from city to city, with substantial private engagement. For example, in Tai'an, Shandong, the government contracts with several private companies to provide care for the disabled. There are hints of true collaboration with at least one of these companies, which has been granted the discretion to experiment with new approaches to service delivery. Illustrating the rich diversity of organizational models in China, interview subjects in Yichun report close collaboration between local officials and a "volunteer association" established in 2011. But upon closer examination the "private" association is revealed to be closely associated with the city government. This revelation, to be clear, does not establish that the Yichun arrangement lacks merit, or even novelty, but it does illustrate the hazards of applying Western labels and concepts uncritically to Chinese contexts. Pudong New District in Shanghai epitomized contracting-out for disabled care with more than 20 projects in 2012 and total expenditures exceeding ¥100 million. In Jiading, another district in Shanghai, spending on private care for the disabled surged from ¥1 million to ¥7 million between 2010 and 2012.[9]

In Shanghai, one of the world's most sophisticated cities, and a true standout city in China itself, local governments have the advantage of large, well-established, thoroughly capable private-sector counterparts. Dealing with such collaborators offers ample room for value-enhancing private discretion. In other sample cities, by contrast, private entities are newer, fewer, and less fully developed. These factors constrain delegation, and especially the complex form of delegation we call collaborative governance. In some cases, the level of funding seemed designed to repel private providers. In Xishui County, Hubei Province, the government subsidy for care for the disabled was ¥3,600 per person per year when we fielded the survey—far too low to support even low-quality operations.

Some Concluding Observations

Private engagement in Chinese social services five years ago, despite some remarkable achievements and many examples of great potential, remained embryonic in most realms and, where it did exist, was hedged about with constraints. With limited exceptions, potential private suppliers were few

9   Data from an interview with officials of the Jiading Association of the Disabled on June 7, 2012.

and unsophisticated, undercutting the appeal of delegation in the eyes of public officials. To complement the 17-community interview project, we conducted a separate survey of 318 local civil servants. Over 93 percent of them endorsed the prospect of greater private provision of publicly funded services in the future, a remarkable statistic given so few existing positive role models. Fewer than half as many of these officials, however, believed that *current* procurement practices in China were very successful. In the intervening years, as these findings suggest, some services have expanded collaboration, while others have not, and variation between localities remains pronounced.

Indeed, delegation remains a secondary counterpoint to today's dominant theme for social services: the state is taking on vastly more responsibilities. As such services become de-coupled from employment at public enterprises, China's government has quickly expanded its role in service provision and has increasingly emphasized the "public-ness" of social services. Such services are expected to offer equal access, guaranteed quality, reliable supply, and assured accountability. In many realms, of course, such as affordable housing or long-term care, the reality is far from the announced expectation.

In addressing the vast demand for expanded and enhanced social services, public responsibility, however, does not necessarily entail public provision. And public provision is highly unlikely to be able to meet the challenge. Admirably alert to these crucial points, China's central and local governments have begun to invite private engagement as they seek to sidestep the sterile debate over the size of the public sector that engages so much political debate in the West (Jing 2008, 2012).

Yet, for many social services, current capabilities fall short of aspirations. The Chinese government has never had the benefit of a well-developed market of private providers for some of these social services. This lack of a history of fruitful cross-sector interaction in social service areas has not prepared officials with the information, experience-nurtured intuition, and institutions required for true collaborations with shared discretion.[10]

Despite great potential, lofty ambitions, and sincerely expressed desires to do much more, the private role in Chinese social services delivery remains limited. One important constraint, of course, is the embryonic form of the private not-for-profit sector in China compared to countries in Europe and particularly the United States, where there are long traditions of social service provision through such organizations. Moreover, China's central authorities appear to harbor doubts about the authenticity and reliability

---

10   See Donahue, Eggleston, and Zeckhauser (2018). For a related discussion from earlier in China's reforms, see Whiting (1998).

of non-governmental organizations and their link to the touchy subject of civil society. Much of what has actually been accomplished in this realm in China owes less to policy pronouncements on high than to pragmatic improvisation by local governments who are actually on the line to arrange for the provision of services. Localities tend to adopt their own approaches to each service. What is surprising is the limited evidence for convergence on any standard delivery model across the localities studied.

We do note a weak and uneven tendency for private involvement in social services to be somewhat higher for both low-income *and* high-income locales and somewhat lower in the middle. One possible interpretation is that in less-developed cities, "delegation by default" occurs when the government lacks the necessary resources. At the other extreme (and perhaps best illustrated by the districts of Shanghai in our sample), local governments in more-developed areas delegate with conscious strategic intent, and have rich ecologies of private counterparts and the institutional capacities to oversee their effort, so as to permit experimentation with collaborative governance, in both simple and complex forms, as well as simple outsourcing. This theory that collaborative governance in China comes in two models, basic and sophisticated, may ultimately prove to be the driving force for today's pattern. Whether or not, a high degree of diversity in the earlier stages of policy development can pay dividends down the road. Best practices advance when the most promising approaches expand and proliferate, while less effective models wither. It is hard to imagine a larger or more fertile laboratory in this regard than today's China.

It is not surprising that both our customized survey and broader official statistics indicate that, at least to date, the private role in China's social services remains limited. One reason to expect this pattern is straightforward: social services are relatively hard to delegate. They tend to be complex, non-standard, and more resistant to definition, measurement, and monitoring than (for example) roads, bridges, or parks. Even in the United States—with its enthusiastic embrace of private-sector solutions and a long history of experimentation—the private role in social services remains constrained by the challenges of structuring collaborative relationships that meet acceptable standards of efficiency and accountability. These challenges can be overcome, of course; they frequently have been in the United States, and we are confident that they frequently will be in China. But it will take time, and the experience that accumulates with time, for this to occur.[11]

---

11   Jing and Hu (2017) provide examples of how contracting over time can evolve into collaborative governance in China, by fostering mutual trust and collaborative accountability.

A second factor inhibiting private social services is more specific to China and will require special efforts to loosen. Theory suggests, and international experience affirms, that for many and indeed most social services, *non*-profit private entities are more suitable providers than *for*-profit entities. The complexity of the services to be delivered in education, healthcare, elder care, and other sectors; the vulnerability of the clients; and the difficulty or impossibility of complete or current monitoring, make the high-powered incentive of the profit motive—such a beneficial force when well-harnessed—somewhat hazardous.

Non-profit organizations, by contrast, are prohibited by law from distributing net revenues to owners, and this non-distribution constraint (when rigorously enforced) severely restricts the scope for manipulation for private benefit. In addition, non-profits can often exploit the motive of mission as well as (or instead of) money to lower the cost, improve the impact, and minimize the management burden of providing social services. There certainly are successful examples of for-profit social services in the United States and elsewhere. But the non-profit model predominates, and generally outperforms in such areas as higher education, hospitals, and welfare services. So the domain of the private sector may increase substantially as China creates its own path to expanding the non-profit private sector (as it has by calling for expansion of non-profits in health and education; see the respective chapters in Donahue, Eggleston, and Zeckhauser [2018]).

One final note warrants emphasis, however. *Within* this limited domain of private involvement, we expect collaborative governance to be especially important. The extremes on the spectrum of discretion are where the constraints bind tightest. Contractual outsourcing, whereby government retains discretion and private agents simply do what they're paid to do, is constrained by the difficulty of writing sufficiently specified contracts for many social services. Voluntary philanthropy, where private parties advance the public good as they define it with little discretion for government, is constrained by the underdevelopment of the non-profit sector in general and philanthropy in particular. Thus we expect China to become a laboratory for that middle ground of collaborative governance, where the public and private sectors experiment with models of shared discretion for the delivery of social services. And the world will watch and learn.

References

Adams, Jennifer, and Emily Hannum. 2005. "Children's Social Welfare in China, 1989-1997: Access to Health Insurance and Education." *China Quarterly* 181 (March): 100–21.

Bloomberg. 2017. "In China, Public-Private Partnerships Are Really Public-Public." February 27, 2017. https://www.bloomberg.com/news/articles/2017-02-27/in-china-public-private-partnerships-are-really-public-public.

Brown, Trevor, Ting Gong, and Yijia Jing. 2012. "Collaborative Governance in Mainland China and Hong Kong: Introductory Essay." *International Public Management Journal* 15 (4): 393–404.

Cook, Sarah. 2011. "Global Discourses, National Policies, Local Outcomes: Reflections on China's Welfare Reforms." In *China's Changing Welfare Mix: Local Perspectives*, edited by Beatriz Carillo and Jane Duckett, 211–22. New York, NY: Routledge.

Croll, Elisabeth J. 1999. "Social Welfare Reform: Trends and Tensions." *China Quarterly* 159 (1): 684–99.

CPCCC (Caizheng bu zhengfu he shehui ziben hezuo zhongxin [China Public Private Partnerships Center]). 2019. "National PPP Comprehensive Information Platform Project Management Database." Last updated September 25, 2019. http://www.cpppc.org:8082/efmisweb/ppp/projectLibrary/toPPPMapEng.do.

CPCCC. 2016a. "Analysis Report on the Third Batch of Demonstration Projects." November 4. http://www.cpppc.org/en/NationalDemonstration/4686.jhtml.

CPCCC. 2016b. "Circular on Further Advancing the Public-Private Partnership in Public Services."

Donahue, John D., and Richard J. Zeckhauser. 2011. *Collaborative Governance: Private Roles for Public Goals in Turbulent Times*. Princeton: Princeton University Press.

Donahue, John D., Karen Eggleston, and Richard J. Zeckhauser. 2018. *Private Roles for Public Goals in China and the United States*. Unpublished book manuscript.

Duckett, Jane. 2011. *The Chinese State's Retreat from Health: Policy and the Politics of Retrenchment*. New York: Routledge.

Eggers, William D., and Paul Macmillan. 2013. *The Solution Revolution: How Government, Business, and Civil Society Are Teaming up to Solve Society's Toughest Problems*. Boston: Harvard Business School Press.

Eggleston, Karen. Forthcoming. "Demographic Challenges: Healthcare and Elder Care." In *Fateful Decisions: Choices That Will Shape China's Future*, edited by Thomas Fingar and Jean C. Oi. Stanford, CA: Stanford University Press.

Eggleston, Karen, Jean Oi, and Yiming Wang. 2017. *Challenges in the Process of China's Urbanization*. Stanford, CA: Shorenstein Asia-Pacific Research Center.

Eggleston, Karen, Jean C. Oi, Scott Rozelle, Ang Sun, Andrew Walder, and Xueguang Zhou. 2013. "Will Demographic Change Slow China's Rise?" *Journal of Asian Studies* 72 (3): 505–18

Fewsmith, Joseph. 2006. "Promotion of Qiu He Raises Questions about Direction of Reform." China Leadership Monitor No. 17. https://www.hoover.org/research/promotion-qiu-he-raises-questions-about-direction-reform.

Francis, Corinna-Barbara. 2001. "Quasi-Public, Quasi-Private Trends in Emerging Market Economies: The Case of China." *Comparative Politics* 33 (3): 275–94.

Guess, George M., and Jun Ma. 2015. "The Risks of Chinese Subnational Debt for Public Financial Management." *Public Administration and Development* 35 (2): 128–39.

Hannum, Emily, Jere Behrman, Meiyan Wang, and Jihong Liu. 2008. "Education in the Reform Era." In *China's Great Economic Transformation*, edited by Loren Brandt and Thomas G. Rawksi , 215–49. Cambridge and New York: Cambridge University Press.

Jing, Yijia. 2008. "Outsourcing in China: An Exploratory Assessment." *Public Administration and Development* 28 (2): 119–28.

Jing, Yijia. 2012. "From Stewards to Agents? A Case of Intergovernmental Management of Public-Nonprofit Partnership in China." *Public Performance and Management Review* 36 (2): 230–52.

Jing, Yijia. 2015. "Between Control and Empowerment: Governmental Strategies Towards the Development of the Non-Profit Sector in China." *Asian Studies Review* 39 (4): 589–608.

Jing, Yijia, and Yefei Hu. 2017. "From Service Contracting to Collaborative Governance: Evolution of Government–Nonprofit Relations." *Public Administration and Development* 37 (3): 191–202.

Jing, Yijia, and E. S. Savas. 2009. "Managing Collaborative Service Delivery: Comparing China and the United States." *Public Administration Review* 69: S101–07.

National Bureau of Statistics of China. 2012. *China Statistical Yearbook 2012*. Beijing: China Statistical Press.

Oi, Jean Chun. 1995. "The Role of the Local State in China's Transitional Economy." *China Quarterly* 144 (December): 1132–49.

Osborne, David, and Ted Gaebler. 1993. *Reinventing Government: How the Entrepreneurial Spirit Is Transforming the Public Sector*. New York: Plume Publishing.

Peng, Xizhe. 2011. "China's Demographic History and Future Challenges." *Science* 333 (6042): 581–87.

Whiting, Susan H. 1998. "The Mobilization of Private Investment as a Problem of Trust in Local Governance Structures." In *Trust and Governance*, edited by Valerie Braithwaite and Margaret Levi, 167–93. New York: Russell Sage Foundation.

Wong, Christine. 1991. "Central–Local Relations in an Era of Fiscal Decline: The Paradox of Fiscal Decentralization in Post-Mao China." *China Quarterly* 128 (1991): 691–715.

Wong, Christine. 2016. "Budget Reform in China: Progress and Prospects in the Xi Jinping Era." *OECD Journal on Budgeting* 15 (3): 27–46.

13 Cancer, Disparities, and Public-Private Roles

Karen Eggleston, Jui-fen Rachel Lu, Christina Ping, and
Nancy Hanzhuo Zhang

I n societies and economies well into the epidemiological and demographic
transitions, cancer is one of the leading causes of death and a major
focus of health policy for extending healthy life expectancy. Cancer also
epitomizes many of the challenges of healthy aging, because although it is
one of the most prominent "chronic" diseases, many cancers are caused by
infection, highlighting the lingering effects of social determinants of health
and associated disparities. Screening programs have varied effectiveness in
diverse groups. Moreover, case-fatality rates are high and treatment can be
very expensive, challenging patients, families, and health systems to finance
therapies, often at the cutting edge of "personalized medicine" (see chapter
5 in this volume for the case of Japan). This chapter provides a case study
of how middle- and high-income economies in Asia with differing health
systems—ranging from rural communities covered by voluntary basic medical insurance in the People's Republic of China (PRC), to high-income cities
such as Guangzhou and Taipei—have been trying to address disparities in
the incidence of different cancers and access to treatment, with a discussion
of public and private roles in financing and delivery.

For the Taiwan portion of this study, we thank Ying Isabel Chen, Pin-Sung Peter Liu, and
Andrew Lee for excellent research assistance; the Stanford Asia Health Policy Program,
National Bureau of Economic Research, Taiwan Ministry of Science and Technology
(MOST105-2410-H-182 -017 -MY2, MOST107-2410-H-182-014-MY3), and Chang
Gung Memorial Hospital and Chang Gung University (BMRP285) for research funding;
and Health and Welfare Data Science Center, Ministry of Health and Welfare (HWDC,
MOHW), and Research Services Center for Health Information, Chang Gung University,
for data analysis support.

The first section overviews the epidemiology of cancer in this region, especially the prevalence of infection-caused cancers and their disproportionate burden on rural residents. We then discuss public and private roles in the gamut of policies to address the personal and social implications of cancer, from personalized medicine discovery, to family and taxpayer financing of care, to the range of ownership of providers. Finally, we discuss recent developments in enhancing access to cancer treatments in the PRC, and remaining challenges for which public and private sectors each have their roles in finding paths forward.

The Epidemiology of Cancer in Chinese

Cancer is a leading cause of morbidity and premature mortality for Chinese, both for those in rural parts of the PRC, along with urban residents, such as those in Shanghai, Hong Kong, Macao, Taiwan, Southeast Asia, or indeed in other parts of the world, such as among Chinese Americans. This section provides an overview of that epidemiology, focusing mostly on the PRC.

Today in China, the top 10 most common causes of death include multiple forms of cancer, with lung, liver, stomach, and esophageal cancers each ranking fourth, sixth, seventh, and tenth, respectively (Institute for Health Metrics and Evaluation 2017). Cancer's prominence as a public health concern in China has risen over the years as the competing risks of other causes of death (such as from communicable diseases) have subsided as a result of improvements in sanitation and advancements in medical technology. Consequently, the primary diseases the country deals with today are conditions often considered ailments of aging: cancer, stroke, Alzheimer's, or ischemic heart disease, the latter three of which were responsible for 16.24%, 20.19%, and 4.69% of all deaths in 2017, respectively (Institute for Health Metrics and Evaluation 2017).

However, such developments in living standards have not necessarily been uniformly distributed across the country. Vast in size and heterogeneously diverse in its makeup, China bears a "double burden": on one hand, rapidly urbanized cities are wracked with the diseases of old age; on the other, rural, underdeveloped regions of the country still find themselves battling infection and communicable diseases. Lying at the intersection of these two epidemiological burdens are infection-based cancers. A study examining infection-related cancer in 13 principal Asian countries found that the percentages of cancer incidence attributable to infection were 19.7% and 19.5% in men and women, respectively, and mortality at 21.9% and 22.1% (Huang et al. 2015). According to the American Cancer Society's Cancer

Atlas, 26.1% of all cancer cases in China are due to infection. The three cancers with the largest proportion of cases attributable to infection are liver (77% of all diagnosed cases), stomach (90%), and cervix (nearly 100%) (American Cancer Society 2014).

Two key trends can be seen among these infection-based cancers in China: (1) geographic disparities between urban and rural patients in terms of incidence and mortality; (2) the subsequent adoption of screening and prevention programs by the Chinese government in order to combat the diseases.

Liver cancer

The hepatitis B virus (HBV) and hepatitis C virus (HCV) both result in viral hepatitis, a type of liver infection; chronic infections increase a person's chance of liver cancer. Unfortunately, China is home to the world's largest burden of HBV, the virus that is the more common cause of cancer among the two. In 2013, 93 million Chinese people carried the infection, associated with 250,000–300,000 HBV liver cancer deaths every year (Center for Global Development 2016). Currently, there only exists a vaccine to protect against HBV infection. In response to the financial barriers that kept this vaccine out of reach for those residing in China's poorer regions, the government has run an HBV prevention campaign since 1992 to administer the vaccine to these populations. As a result of these efforts, approximately 3.8 million chronic HBV infections were prevented between 2003 and 2009 in program areas, thereby avoiding an estimated 680,000 future deaths from HBV infection (Center for Global Development 2016).

New liver cancer diagnoses in China account for 55% of the world's annual total, and the mortality rate of liver cancer makes it the second-most deadly cancer in the nation (after lung cancer) (Yan 2018). Fan et al. (2013) estimate that HBV infection is responsible for 65.9% of liver cancer deaths in men and 58.4% in women. This is in comparison to the 23.4% and 2.2% (in men and women, respectively) of deaths that are attributed to alcohol consumption, another common risk factor for liver cancer.

As a condition predicated upon infection, it is unsurprising that disparities exist between urban and rural areas in China in incidence and mortality rates of liver cancer. These disparities can be traced to differences in sanitation, living standards, and disease prevention measures. The mortality rate for liver cancer is much higher in rural areas than in urban areas, although rural residents have exhibited larger declines in recent years (figure 13.1). Broadly, liver cancer mortality is relatively low and stable in younger age cohorts, then exhibits an explosive growth in midlife, before finally decelerating or leveling off by old age. However, the decreasing trend is observed earlier in urban birth cohorts than in rural ones, indicating that rural patients are at an increased risk for liver cancer for a longer duration of their lives. As shown in table 13.1, there are substantial differences in mortality rate between male and female patients, and between urban and rural regions, with a decline in mortality over time. In rural areas, liver cancer has become the leading cause of death among cancers, with a mortality rate of 36.58 (or 28.17 due to HBV) per 100,000 in men and 11.65 (or 8.97 due to HBV) per 100,000 in women; in urban areas, it is the second leading cause of death at a rate of 30.97 (or 23.85 due to HBV) in men and 10.22 (or 7.87 due to HBV) in women (Chen and Zhang 2011).

FIGURE 13.1 Disparities in Chinese mortality rates for infection-based liver cancer, urban vs. rural, 1991–2014

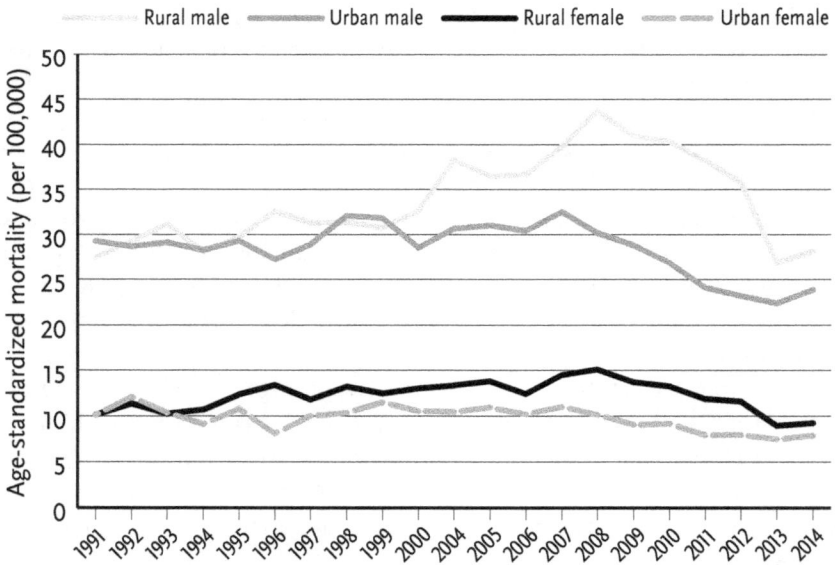

TABLE 13.1 Crude mortality rates (per 100,000) for liver cancer in China, 1990–92 and 2004

Province	Male		Female	
	1990–92	2004	1990–92	2004
Anhui	28.7	—	11.9	—
Beijing	18.9	24.1	8.5	9.35
Fujian	41.2		13.9	
Changle	—	28.67	—	8.35
Gansu	25.0	—	12.6	—
Guangdong	35.2	—	10.7	—
Guangzhou*	—	39.05	—	12.6
Shenzhen	—	12.46	—	2.78
Guangxi	41.8	—	11.7	—
Fusui	—	92.3	—	17.29
Guizhou	14.5	—	4.7	—
Hainan	32.8	—	6.6	—
Hebei	24.2	—	10.3	—
Cixian	—	32.31	—	12.9
Heilongjiang	33.1	—	16.6	—
Harbin*	—	29.09	—	11.37
Henan	22.6	—	11.5	—
Linzhou	—	10.43	—	6.17
Hubei	26.1	—	8.9	—
Wuhan*	—	26.3	—	10.18
Hunan	19.5	—	7.3	—
Inner Mongolia	21.9	—	8.9	—
Jiangsu	52.4	—	20.7	—
Qidong	—	117.08	—	39.06
Haimen	—	97.8	—	25.24
Yangzhong	—	52.59	—	36.4
Jiangxi	23.1	—	8.2	—
Jilin	33.3	—	11.5	—
Liaoning	28.3	—	11.3	—
Shenyang*	—	29.4	—	12.77
Ningxia	18.1	—	6.8	—
Shaanxi	24.7	—	10.8	—
Shandong	30.2	—	12.8	—
Linqu	—	39.01	—	16.76
Shanghai	39.7	33.59	16.3	13.39
Shanxi	21.4	—	11.7	—
Sichuan	26.3	—	9.1	—
Chongqing*	—	31.03	—	12.77
Yanting	—	60.92	—	24.97
Tianjin	21.5	13.22	8.7	8.39
Yunan	13.7	—	6.2	—
Zhejiang	34.9	—	128.0	—
Hangzhou*	—	38.09	—	14.21
Jiashan	—	45.35	—	16.78

SOURCE: Chen and Zhang 2011.
NOTE: *Urban areas; italicized place names are cities/towns belonging to the province above.

Stomach cancer

As one of the few cancers caused by a bacterium, stomach cancer arises from *Helicobacter pylori*, a pathogen known to cause stomach ulcers. *H. pylori* is most commonly transmitted through the fecal-oral route, such as through contaminated food or water sources, or from one person to another via mouth to mouth; thus, it is particularly problematic in areas of the world with low sanitation and hygiene, such as rural China. Using 2012 data, approximately 64.91 percent of all gastric cancer deaths were due to *H. pylori* (Huang et al. 2015).

In 2014, there were approximately 410,000 new cases of stomach cancer documented in China, accounting for 10.79 percent of all cancer cases (Yang et al. 2018). Using the Chinese standard population, this translates to an age-standardized incidence rate (ASIRC) of 19.62 per 100,000, with a marked difference between rural and urban areas (ASIRC of 22.82 vs. 17.29 per 100,000, respectively) (Yang et al. 2018). Evidence suggests that 90 percent of all stomach cancers are infection-based in cause (American Cancer Society 2014). Overall, stomach cancer incidence rates in rural parts of the country have been found to be 1.3 times higher than those in urban areas (Yang et al. 2018).

An often-noted characteristic of the disease is its disproportionate presentation between the two genders; from the age of 45 onward, rates among men are significantly higher than those among women. It has been found that the incidence sex ratio for males to females is 2.4, indicating that Chinese men are at more than double the risk of stomach cancer (Yang et al. 2018).

Unfortunately, stomach cancer has a high case-fatality rate, and the patterns of age-specific mortality rates closely mirror the age-specific incidence rates. In 2014, estimates count approximately 293,800 stomach-cancer-associated deaths occurring in China, amounting to 12.80 percent of all cancer-related deaths. The age-standardized mortality rate of stomach cancer that year was 16.12 per 100,000 and 11.51 per 100,000 in rural and urban areas, respectively (14.51 per 100,000 and 10.36 per 100,000 for infection-based stomach cancer mortality rates in rural and urban areas, respectively) (Yang et al. 2018).

In recent years, national stomach cancer incidence rates in China have been declining, a positive trend for healthy aging that experts have attributed to a "reduction in the prevalence of *H. pylori*, improvements in sanitation and in the preservation and storage of foods and increasing consumption of fresh fruit and vegetables" (Yang et al. 2018). However, the prognosis for patients diagnosed with stomach cancer in China remains poor, with a five-year relative survival rate of 35.9% between 2010 and 2014. This is in stark contrast with the higher survival rates observed in South Korea (68.9%) and Japan (60.3%) during this same four-year period (Yang et al. 2018).

Cervical cancer

Almost all cases of cervical cancer are caused by the human papilloma virus (HPV), a virus that is primarily passed through sexual contact. Research has identified at least a dozen types known to cause cancer, with HPV-16 and HPV-18 being the most prevalent among the Chinese population. Additionally, HPV prevalence within patient tumor samples appears to increase as lesions progressed to higher grades. Fortunately, although most sexually active people are infected with at least one type of HPV at some point in their lives, most do not develop cancer as a result of the infection. At the current moment, there is no direct treatment available for HPV itself, though a vaccine (Gardasil 9) has been developed which confers immunity to up to 90 percent of the HPVs that can cause cervical cancer (Li 2017).

Cervical cancer ranks as the eighth-most common cancer among Chinese women, and second-most common among women between the ages of 15 and 44. The related disease burden in China has increased drastically in recent years; the national incidence of cervical cancer swelled 200 percent, from 3.8 per 100,000 people in 2003 to 11.4 per 100,000 in 2012 (Di 2017). During this same period, the national mortality rate also grew by 116.7 percent (Di 2017). In 2013, there were 100,700 new cases and 26,400 documented deaths due to cervical cancer (Song et al. 2017).

As was observed with the previous two cancers, this urban versus rural divide characterizes cervical cancer outcomes as well. Whereas the age-standardized incidence rate in urban areas was 11.12 per 100,000, and the mortality rate was 3.85 per 100,000, these numbers were 11.47 per 100,000 and 4.14 per 100,000, respectively, in rural China (Song et al. 2017). Unlike other cancers, cervical cancer presents in younger patients, with incidence reaching a peak at age ≥ 45 years (34.24 per 100,000) and ≥ 50 years (32.05 per 100,000) in rural areas (Song et al. 2017). Age-specific mortality rates of cervical cancer in urban areas are lower than those in rural areas between the ages of 55 to 75 (Song et al. 2017).

To reduce the cancer burden and address disparities, Chinese authorities have implemented HPV prevention and screening, with a program targeting rural women. These efforts led to increased diagnosis and awareness of the disease. Between 2012 and 2014, 31.20 million rural women aged 35–64 received free cervical cancer screenings, with 13 provinces (41.9 percent of all provinces) carrying out cervical cancer screening in their entire province (Di 2017). However, while such efforts have positively impacted these communities, they have only been able to capture 19.99 percent of the entire at-risk population (Di 2017).

Breast cancer

Cancers of the lung and female breast are the leading types worldwide in terms of the number of new cases. Breast cancer is the most commonly diagnosed cancer in women (24.2 percent, i.e., about one in four of all new cancer cases diagnosed in women worldwide are breast cancer), and the cancer is the most common in 154 of the 185 countries included in the Global Cancer statistics (GlobalCan) published by the International Agency for Research on Cancer in 2018 (IARC 2019). More specifically, 2,088,849 new cases were diagnosed in 2018, contributing about 11.6% of the total cancer incidence burden. Breast cancer is also the leading cause of cancer deaths in women (15.0%), followed by lung cancer (13.8%) and colorectal cancer (9.5%). Looking at the regional distribution of breast cancer cases in 2018, Australia and New Zealand have the highest breast cancer incidence rate, i.e., 94.2 per 100,000, followed by Western Europe and Northern Europe with respectively 92.6 and 90.1 per 100,000.[1] The mortality rate for breast cancer is the highest in Melanesia and Polynesia,[2] with respectively 25.5 and 21.6 per 100,000 (IARC 2019).

More specifically in China, 367,900 new cases of breast cancer arose— 8.6% of all cancer cases or 19.2% of new cancer cases among women—in 2018 (IARC 2019; WHO 2019). More alarmingly, mortality-to-incidence ratios of breast cancer are higher in Asia than in Western countries.

In order to develop or identify an effective policy model that targets breast cancer, we next turn to a successful approach taken in Taiwan as a comparative case study for Chinese women living in a high-income economy in the region.

In Taiwan, between 1960 and 1990, breast cancer mortality rates doubled. More recently, in 2009–12, female breast cancer in Taiwan accounted for 16.49% of use and 27.18% of costs for targeted therapies. Starting from 2004, Taiwan has provided nationwide free biennial mammographic screening. A total of 2,392,789 consecutive screening mammography exams were

---

1   These incidence rates and mortality rates are age standardized.

2   Melanesia and Polynesia are subregions of Oceania; the former includes, among other countries, Papua New Guinea, Fiji, the Solomon Islands, and Vanuatu; the latter consists of more than 1,000 islands throughout the central and southern Pacific.

performed for women aged 50–69 years (2006–09) and 45–69 years (from December 2009 onward)—33.2% of the target population in 2013–14. Overall, the cancer detection rate (CDR) and cancer incidence rate (CIR) have increased from 3.94% and 4.8% to 4.71% and 5.71%. The sensitivity of the mammography is slightly lower than the American College of Radiology's recommended level (>85%), but the overall quality outcome of the screening program was decent (Pan et al. 2014). Taiwan has also increased organized financing and reduced patient burden for treatment and moved to finance target therapy for both poor and rich by including it within the National Health Insurance (NHI) benefit package.

In the next section, we continue the Taiwan case study of breast cancer as we discuss the varied public and private roles in addressing cancer.

Public and Private Roles, from Financing to Delivery

As a "dread disease," cancer inspires fear and social pressures for innovation in prevention and treatment. Both the public and private sectors play a role in policies for healthy aging to reduce the burden of cancer. For example, in almost all economies, private firms take the lead in drug discovery and therapy development, including conventional biomedicine, traditional Chinese medicine (discussed more in the section on the essential medication system, below), and new molecularly targeted therapies. In the PRC, corporatized state-owned enterprises also play a large role in the evolving biotechnology sector. Governments in turn regulate the sector and approve therapies before they are allowed to be given to patients. Governments also often promote innovative public-private approaches to enhance innovation and/or improve access to therapies.

China launched a precision medicine initiative in 2016 with over US$9 billion in funding, and other countries in the region also aim to become global leaders in the field. Continuing our focus on breast cancer treatments as an example, the first biosimilar to Herceptin, developed by Biocon and Mylan, received market authorization in India in 2013; and biosimilar Herzuma, produced by the South Korean biotech company Celltrion, was approved by the Korean Ministry of Food and Drug Safety in 2014 (Lu, Eggleston, and Chang 2019). Private-sector developments in cancer therapies also frequently cross national boundaries. For example, the Korean firm Alteogen contracted with a Chinese firm, Qilu, in the process of developing another Herceptin biosimilar (Park 2017).

The private and public sector roles in cancer prevention and control extend beyond the biomedical industry. Individuals and households make decisions about vaccination, lifestyle (e.g., smoking), and participation in screening, although many factors (e.g., environmental exposure) lie outside their control. Patients and their families also bear a large share of the economic burden from cancer, including direct and indirect costs of treatment, caregivers' time, and difficult trade-offs when expensive therapies must be paid for out of their own pockets.

The public sector steps in to help patients in health systems with universal coverage. Taiwan has adopted a single-payer system for residents since 1995, including cancer treatments with no copayments. The NHI administration is the sole responsible entity for paying the cancer treatment fees—cancer patients pay zero copayments under this health insurance. NHI finances treatment from compulsory payroll taxes, as well as a supplementary tax introduced in 2013 and levied on six categories of non-payroll income. Other funding sources include direct government subsidies (25 percent) and employer contributions (38 percent). The NHI offers comprehensive service coverage and complete freedom of choice, that is, all patients are free to use any provider of choice.

In high-income economies with communicable disease well under control and people living longer, more people survive other causes of death to go on to develop cancer. In recent years, the increasing number of cancer patients in Taiwan has caused NHI's expenditures for cancer treatments to increase significantly. According to the overall mean annual growth rate, the medical care expenditure on cancer patients has grown by 5.4%, drug costs by 6.6%, and the number of patients by 4.9% (National Health Insurance Administration 2016).

Public financing of health insurance spreads these costs across taxpayers and helps patients obtain access to care. The organization of the health system also matters for the sustainability of affordable care. In Taiwan (and in many other single-payer or other universal health coverage systems), the increasing burden in costs could be alleviated to some extent by the market power of the public purchaser—the monopoly and monopsony power of NHI in Taiwan. Indeed, as a single payer, NHI enjoys direct savings due to its market power. For some cancers, NHI requires drug companies to cover the costs of companion diagnostic tests in exchange for a better NHI reimbursement rate for the therapy (Lu, Eggleston, and Chang 2019). The NHI's operational efficiency is also enhanced through a universal, uniform claim filing system that substantially reduces administrative costs and achieves economies of scale. The single-payer system also offers the information and tools to effectively manage healthcare costs through a stringent claim review process, avoiding large shifts in costs and adverse selection.[3]

However, even a strong government purchaser cannot erase the life-course implications of social disparities. Despite its universal health coverage, there remain concerns about geographical and income disparities in Taiwan. A case study, specifically looking at the impact of NHI coverage on HER2-positive breast cancer in Taiwan in the period 2004–15, studies Taiwan's policy response. The results show that NHI coverage of target therapy is pro-poor even before coverage of the companion diagnostic test. Although lower-income patients are more likely to be diagnosed with later stages of breast cancer, they also receive coverage of the target therapy designed for metastatic cancer, outweighing the presumed previous access advantage of the rich (Lu, Eggleston, and Chang 2019).

A final dimension of public and private roles in cancer treatment—and other challenges of healthy aging—lies in the ownership of health service providers. Many health systems feature a mix of ownership forms for clinics and hospitals, with a differing balance of public and private. For example, Taiwan's system has a large share of private providers, while in most provinces of the PRC the role of government-owned hospitals remains dominant, especially among urban tertiary-care hospitals. Figure 13.2 shows the distribution of hospitals by organizational form for breast cancer patients in Taiwan in the period 2004–15, while figure 13.3 shows the rate of admissions to private hospitals for all patients seeking inpatient care in China between 2011 and 2016.

Another growing area of public-private collaboration in China is in innovative service modalities, including telemedicine and e-health services. In an effort to reduce costs and boost the overall efficiency of its medical system in coming decades, the nation has been expanding its telemedicine/e-healthcare services and resources—including in controversial areas such as facial scanning of physicians and patients—and the government has been fleshing out relevant regulation (e.g., State Council 2018a).

We next return to our specific focus on cancer to examine how China's authorities are trying to make cancer treatments more affordable through subsidized health insurance schemes and other policies.

---

3   See Lu and Eggleston (2018) and Lu et al. (2019) for further details.

FIGURE 13.2 Main care hospitals for breast cancer patients in Taiwan, by type, 2004–15

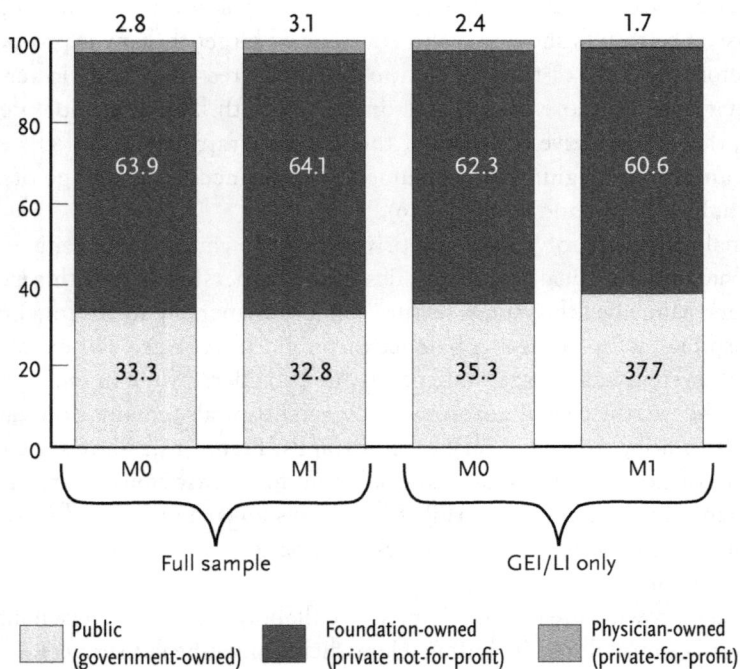

SOURCE: Analysis of patient-level data for 2004–15 by Eggleston and Lu, based on NHI claims data as described in Lu, Eggleston, and Chang (2019).

NOTE: M0 = No metastasis (i.e., no evidence at time of diagnosis that the cancer had traveled to other parts of the body); M1 = metastatic breast cancer; GEI = government employee insurance; LI = labor insurance; "Full" means the full sample including both GEI and LI sample patients.

FIGURE 13.3 Rate of inpatient admissions to private hospitals by province, PRC, 2011–16

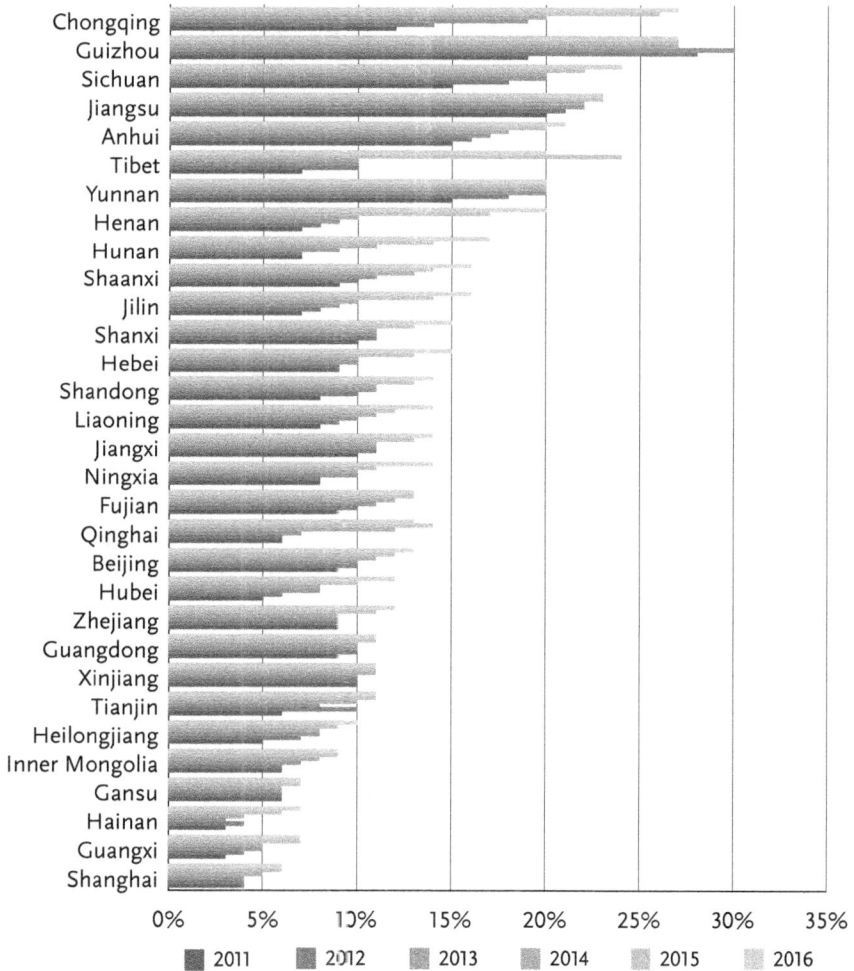

SOURCE: Authors' compilation of data from PRC Health Statistical Yearbooks, various years.

Making Cancer Treatment More Affordable: Recent Developments

China's cancer rates have increased, driven mostly by reduction in competing risks (e.g., lower infant and under-five mortality, control of other communicable diseases), continued heavy male smoking, other unhealthy lifestyles, and exposure to pollution.

To make cancer drugs more affordable, new anti-cancer drugs were added to China's public medical insurance system in November 2018, as noted in Xi Jinping's New Year's speech at the end of 2018 (CGTN America 2018).

The National Healthcare Security Administration (Guojia yiliao baozhang ju, or NHSA), which was set up in 2018 and which consolidated a number of related functions and roles, negotiated with domestic and international pharmaceutical companies to lower prices, with the new reimbursements scheduled for review in November 2020 (EIU 2018). Of course, patients still bear deductibles and copayments according to their insurance coverage (which is more generous for formal sector employees, and more limited for voluntary insurance programs for urban non-employed and rural residents).

The prices of the 17 newly covered drugs have reportedly fallen by 57 percent on average compared to the average retail price. According to Xiong Xianping, an NHSA division director, 2018 purchases of these drugs came to ¥562 million, a savings of ¥918 million compared to pre-negotiation prices. A total of 44,600 people received reimbursements for those 17 drugs in 2018 (Wu 2019).

Additional endeavors have been undertaken by the government to make medical treatment more affordable. The country is trying to open up its market to more innovative cancer medicines. In May, the government lifted import tariffs on 103 of the 138 anti-cancer drugs available on the market, and also lifted the value-added tax levied on these drugs. Of the 103 drugs affected, 82 are included in the government's basic medical insurance programs. More tariff cuts kicked in at the start of 2018 (Stanway and Perry 2018). Furthermore, 18 new anti-cancer drugs were approved by the National Medical Products Administration and made available immediately on the market, compared to seven in the previous year. These included new drugs from overseas markets, as well as some products from Chinese companies. The average approval time has also been expedited from 24 to 12 months, boosting the availability of more "innovative" cures (Wu 2019).

Conclusion

Cancer provides a lens for understanding the many pressing challenges for societies and economies adjusting the financing and delivery of healthcare to the demographic and epidemiological reality of longer lives and older population age structures. Healthy aging begins early in the life course with immunization and protection against infections that cause cancer, and continues with public and private organizations influencing prevention, control, screening, treatment, and end-of-life care. Policymakers must continually seek evidence to help improve health system financing mechanisms, update insurance coverage, and enhance health service access and responsiveness in caring for their many citizens impacted by cancer. The examples we have discussed provide a window into how health systems have been grappling with these challenges.

References

American Cancer Society. 2014. "Many of the Most Common Cancers Are Attributable to Infection." Accessed May 4, 2019. http://cancerat-las.cancer.org/risk-factors/infection/.

Barber, Sarah L., Baobin Huang, Budiono Santoso, Richard Laing, Valerie Paris, and Chunfu Wu. 2013. "The Reform of the Essential Medicines System in China: A Comprehensive Approach to Universal Coverage." *Journal of Global Health* 3 (1): 010303.

Cai, Muyu, Yanping Li, Senmao Dai, and Chaoxian Lin. 2017. "Investigation on Implementation of National Essential Medicine System in Primary Health Care Institutions of Shantou Region." [In Chinese.] *Evaluation and Analysis of Drug Use in Hospitals of China* 17 (2): 254–56.

Center for Global Development. 2016. "Reducing Cancer Risk in China." http://millionssaved.cgdev.org/case-studies/reducing-cancer-risk-in-china.

CCCPC (Central Committee of the Communist Party of China). 2016. Zhonghua Renmin "Gongheguo guomin jingji he shehui fazhan di shisan ge wunian guihua gangyao" [The 13th five-year plan for economic and social development of the People's Republic of China]. http://www.china.com.cn/lianghui/news/2016-03/17/content_3805301. htm.

Chen, Jian Guo, and Si Wei Zhang. 2011. "Liver Cancer Epidemic in China: Past, Present and Future." *Seminars in Cancer Biology* 21 (1): 59–69.

CGTN America. 2018. "Full Text: 2019 New Year Speech by President Xi Jinping." December 31. https://america.cgtn.com/2018/12/31/full-text-2019-new-year-speech-by-president-xi-jinping.

Di, Jiangli. 2017. "Opportunities and Challenges in Cervical Cancer Screening Program in China: SWOT Analysis for Implementation of Program." *Quality in Primary Care* 25 (5): 282–88.

Dong, C., and Y. Song. 2009. "Impacts of Different Insurance Schemes on Non-Communicable Diseases Services Utilization." World Bank, Beijing .

EIU (Economist Intelligence Unit). 2018. "China to Add to Its Essential Drugs List." *Economist*, September 6, 2018. http://www.eiu.com/industry/article/1627163346/china-to-add-to-its-essential-drugs-list /2018-09-06.

Fan, Jian-Hu, Jian-Bing Wang, Yong Jiang, Wang Xiang, Hao Liang, Wen-Qiang Wei, You-Lin Qiao, and Paolo Boffetta. 2013. "Attributable Causes of Liver Cancer Mortality and Incidence in China." *Asian Pacific Journal of Cancer Prevention* 14 (12): 7251–56.

He, Jiangjiang, Mi Tang, Ziping Ye, Xiaotong Jiang, Duo Chen, Peipei Song, and Chunlin Jin. 2018. "China Issues the National Essential Medicines List (2018 Edition): Background, Differences from Previous Editions, and Potential Issues." *BioScience Trends* 12 (5): 445–49.

Huang, He, Xiao-Feng Hu, Fang-Hui Zhao, Suzanne M. Garland, Neerja Bhatla, and You-Lin Qiao. 2015. "Estimation of Cancer Burden Attributable to Infection in Asia." *Journal of Epidemiology* 25 (10): 626–38.

IARC (International Agency for Research on Cancer, World Health Organization). 2019. "The Global Cancer Observatory. Global Cancer Statistics (GlobalCan)." http://gco.iarc.fr/today/home and https://gco.iarc.fr/today/data/factsheets/cancers/20-Breast-fact-sheet.pdf.

Institute for Health Metrics and Evaluation. 2017. "Global Burden of Disease—China." Accessed May 5, 2019. http://www.healthdata.org/china.

Li, Shadow. 2017. "In HK, Women Must Wait for Vaccine against HPV." *China Daily Hong Kong*, November 3, 2017. https://www.chinadailyhk.com/articles/188/147/174/1509693260205.html.

Liu, D., and Z. Yu. 2017. "The Status and Effect Study of the Policy Implementation of Essential Drug in Chinese City Community Health Institutions." [In Chinese]. *China Practical Medicine* 12: 182–83.

Lu, Jui-fen Rachel, Karen Eggleston, and Joseph Tung-Chieh Chang. 2019. "Economic Dimensions of Personalized and Precision Medicine in Asia: Evidence from Breast Cancer Treatment in Taiwan." In *Economic Dimensions of Personalized and Precision Medicine*, edited by Ernst R. Berndt, Danan P. Goldman, and John W. Rowe. Chicago: University of Chicago Press.

Lu, Jui-fen Rachel, and Karen Eggleston. 2018. "Organizational Form and Provider Incentives in Cancer Care: Evidence from Breast Cancer Target Therapy in Taiwan." Presentation at the EuHEA health economics conference, part of organized session "Service Delivery Organizational Forms of Chronic Care and Net Value: Evidence from Europe and East Asia." July 14, 2018.

National Health Commission of the People's Republic of China. 2009. "Notice on Issuance of the Opinions on Establishment of a National Essential Medicines System." [In Chinese.]

National Health Insurance Administration. 2016. "Targeted Drugs Intro-
duced by NHI to Benefit Cancer Patients." Ministry of Health and
Wealthfare, October 12, 2016. https://www.nhi.gov.tw/english/News_
Content.aspx?n=996D1B4B5DC48343&sms=F0EAFEB716DE7F-
FA&s=49450AC9AB9E173C.

NHSA (National Healthcare Security Administration, China). 2018.
"Guojia yiliao baozhang ju guanyu jiang 17 zhong kang ai yao naru
guojia jiben yiliao baoxian, gongshang baoxian he shengyu baoxian
yaopin mulu yi lei fanwei de tongzhi" [National Healthcare Security
Administration notice on the inclusion of 17 anticancer drugs in
national basic medical insurance, work injury insurance, and maternity insurance drug catalogs in the range of category B]. Notice no.
17, October 10, 2018. http://www.gov.cn/xinwen/2018-10/10/con-
tent_5328891.htm.

OECD (Organisation for Economic Cooperation and Development).
2008. *Pharmaceutical Pricing Policies in a Global Market*. Paris:
OECD.

Pan, Huay-Ben, Kam-Fai Wong, Tsung-Lung Yang, Giu-Cheng Hsu,
Chen-Pin Chou, Jer-Shyung Huang, San-Kan Lee, Yi-Hong Chou,
Chia-Ling Chiang, and Huei-Lung Liang. 2014. "The Outcome of a
Quality-Controlled Mammography Screening Program: Experience
from a Population-Based Study in Taiwan." *Journal of the Chinese
Medical Association* 77 (10): 531–34.

Park, Han-na. 2017. "Alteogen Partners with China's Qilu for Herceptin
Biosimilar." *The Investor*, March 30, 2017. http://www.theinvestor.
co.kr/view.php?ud=20170330000590.

Song, Bingbing, Chao Ding, Wangyang Chen, Huixin Sun, Maoxiang
Zhang, and Wanqing Chen. 2017. "Incidence and Mortality of Cervical Cancer in China, 2013." *Chinese Journal of Cancer Research* 29
(6): 471–76.

Stanway, David, and Michael Perry. 2018. "China Approves 17 Anti-Cancer Drugs for Medical Insurance Coverage." Reuters, October 9,
2018. https://www.reuters.com/article/us-china-health-cancer/
china-approves-17-anti-cancer-drugs-for-medical-insurance-cover-
age-idUSKCN1MK028.

State Council (Zhonghua renmin gongheguo zhongyang renmin zhengfu).
2018a. "Guowuyuan bangongting guanyu cuijin 'hulianwang + yiliao
jiankang' fazhan de yijian" [State Council opinions on improving the
development of the "e-Healthcare" industry]. State Council issuance
no. 26, April 25, 2018. http://www.gov.cn/zhengce/content/2018-04/28/

content_5286645.htm.

State Council. 2018b. "Guowuyuan bangongting guanyu wanshang guojia jiben yaowu zhidu de yijian" [State Council opinions on improving
the national essential medicines system]. State Council issuance no. 88,
September 19, 2018. http://www.gov.cn/zhengce/content/2018-09/19/
content_5323459.htm.

Sun, Yuanyuan, Yanhong Wang, Mengmeng Li, Kailiang Cheng, Xinyu
Zhao, Yuan Zheng, Yan Liu, Shaoyuan Lei, and Li Wang. 2018. "Long-
term Trends of Liver Cancer Mortality by Gender in Urban and Rural
Areas in China: An Age-period-cohort Analysis." *BMJ Open* 8 (2):
e020490.

Wang, Li, Chuan Zhang, Qiang Yuan, Wei Zhang, and Youping Li. 2009.
"A Comparative Study between the Newest Essential Medicine Lists
of China and the WHO in 2009." *Chinese Journal of Evidence-Based
Medicine* 9 (11): 1173–84.

WHO (World Health Organization). 2019. *International Agency for
Research on Cancer: Cancer in China.* The Global Cancer Observatory, May, 2019. http://gco.iarc.fr/today/data/factsheets/popula-
tions/160-china-fact-sheets.pdf.

Wu, Guoxiu. 2019. "Lightening the Load: China to Include More
Anti-Cancer Drugs in Medical Insurance" *CGTN*, February 20, 2019.
https://news.cgtn.com/news/306b7a4e31494464776c6d636a4e6e626
84a4856/share_p.html.

Xinhua. 2017. "Full Text: Development of China's Public Health as an
Essential Element of Human Rights (2)." Xinhuanet, September 29.
http://www.xinhuanet.com/english/2017-09/29/c_136648780.htm.

Yan, Li. 2018. "New Technology Developed for Early Liver Cancer Detection." *ECNS*, January 2, 2018. http://www.ecns.cn/2018/02-01/291117.
shtml.

Yang, Lei, Rongshou Zheng, Ning Wang, Yannan Yuan, Suo Liu, Huichao
Li, Siwei Zhang, Hongmei Zeng, and Wanqing Chen. 2018. "Incidence
and Mortality of Stomach Cancer in China, 2014." *Chinese Journal of
Cancer Research* 30 (3): 291–98.

14 Healthy Aging Policies in India

Kavita Singh and Dorairaj Prabhakaran

The unprecedented increase in global population aging over the last two decades is a conquest and a challenge (WHO 2015). The pace at which demographic transition (declining fertility, reduction in mortality, and increasing survival at older ages) occurs varies across countries of the world, but most developing nations are now challenged by increased elderly populations (WHO 2015; Gorman 1999; UN 2015). In 2000, there were more than 400 million people (11.5% of the total population) aged 65 and over in the world—projected to increase to almost 1.5 billion (22% of the world population) by the year 2050—nearly a fourfold increase compared to the 50% increase for the global population as a whole (UN 2015). From 1990 to 2025, the elderly population in Asia will rise from 50% of the world's elderly to 58%, while Europe's share of the world's elderly will decline from 19% to 12% (WHO 2015; UN 2015). In general, health-related morbidity and disability are high in old age. Acute and chronic diseases increase with age, and the associated costs of treatment impose a significant burden on individuals, families, and societies, and even more so in the absence of health insurance or social security (Gorman 1999; UN 2015; WHO n.d.)

Given the rapid rise in population aging, governments and health systems, particularly in developing countries such as India, are often unprepared to mitigate the adverse consequences, which has implications for the socio-economic and health status of the elderly (WHO n.d.; Kumar 1997). In this chapter, we provide a situational analysis of population aging in India (current status and trends over 2011–50). In addition, we describe the challenges of population aging in India and the government policies and schemes that address those challenges. Lastly, we also make government recommendations on ways to improve elderly care services in India.

Population Aging in India:
Status and Future Trends, 2011–50

According to Census 2011, India had 104 million elderly people[1] (those 60 years old and over), constituting 8.6 percent of the total population (ORGI 2011a, 2011b). Within India's elderly population, females outnumber males and a greater number still live in rural areas than in urban. According to a 2014 United Nations report, the number of elderly people in India is expected to surpass 300 million by 2050, accounting for around 20 percent of the population (UN 2015). By the end of the century, the elderly will constitute around 34 percent of India's total population (ORGI 2011a).

According to HelpAge India (2015), India's level of demographic transition and fertility rates display significant disparity across states and regions. Consequently, there are considerable variations in the age structure of the population across the nation, and as a result variation in the aging experience as well. For example, the southern states in India are the front-runners in population aging, along with Himachal Pradesh, Maharashtra, Odisha, and Punjab (see figure 14.1). According to Census 2011, there is an overall old-age dependency ratio of about 14 elderly per 100 working-age population, with significant variations across states (ORGI 2011a). India's life expectancy had increased from 32 years in 1947 to more than 62 years as of 2019. According to recent data from the Sample Registration System (SRS), life expectancy at the age of 60 increased from 14 years in 1970–75 to 18 years in 2010–14, with women living about two years longer than men (ORGI 2011b).

Health Status, Morbidity, and Mortality in the Elderly

The Global AgeWatch Index ranks 96 countries by how well their older populations (60 years and over) are performing across four domains: health status, income security, capability, and enabling environment. India was ranked at 71, lowest among South Asian countries, barring Afghanistan, on the Global AgeWatch Index 2015 (HelpAge International Global Network 2015). This index signifies not only how older people are faring but also how much needs to be done to achieve sustainable development goals. A recent survey assessed the mental health status of a sample of elderly persons in India using the 12-item General Health Questionnaire and found that nearly half of respondents experienced some form of psychological distress (Sell

[1]   This chapter uses the terms "older people," "the elderly," and "senior citizens" interchangeably.

FIGURE 14.1 Percentage of elderly people across states in India, 1991–2011

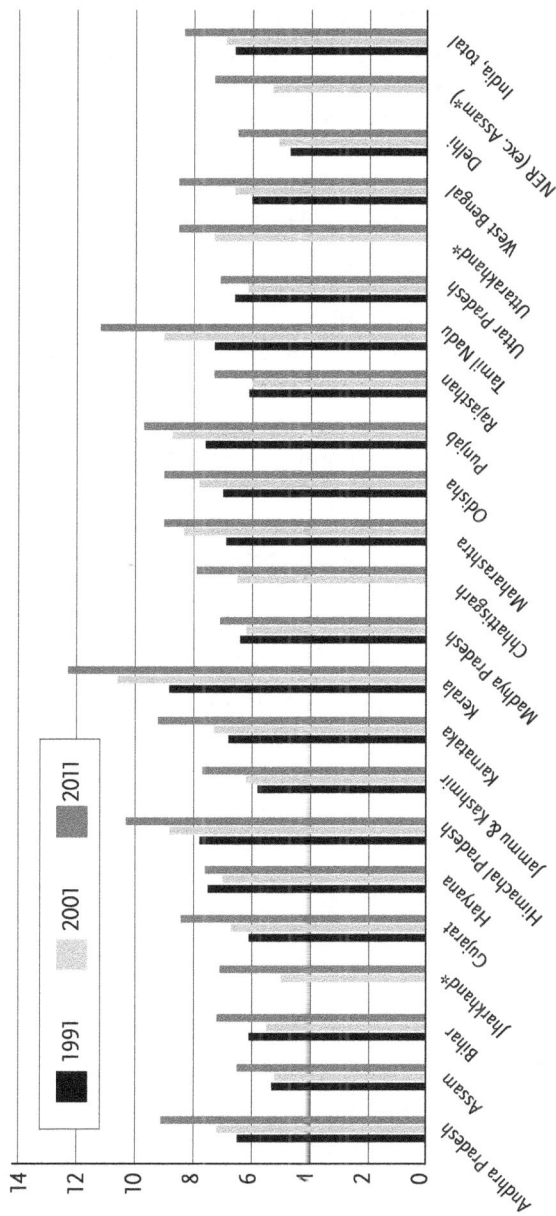

SOURCE: Compiled from Office of the Registrar General India (ORGI) and the Census Commissioner of India, Ministry of Home Affairs, Government of India (various years), Census of India, http://www.censusindia.gov.in.

NOTE: * No 1991 data are available for states that were formed in 2000; NER=the states of India's North Eastern Region, excluding Assam (Arunachal Pradesh, Manipur, Meghalaya, Mizoram, Nagaland, Sikkim, and Tripura).

and Nagpal 1992; Goldberg and Blackwell 1970). Further, mental health status worsened with advancing age, indicating higher mental health vulnerabilities among the very elderly population (Shaji et al. 2010). Mental health problems were higher among women, the less-educated, low-income classes, and those living in rural areas (Goldberg and Blackwell 1970). The SAGE Wave 1 survey shows that 75 percent of elderly women reported their current health as moderate or bad versus 64 percent of men (Arokiasamy, et al. 2013).

Infections are still the predominant form of illness among the elderly apart from degenerative disorders. Nutritional deficiencies are also prevalent but often remain subclinical, thus escaping the desired interventions. Recent surveys suggest that more than 50 percent of the elderly in India have chronic diseases and 5 percent suffer from immobility.

According to a 2015 report from the National Sample Survey Office, the prevalence of acute morbidity was 30 percent in the age group 60–69 years, which increased to 37 percent for the 80+ age group (NSSO 2015). Further, as shown in table 14.1, it was marginally higher among women than men. Further, the rate of hospitalization among the elderly was much higher than the general population. While the morbidity prevalence rate was higher among elderly women, their hospitalization rate was lower than that of men, indicating gender differentials in healthcare utilization.

TABLE 14.1 Prevalence of acute morbidities among the elderly (by age and sex), 2015

Sub-groups	Prevalence of acute morbidities
Age strata	
60–69 years	29.5
70–79 years	34.9
80 years and over	36.9
Gender	
Male	31.1
Female	32.3

SOURCE: NSSO (2015), Key Indicators of Social Consumption in India, Health (January–June 2014). 71st Round, National Sample Survey Office, Ministry of Statistics & Programme Implementation, Government of India.

According to Census 2011, the disability rate was 51.8 per 1,000 for the elderly and 84.1 per 1,000 for the 80-plus population as compared to 22.1 per 1,000 of the general population (ORGI 2011a). A breakdown of disabilities is shown in figure 14.2. Women 80 years old and over have higher levels of disability compared to elderly men, indicating that women face greater disadvantages. The HelpAge India 2014 survey found that about half of the elderly population in India face some form of abuse, a rate higher for women than men (2015).

FIGURE 14.2 Disabilities among India's elderly (60 years and over) by gender, 2011

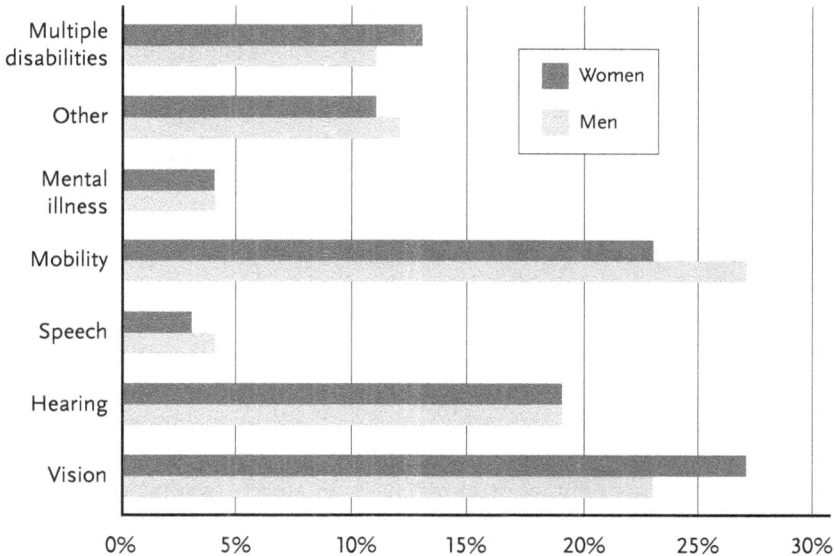

SOURCE: ORGI (2011), Census of India, 2011, Office of the Registrar General and the Census Commissioner of India, Ministry of Home Affairs, Government of India. http://www.censusin-dia.gov.in/2011-common/census_2011.html.

Chronic diseases are a leading cause of death among the elderly in India, and increasingly so over the past two decades. The proportion of elderly with any chronic condition, as estimated by the SAGE Wave 1 survey, was 41.8 percent in 2007 (Arokiasamy et al. 2012). In 2011, the corresponding figure, according to the estimates of the Building Knowledge Base on Population Ageing in India (BKPAI) survey, was 64.8 percent. Chronic conditions are more prevalent among elderly women (674 per 1,000) than elderly men (619 per 1,000) and are also higher in those living in rural areas (658 out of 1,000) than urban (621 out of 1,000) (United Nations Population Fund 2011; Alam et al. 2012). Chronic conditions such as arthritis, hypertension, cataracts, and type 2 diabetes are more prevalent among women, whereas conditions like asthma and heart diseases are more prevalent in men.

The BKPAI 2014 survey found that of the elderly hospitalized, 47 percent were admitted to government hospitals and the rest utilized private facilities. Increasingly, more elderly from urban areas preferred private facilities compared to the rural elderly (United Nations Population Fund 2011; Alam et al. 2012). The cost of healthcare is disproportionately higher for the elderly, which increases their out-of-pocket expenditure in the absence of health insurance and social security (Gorman 1999). Moreover, when the elderly are economically dependent on others, higher health expenditure adds to their families' economic burdens. Therefore, it is important to predetermine the factors that can prevent or reduce the burden of morbidity, disability, and mortality among the Indian elderly.

Population Aging Challenges in India

The increase in longevity and the decline of the joint family structure often drives older people into isolation and neglect. There are four aspects of aging particularly relevant in the Indian context that present challenges to elderly care policies and programs: ruralization (a large proportion of elderly living in rural areas), feminization (a higher number of elderly women), migration, and income insecurity (Sathyanarayana, Kumar, and James 2012).

According to Census 2011, 71 percent of the Indian elderly live in rural areas. In almost all Indian states (with the exceptions of Goa and Mizoram, two smaller states), a higher proportion of elderly live in rural areas than in urban areas (ORGI 2011). Many rural areas are still remote, with poor road and transport access. Isolation and inadequate access to quality healthcare are more severe problems for the rural elderly than their urban counterparts.

Aging is also likely to become a gender issue, essentially becoming "feminized," with a large number of women surviving into very old age in most countries of the world. Elderly women, especially in low-income countries like India, face a number of difficulties (Prakash 1997). They are most likely to be illiterate or less educated, widowed, unemployed, and dependent on others. Consequently, they are more likely to suffer from malnourishment, debilitating symptoms, and higher psychological distress (Giridhar, Subaiya, and Verma 2015).

The migration of younger working-age persons from rural areas can have both positive and negative impacts on the elderly. The phenomenon of elderly people living alone, or with only a spouse, is usually discussed in terms of social isolation, poverty, and distress. However, older people in rural areas often prefer to live in their own homes and communities. While the majority of India's elderly are still living with their children, about one-fifth either live alone or only with a spouse and hence have to manage their material and physical needs on their own. Recent survey data (BKPAI 2011) showed that the highest proportion of elderly living alone—26 percent—was in Tamil

Nadu (Sathyanarayana, Kumar, and James 2012).

Income insecurity is one of the major causes of vulnerability among the elderly. In India, it is typical for families to take care of the needs of older persons, including their economic and social needs. With India's changing socioeconomic, demographic, and development scenarios, financial security arising from personal income and asset ownership has become a major determinant of the well-being of the elderly (NSSO 2013). The BKPAI survey data indicate that 26 percent of older men and around 60 percent of older women do not have any personal income (Alam et al. 2012). About one-third of older men and women receive income from employers or social pensions. Although around 50 percent of the elderly have some type of personal income, it is insufficient to fulfill their basic needs and, therefore, they are financially dependent on others.

Healthy Aging Policies and Programs in India

Over the years, the Indian government has launched various schemes and policies to improve the quality of life of the elderly (Ministry of Health & Family Welfare 2018). We summarize below the schemes and programs initiated by the Indian government to promote the health, well-being, and independence of older persons in the country.

The central government introduced the National Policy for Older Persons (NPOP) in 1999 to promote the health and welfare of senior citizens in India. This policy aims to encourage individuals to make provision for their own as well as a spouse's old age. It also strives to encourage families to take care of their older family members. The policy enables and supports voluntary and non-governmental organizations (NGOs) to supplement the care provided by the family and provide care and protection to vulnerable elderly people. The main objective of this policy is to make older people fully independent citizens. This policy has also resulted in the launch of new schemes, such as the strengthening of the primary healthcare system to enable it to meet the healthcare needs of older persons, training of medical and paramedical personnel to provide healthcare to the elderly, promotion of the healthy aging concept, and provision of separate queues and reserved beds for elderly patients in hospitals (MSJE 1999).

The Integrated Programme for Older Persons is a government scheme that provides NGOs with financial assistance for projects, up to 90 percent of the total project cost. The funded projects establish and maintain old age homes, daycare centers, and mobile Medicare units, and provide non-institutional services to older persons. Another program is the Scheme of Assistance to

Panchayati Raj Institutions, which provides a one-time construction grant to voluntary organizations and self-help groups for the construction of old age homes and multi-service centers for older persons (MSJE 2016).

The Central Government Health Scheme provides pensioners of central government offices the facility to obtain medicines for chronic ailments up to three months at a stretch. The National Mental Health Programme focuses on the needs of senior citizens who are affected with Alzheimer's and other dementias, Parkinson's disease, depression, and psychogeriatric disorders (National Health Portal 2019). The Annapurna Yojana, launched in 2000, is a plan that aims to provide food security to meet the requirements of those senior citizens who, though eligible, have remained outside the old-age pension scheme. It provides 10 kilograms of free rice every month to each beneficiary. In 2007, the old-age pension scheme was renamed as the Indira Gandhi National Old Age Pension Scheme (IGNOAPS) and covered all families below the poverty line (BPL) (NSAP 2019).

Subsequently, in 2009, the National Social Assistance Program was expanded to include the Indira Gandhi National Widow Pension Scheme, covering widows aged 40–64 years, and the Indira Gandhi National Disability Pension Scheme, for persons with multiple or severe disabilities aged 18–64 years and living below the poverty line (NSAP 2019; SWD 2017a, 2017b). In 2011, the age limit for IGNOAPS was lowered from 65 to 60 years and the monthly pension amount for those 80 years and above was increased from ₹200 to ₹500. The Ministry of Health and Family Welfare launched the National Programme for Health Care of the Elderly (NPHCE) during the year 2010–11, to address various health-related problems of the elderly (Ministry of Health & Family Welfare 2018).

Furthermore, the draft revision of the National Policy for Senior Citizens (NPSC) was submitted in 2011 but still awaits cabinet approval. The NPSC follows a rights perspective and calls for special attention to elderly women and the rural poor. It identifies income security as a key intervention, as more than two-thirds of elderly live below the poverty line. Hence, the draft policy recommends a monthly pension of ₹1,000 per person to be revised periodically for inflation adjustment. It also calls for expanded implementation of the NPHCE and lays specific emphasis on support for productive aging (MSJE 2011).

Health insurance for senior citizens

Health insurance for the elderly is seen as a logical extension of the ongoing low-premium life insurance (Pradhan Mantri Jeevan Jyoti Bima Yojana), general insurance (Pradhan Mantri Suraksha Bima Yojana), and the pension plan (Atal Pension Yojana, or APY). Under APY, for every contribution made to the pension fund, the central government also co-contributes 50 percent of the total contribution or ₹1,000 (US$14) per annum, whichever is lower, to each eligible subscriber account, for a period of five years. The minimum age to join APY is 18 years and maximum age is 40 years. The age of exit and the start of pension is 60 years. Therefore, the minimum period of contribution by the subscriber under APY is 20 years (NSDL 2017).

Varishtha Pension Bima Yojana 2017 is a scheme that is part of the government's commitment to financial inclusion and social security during old age, and to protect those aged 60+ years (LIC n.d.). Senior citizens will be able to make investments of up to ₹750,000 in the scheme, which provides an assured pension based on a guaranteed rate of return of 8 percent per annum for 10 years, with an option to receive the pension on a monthly, quarterly, biannual, or annual basis. The scheme is implemented through the Life Insurance Corporation in India.

Scheme for providing aid and assisted living devices to senior citizens

The scheme aims to provide assisted living devices to BPL senior citizens who suffer from any age-related disability or infirmity, such as low vision, hearing impairment, loss of teeth, or locomotor disability. The assistive devices provided through this scheme are of high quality and conform to the standards laid down by the Bureau of Indian Standards (Ministry of Social Justice and Empowerment 2019).

While there are many beneficial schemes aimed at improving the quality of life for older persons, an equally important concern is the extent to which the elderly are aware of these schemes and actually use them. The BKPAI survey, conducted in seven states in India, found that among BPL households the overall awareness of these social security schemes is around 70 percent, with awareness levels generally higher among older men than women, and generally decreasing with increasing age (Bhat, James, and Giridhar 2014). The problem, however, is with the utilization of these schemes: only 17–20 percent of BPL elderly take advantage of them, with significant variations across states. About 10 percent and 15 percent of non-BPL elderly persons were beneficiaries of old-age pension schemes and widow pension schemes, respectively. These findings suggest administrative access hurdles that should be removed or minimized by state governments, with active support from NGOs (Rajan 2014). In addition to government schemes, a large number of NGOs are providing elderly care services in India, as shown in table 14.2.

TABLE 14.2 Elderly care services in India

Public sector services (policies/programs)	Non-governmental sector services
National Program for Health Care of the Elderly	Integrated Plan for Older Persons
Integrated Plan for Older Persons	National Programme for Health Care of the Elderly
National Programme for Health Care of the Elderly	National Mental Health Program
National Mental Health Program	Central Government Health Scheme
Central Government Health Scheme	National Old Age Pension Scheme
National Old Age Pension Scheme	Indira Gandhi National Old Age Pension Scheme
Indira Gandhi National Old Age Pension Scheme	Varishtha Pension Bima Yojana 2017
Varishtha Pension Bima Yojana 2017	

SOURCE: Authors.

Elderly care services that need special attention

A recent survey showed that more than 50 percent of the elderly believed that the government should provide additional support during old age. In particular, there is a need to have community-based daycare centers for the elderly, which could provide services such as skill building, financial and legal advice, entertainment, exercise, and other ways of encouraging active aging, with effective linkages to the public health system (Shakti 2016). At the family level, stronger inter-generational bonding is recommended, while at the community level, greater participation and involvement of the elderly is important.

Broadly, healthy aging would require the establishment of a national framework (a multi-sectoral approach and partnership involving social welfare, finance, health, education, and urban planning) for productive aging (WHO 2014, 2016). Measurement, monitoring, and research for healthy aging should also be an important part of this national framework (Liebig and Rajan 2005). Furthermore, there is a need to enhance the engagement of older persons in policy decisions so that the elderly are not relegated to being passive recipients of welfare schemes (Ramkumar 2014). Collective efforts by the government and NGOs as well as the active engagement of the elderly in policy decisions and welfare schemes would promote an overall age-friendly environment and foster the autonomy of older persons (through various financial resources and opportunities) (Narayana 2014).

The Way Forward

As we move ahead in the twenty-first century, population aging will put increased economic and social demands on all countries, particularly on developing countries such as India. However, if a greater number of individuals reach older age in good health—and remain healthy for longer—the benefits will be shared by all. Therefore, the promotion of healthy aging and the prevention of disability in the elderly must assume a central role in medical care and research, as well as in the formulation of national health and social policies. Additionally, India must add new priorities for their scarce resources, for social programs for the elderly, while still managing the problems of the younger population. Women's issues are extremely important when considering social policies for the elderly population. The feminization of poverty and poor health during old age is, in fact, a result of exacerbated risks for women across the life course. Therefore, appropriate care and support for aging women and all elderly should be a government priority. In conclusion, leading a healthy life, with regular physical activity, adequate intake of fruits and vegetables, reduced consumption of salt, sugar, and trans fats; avoiding tobacco and alcohol; and maintaining a positive attitude and healthy mental well-being are attributes that will enhance quality of life, even in old age.

References

Alam, Moneer, K. S. James, G. Giridhar, K. M. Sathyanarayana, Sanjay Kumar, S. Siva Raju, T. S. Syamala, Lekha Subaiya, and Dhananjay W. Bansod. 2012. *Report on the Status of Elderly in Select States of India 2011*. Building Knowledge Base on Population Ageing in India. New Delhi: United Nations Population Fund.

Arokiasamy, P., David Bloom, Jinkook Lee, Kevin Feeney, and Marija Ozolins. 2012. "Longitudinal Aging Study in India: Vision, Design, Implementation, and Preliminary Findings." In *Aging in Asia: Findings from New and Emerging Data Initiatives*, edited by James P. Smith and Malay Majmundar. Washington, DC: National Academies Press.

Arokiasamy, P., Sulabha Parasuraman, T. V. Sekher, and H. Lhungdim. 2013. *Study on Global AGEing and Adult Health (SAGE) Wave 1: India National Report*. Mumbai: International Institute for Population Sciences.

Bhat, T. N., K. S. James, and G. Giridhar. 2014. "An Appraisal of the Functioning of the National Programme for the Health Care of the Elderly (NPHCE) in Karnataka and Odisha." Working Paper 7, Series II, Building a Knowledge Base on Population Ageing in India, Institute for Social and Economic Change, Bangalore; United Nations Population Fund; and Institute of Economic Growth, Delhi.

Giridhar, G., Lekha Subaiya, and Supriya Verma. 2015. "Older Women in India: Economic, Social and Health Concerns." Building Knowledge Base on Ageing in India: Increased Awareness, Access and Quality of Elderly Services Thematic Paper 2, United Nations Population Fund.

Goldberg, David P., and Barry Blackwell. 1970. "Psychiatric Illness in General Practice: A Detailed Study Using a New Method of Case Identification." *British Medical Journal* 2 (5707): 439–43.

Gorman, Mark. 1999. "Development and the Rights of Older People." In *The Ageing and Development Report: Poverty, Independence and the World's Older People*, edited by Judith Randel, Tony German, and Deborah Ewing. London: Earthscan Publications Ltd.

HelpAge India. 2015. *The State of Elderly in India, 2014*. New Delhi: HelpAge India. https://www.helpageindia.org/wp-content/themes/helpageindia/pdf/state-elderly-india-2014.pdf.

HelpAge International Global Network. 2015. *Global Health Watch Index 2015: Insight Report*. http://globalagewatch.org/reports/global-agewatch-index-2015-insight-report-summary-and-methodology.

Kumar, Vinod. 1997. "Ageing in India—An Overview." *Indian Journal of Medical Research* 106 (October): 257–64.

LIC (Life Insurance Corporation of India). n.d. "Varishtha Pension Bima Yojana." Government of India. Accessed June 5, 2019. https://www.licindia.in/Products/Withdrawn-Plans/VARISHTHA-PENSION-BIMA-YOJANA-(UIN-512G291V01).

Liebig, Phoebe S., and S. Irudaya Rajan. 2005. "An Ageing India: Perspectives, Prospects and Policies." *Journal of Aging & Social Policy* 15 (2–3): 1–9.

Ministry of Health & Family Welfare. 2018. "National Programme for Health Care of the Elderly (NPHCE)." Government of India. https://mohfw.gov.in/major-programmes/other-national-health-programmes/national-programme-health-care-elderlynphce.

MSJE (Ministry of Social Justice and Empowerment). 1999. "National Policy on Older Persons." Government of India, New Delhi. http://socialjustice.nic.in/writereaddata/UploadFile/National%20Policy%20for%20Older%20Persons%20Year%201999.pdf.

MSJE. 2011. "National Policy for Senior Citizens: March 2011." Government of India. http://socialjustice.nic.in/writereaddata/UploadFile/dnpsc.pdf.

MSJE. 2016. "Integrated Programme for Older Persons." Government of India. http://www.socialjustice.nic.in/writereaddata/UploadFile/IPOP%202016%20pdf%20document.pdf.

MSJE. 2019. "'Rashtriya Vayoshri Yojana' launched in 2017." Government of India. http://vikaspedia.in/social-welfare/senior-citizens-welfare/rashtriya-vayoshri-yojana.

Narayana, Muttur Ranganathan. 2014. "Impact of Population Ageing on Sustainability of India's Current Fiscal Policies: A Generational Accounting Approach." *Journal of the Economics of Ageing* 3 (April) : 71–83.

National Health Portal. 2019. "National Mental Health Programme." Government of India. https://www.nhp.gov.in/national-mental-health-programme_pg.

NSAP (National Social Assistance Program). 2019. "National Social Assistance Program." Accessed June 5, 2019. http://nsap.nic.in/.

NSDL (National Securities Depository Ltd). 2017. "Atal Pension Yojana (APY)." https://www.npscra.nsdl.co.in/scheme-details.php.

NSSO (National Sample Survey Office). 2013. *Key Indicators of Employment and Unemployment in India, NSS 68th Round (July 2011–June 2012).* New Delhi: Ministry of Statistics and Programme

Implementation, Government of India.

NSSO. 2015. *Key Indicators of Social Consumption in India, Health (January–June 2014)*. 71st Round. New Delhi: National Sample Survey Office, Ministry of Statistics and Programme Implementation, Government of India.

ORGI (Office of Registrar General of India). 2011a. "Census of India, 2011." New Delhi: Office of the Registrar General and the Census Commissioner of India, Ministry of Home Affairs, Government of India.

ORGI. 2011b. "Provisional Population Totals, Paper-1 of 2011." New Delhi: Office of the Registrar General and the Census Commissioner of India, Ministry of Home Affairs, Government of India.

Prakash, Indira Jai. 1997. "Women & Ageing." *Indian Journal of Medical Research* 106 (October): 396–408.

Rajan, Irudaya, and Udaya Mishra. 2014. "The National Policy for Older Persons: Critical Issues in Implementation." In *Population Ageing in India*, edited by G. Giridhar, K. M. Sathyanarayana, Sanjay Kumar, K. S. James, and Moneer Alam. New Delhi: Cambridge University Press.

Ramkumar, R. 2014. "Financing of Old Age Pensions in Maharashtra: A Note." Tata Institute of Social Sciences, Mumbai.

Sathyanarayana K.M., Sanjay Kumar, and K.S. James. 2012. "Living Arrangements of Elderly in India: Policy and Programmatic Implication." Working paper no. 7, Building a Knowledge Base on Population Ageing in India, Institute for Social and Economic Change, Bangalore; United Nations Population Fund; and Institute of Economic Growth, New Delhi.

Sell, Helmut, and R. Nagpal. 1992. "Assessment of Subjective Well-Being: The Subjective Well-Being Inventory." Regional Health Paper, SEARO, no. 24, World Health Organization, Regional Office for South-East Asia, New Delhi.

Shaji K.S., A.T. Jotheeswaran, N. Girish, Srikala Bharath, Amit Dias, Meera Pattabiraman, and Mathew Varghese. 2010. *The Dementia India Report 2010: Prevalence, Impact, Costs and Services for Dementia*. Alzheimer's and Related Disorders Society of India. http://ardsi.org/downloads/main%20report.pdf.

Shakti, Stree. 2016. *Innovative Practices for Care of Elderly Women in India*. United Nations Population Fund. http://india.unfpa.org/publications/innovative-practices-care-elderly-women-india-stree-shakti.

SWD (Social Welfare Department, Government of Chhattisgarh). 2017a. "Indira Gandhi National Widow Pension Scheme." https://sw.cg.gov.in/en/indira-gandhi-national-widow-pension-scheme.

SWD. 2017b. "Indira Gandhi National Disability Pension Scheme." https //sw.cg.gov.in/en/indira-gandhi-national-disability-pension-scheme.

UN (United Nations, Department of Economic and Social Affairs, Population Division). 2015. *World Population Prospects: The 2015 Revision.* https://www.un.org/en/development/desa/publications/world-population-prospects-2015-revision.html.

United Nations Population Fund (UNFPA). 2011. *Delivering Results in a World of 7 Billion. 2011 Annual Report.* https://www.unfpa.org/sites/default/files/pub-pdf/16434%20UNFPA%20AR_FINAL_Ev11.pdf.

WHO (World Health Organization). 2014. "Regional Strategy for Healthy Ageing (2013–18)." http://www.searo.who.int/entity/healthy_ageing/documents/regional-strate- gy-2013-2018.pdf?ua=1.

WHO. 2015. *World Report on Ageing and Health.* Geneva: World Health Organization.

WHO. 2016. "Multisectoral Action for Life Course Approach to Healthy Ageing: Global Strategy and Plan of Action on Ageing and Health." World Health Assembly, Geneva, April 2016.

WHO. N.d. "Healthy Ageing." https://www.who.int/ageing/healthy -ageing/en/.

Appendix

Methods for Estimating
Net Value of Chronic Disease Management

Several chapters in this book, such as chapter 7 by Lam, Wong, and Quan, or chapter 3 by Hashimoto and Eggleston, describe economics research on the net value of chronic disease management. While the technical details of those studies are published in economics journal articles, we wish to make the methods description generally available to any researchers interested in applying this approach. The framework, modified from the seminal work of Cutler et al. (1998) on acute myocardial infarction (AMI), can be applied to many different chronic conditions. This appendix describes the methods for net value analysis of healthcare for patients with type 2 diabetes mellitus (DM) based on longitudinal patient-level data on resource use and quality outcomes, as measured by clinical markers and predicted risk of complications and death.

The Stanford Asia Health Policy Program, directed by Karen Eggleston, coordinates a comparative research project on the net value of diabetes management focusing on Asia in an international comparative perspective. Participating research teams of health economists, epidemiologists, and clinicians apply similar methods for assessing net value developed originally in Eggleston et al. (2009), a study using U.S. Mayo Clinic data. Most samples in this collaboration include several thousand patients each year for at least four years between 2005 and 2019. Some of the studies, such as that of the Taiwan team, apply the method within a difference-in-difference framework to assess a pay-for-performance program, or combine it with a regression discontinuity approach (Japan team) or other design to determine the causal effects of specific programs. This appendix intends to inform researchers who are interested in estimating the net value of diabetes management within similar frameworks to inform policy choices in any country and any provider setting.

Preparing for Net Value Analyses

"Checklist" of sample characteristics to examine before specifying study cohort(s) and study period

- Number of diabetes cases per year—prevalence and incidence in the study population
- Availability of a risk prediction model appropriate for the study population with primary endpoint all-cause mortality. Examples include the UK Prospective Diabetes Study (UKPDS) risk equations, the Japan risk engine "JJRE" (Tanaka et al. 2013), and other tailored models such as those developed by our Hong Kong and Singapore teams (Quan et al. 2019).
- Number of deaths per year (to decide about using an available risk prediction model or the feasibility of developing such a model specific for the sample patient population)
- Average follow-up time per patient
- Completeness of clinical/biomarker data among the study population (e.g., blood pressure, HbA1c, other risk factors used in chosen risk prediction model)

Defining the study population[1]

Inclusion criteria
- Diagnosis of type 2 diabetes (ICD 9 code: 250.*2, 250.*4 / ICD 10 code: E11.**, E14.**)—at least two outpatient visits, and/or one inpatient admission, with diabetes as the primary diagnosis
- Over 18 years old
- Complete demographic and biomarker/laboratory data at baseline (or the time of diagnosis, for those newly diagnosed and entering the study sample during the study period)

Exclusion criteria
- Secondary diabetes (ICD 10 code: E08.*, E09.*, E13.*, unless many type 2 patients may be classified as "other specified diabetes" during the study period)
- Type I diabetes (ICD 9 codes: 250.*1, 250.*3 / ICD 10 code: E10.**). Or can exclude based on age less than 30 at diagnosis and taking insulin.
- Missing data at the baseline time window

---

1 See page 242 for an addendum on notation.

These criteria identify type II diabetic patients who have been diagnosed and potentially obtained management over the defined study period. In order to group patients with similar duration of diabetes, the study population could be further stratified based on the year(s) since diagnosis (i.e., duration of diagnosis >10 years, 5–9 years, 3–4 years, 1–2 years before the baseline period; incident cases in years 1–2, years 3–4, etc., excluding incident cases in the final study period because the method requires some follow-up period).

We code Elixhauser comorbidities (excluding diabetes) at baseline for all patients (see Quan et al. [2005] for coding algorithms).

Health outcomes

We use a diabetes risk prediction model to estimate change in health outcomes of the sample population. Specifically, we measure the change in risk of all-cause mortality as the primary outcome. Other outcomes for sensitivity analyses include (1) major diabetes complications such as non-fatal and fatal coronary heart disease (CHD) and strokes, and (2) remaining life expectancy (LE) and quality-adjusted life years (QALYs) as estimated in models taking account of more sequelae, such as the UKPDS Outcomes Model 2. Previous studies in European countries and North America have used the UKPDS model both for predicting mortality and for applying the outcomes model (see the appendix of Eggleston et al. 2009).

Extracting demographic and biomarker data from the data precedes their use as inputs for the risk prediction model(s). Types and details of required data vary according to the chosen model(s).

In calculating five-year risks of mortality and diabetes complications, we will focus on "modifiable" risks by holding at the baseline value the patient's age and duration of diagnosis (the latter only for teams/samples that have the data). In this way, the net value analyses focus on the change in risks that are plausibly attributable to clinical care, rather than a natural part of the aging process and number of years the patient has lived with diabetes.

Data permitting, measured change in LEs and QALYs can capture the long-term effects of management among type 2 diabetes patients exposed to different treatment modes or changing technologies of treatment that may impact the development of complications including cardiovascular disease (CVD), strokes, renal failure, amputation, and blindness.

Spending

1. Convert nominal spending into real spending in local currency units, using the gross domestic product (GDP) deflator.
2. Include all spending for a given individual, with no attempt to isolate DM-specific spending.
3. Aggregate up to total annual spending, for each year in the study period (using fraction of year enrolled/observed, for individuals in the sample for only part of a year).
4. However, in year of death for decedents, include total spending and count as a full year.

For samples that lack data at the patient level on actual spending in nominal or real currency (e.g., in whole or in part a national health service such as in Hong Kong, other parts of China, India), we use a standardized price vector applied to utilization data.

Net Value Analyses

Net value is estimated as the present discounted monetary value of improved survival (and, in a secondary analysis, improved survival plus avoided treatment spending for stroke and coronary heart disease), holding age and duration of diagnosis constant at baseline ("modifiable risk"), net of the increase in annual inflation-adjusted spending per patient. To accomplish this, we will estimate two different risk predictions for each patient-year, for those who survive from the baseline through the final period: actual (non-modifiable) risk, and modifiable risk. The two measures coincide only for the initial observation (i.e., in the baseline period or at the year of cohort entry). In other words, for each year a DM patient is in the sample from the baseline period to the final period, we compute actual risk and modifiable risk (holding age and duration of DM at their levels in the baseline period but allowing other risk factors to change between years/periods).

This cost-of-living approach is analogous to a cost-benefit analysis, or a cost-effectiveness analysis in which outcomes and costs for two interventions (e.g., medical care in the baseline period and in the final period) are compared, but instead of a threshold, we assign a monetary value to life-years gained as a result of improvements in health status between the two periods, and then subtract the added costs of care (see discussion in Eggleston et al. 2009, 388).

Each team used a life table most applicable to that population (i.e., national or regional/state life table estimates for a year within the study period). None had access to life tables estimated for individuals with diagnosed diabetes, although in the future that would be a desired refinement of the net value estimates. Each research team applied the age- and sex-specific remaining life expectancy from that life table to the individual patient-level estimate of value, to estimate survival if the individual survives beyond the five years predicted by the mortality model. Following is the approach that we use.

I. Primary analyses:

    a. Baseline (or year of cohort entry) vs. final period

    b. Among patients who survive to the final period, change in modifiable predicted risk of all-cause mortality (i.e., holding age and duration of diagnosis at the same values as baseline)

    c. Spending in baseline and final periods, including all spending in year of death for decedents, and no attempt to isolate DM-specific spending

    d. Value

        i. Estimate individual actual five-year mortality risk using risk factors for the baseline period, and then do the same for the final period.

        ii. Estimate individual *modifiable* mortality risk in the final period, replacing the individual's actual age with the baseline period age (and duration of diagnosis).

        iii. In estimating the value of (any) improved survival, use estimated modifiable all-cause mortality for the next five-year period based on the risk model, and for survivors beyond that period, *assume remaining age- and sex-specific life expectancy from the life table for that country/region/year.*

    e. Spending

        i. Estimate the generalized linear model (GLM) regression of medical spending for all patients in the baseline period (empirical specification below).

        ii. Predict each individual's medical spending in the baseline period.

        iii. Estimate medical spending for all patients in the final period in the same way.

        iv. Predict each individual survivor's *modifiable* spending in the final period by predicting spending from the final period regression BUT keeping the age and duration of diagnosis at the same value as for that individual in the baseline period.

        v. Change in spending is the additional annual spending between the baseline and final periods, that is, the difference between predicted annual real spending in the baseline period and predicted annual real *modifiable* spending in the final period.

f. Net value

 i. Net Value 1

  1. At the individual patient level, for each survivor, subtract the change in spending from the change in the modifiable risk of all-cause mortality.

  2. Summarize net value by five-year age group as specified in the reference populations.

 ii. Net Value 2: Age- and sex-standardized population, using World Health Organization world population standard reference population (modified for adult population 15–85+ years old)

  1. Separately for men and for women, multiply the mean net value of each five-year age group by the weight assigned to that group in the reference population.

  2. Summarize the overall weighted average net value.

II. Secondary analyses: All-cause mortality, plus avoid treatment spending for stroke and CHD; and accounting for decedents, as described below.

Primary analyses: Protocol for survivor panel

Each team defines the relevant baseline and final periods. The baseline period may include one, two, or three years; the final period similarly. For large, short panels, one year is appropriate; for small, long panels, three years is appropriate. We will summarize in this document assuming two years in the baseline period (Baseline Year 1 [BY1] and Baseline Year 2 [BY2]) and two years in the final period (Final Year 1 [FY1] and Final Year 2 [FY2])

Denote the five-year risk of all-cause mortality for individual j in period t as P_{jt}. We calculate the value of reductions in fatal risk as follows: Assuming a 3 percent annual real discount rate applied halfway through each year and a given value of one life-year (ranging from US$50,000 to $150,000), estimate the present discounted value of remaining life for two time points: the baseline and final observation periods.

To do so, we approximate the predicted probability of death in the next five years by giving one-fifth of the predicted probability ($0.2\,P_{jt}$) to each of the first five years, and assume that all patients surviving beyond year five (with probability $1 - P_{jt}$) have the same age- and sex-specific remaining life expectancy as a general individual from the life table of that population. In calculating the present discounted value of remaining life from the model simulations, we assume a 3 percent real annual discount rate.

We calculate a monetary value for changes in life expectancy for a given assumed value of one life-year (LE value) and calculate a net value for each individual j as follows:

net value$_j$ = LE value$_j$ − cost increase$_j$,

in which

cost increase = C_{Final} − $C_{Baseline}$,

with

C_{Final} = (total predicted individual spending in FY1 and FY2)/2

and

$C_{Baseline}$ = (total predicted individual spending in BY1 and BY2)/2.

We estimate predicted spending rather than actual spending to smooth variation in individual observations of actual spending, as well as to predict what individuals would probably spend if they were the same age and had the same duration of diabetes they had at the baseline. We estimated the total predicted medical spending by using administrative claims data for the first and last period of the study for each patient. To account for differences in how risk factors affect spending, we estimated a multivariate regression model by using generalized linear models as suggested by Manning and Mullahy. Using the modified Park test, as suggested by Manning and Mullahy, we assumed a log link and gamma distribution. All medical and pharmaceutical spending are included in the dependent variable: total two-year spending for each patient. The independent variables in the model were age, sex, and Elixhauser comorbid conditions except diabetes (included as a vector of indicator variables for the presence of each comorbidity at baseline). For teams/samples having information on duration of diabetes, duration (years with diagnosis) is included, as well as an interaction term of age with duration. For teams/samples lacking the duration of diabetes variable, age-squared is included in the regression model. By using the estimated coefficients from the model, we predict total spending for each patient in the baseline and final periods, and then predict total spending while holding age (and duration of diagnosis) constant at their baseline values.

The increase in predicted spending between the baseline and final periods is then compared with the value of health status improvement to calculate the net value of additional spending.

We performed non-parametric bootstrapping with a large number of samples (e.g., 1,000) to calculate 95 percent confidence intervals (CIs) (using the percentile method) for patient risk factors, spending, and net value.

Net value methods to account for
selective survival and expense in the last year of life

We started with method (1), the survivor panel. This section describes the methods for the method (2) robustness check including half a value of a life-year for every year survived by both decedents and survivors, using the example of four years of data (such as the Netherlands sample), with year 1 (Y1) as the baseline and Y4 as the final period.

We account for deaths using data on spending and mortality for those who died during our study period (i.e., decedents) in the following way:

Our analytic dataset includes a cohort that enters the data in the baseline year (Y1 cohort), some of whom survive to the end of the study period (e.g., Y4), and some of whom die during the study period. We ignore the incident cohorts who joined the sample after the baseline year, for lack of a sufficient follow-up period.

Analysts do the net value analyses on the panel of survivors between the baseline and final periods, method (1). That yields the net value for the age-constant survivor panel (i.e., based on modifiable risk as predicted by biomarkers in the baseline and final years). Call this NV_s. This receives a weight in the overall net value that is proportional to the fraction of the baseline cohort that survives through the end of the study period.

Then we estimate the net value of decedents, NV_D; this receives a weight in the overall net value that is proportional to the fraction of the baseline cohort that dies before the end of the study period. NV_D is estimated in a different way from that of survivors, because it is based on cumulative spending and cumulative life-years, not subtracting the baseline from final period values. As described in the main text, to this NV_D we add half the value of a life-year for every year survived by individuals who survived to the final period, net of mean expenditures among survivors and weighted by the percentage of survivors in the sample.

We denote the average total spending of the decedents in the year that they died as M^D_t. To do this, we, sum all the spending of all those who died at any point in the year, and divide the result by the number who died in that year. If there are data on spending and mortality in each of the four years, we give the decedents the full assumed value for the years they actually survive and their spending up to the time they died. If the intermediate year data are not available but the year of death is known, we give the decedents the average spending for survivors for the years they survive in full (we can interpolate spending if necessary) and the average spending among decedents for the year they died. We assume they lived on average 0.5 years in the year they died, on the assumption of a uniform distribution of dates of death during the year. We give the decedents 0.5*(assumed value of life-year) for the year they died. With exact dates of death we can compute the average fraction of the year survived, which should be close to 0.5.

Using this method, Eggleston et al. (2019) also explore the sensitivity of net value to the assumed degree of survival attributable to medical care. One way to do this is to include a parameter α representing the fraction of a life-year attributable to medical care, with $0 < \alpha \leq 1$. Dubbed the "Cutler coefficient," the default is set to 0.5 following Cutler, Rosen, and Vijan (2006) in assuming that medical care accounts for half of health gains, with non-medical factors playing an equally important role in health improvement (Eggleston et al. 2019). We subtract decedents' actual (or, if not available, assumed average) spending, and express this as a per-decedent net value ((Total value − total spending)/(# of decedents)). This gives the average net value of a life-year for the decedents in a given year:

$$NV_{D1} = \text{Per-decedent net value for decedents in Y1}$$
$$= \{(0.5LY) * \alpha * \$perLY\} - M^D_b$$

For people who die in Y2, Y3, and Y4, we give them 1.5, 2.5, and 3.5 years of life, respectively, and tabulate their expenses for each year (M_{Y1}, M_{Y2}, M_{Y3}). Then the average per-decedent net value for Y1 cohort decedents in Y2, Y3, and Y4 can be estimated as follows:

$$NV_{D2} = \{(1.5LY) * \alpha * \$perLY\} - M_{Y1} - M^D_{Y2}$$
$$NV_{D3} = \{(2.5LY) * \alpha * \$perLY\} - M_{Y1} - M_{Y2} - M^D_{Y3}$$
$$NV_{D4} = \{(3.5LY) * \alpha * \$perLY\} - M_{Y1} - M_{Y2} - M_{Y3} - M^D_{Y4}$$

We then compute a weighted average net value for decedents of the Y1 cohort as follows:

$$NV_D = \sum_{(t=1)}^{4} \frac{D_{Yt}}{D} * NV_{Dt}$$

Where D = Total Y1 cohort decedents who died in the Y1–Y4 study period; and D_Y = Decedents in year Y, where $D = D_{Y1} + D_{Y2} + D_{Y3} + D_{Y4}$.

Finally, compute a weighted average net value for the panel of survivors and the decedents as follows:

$$NV = \left(\frac{D}{S+D}\right) NV_D + \left(\frac{S}{S+D}\right) [NV_S + \frac{1}{2}\$QALY - mean\ spending]$$

Where S = Total Y1 cohort of survivors, the survivor panel.

Addendum on notation

BY1	Baseline period Year 1	E10	Insulin-dependent diabetes mellitus
BY2	Baseline period Year 2	E11	Non-insulin-dependent diabetes mellitus
FY1	Final period Year 1	E12	Malnutrition-related diabetes mellitus
FY2	Final period Year 2	E13	Other specified diabetes mellitus
		E14	Unspecified diabetes mellitus
		O24	Diabetes mellitus in pregnancy

References

Cutler, David M., Mark McClellan, Joseph P. Newhouse, and Dahlia Remler. 1998. "Are Medical Prices Declining? Evidence from Heart Attack Treatments." *Quarterly Journal of Economics* 113 (4): 991–1024.

Cutler, David M., Allison B. Rosen, and Sandeep Vijan. 2006. "The Value of Medical Spending in the United States, 1960–2000." *New England Journal of Medicine* 355 (9): 920–27.

Eggleston, Karen N., Nilay D. Shah, Steven A. Smith, Amy E. Wagie, Arthur R. Williams, Jerome H. Grossman, Ernst R. Berndt, Kirsten Hall Long, Ritesh Banerjee, and Joseph P. Newhouse. 2009. "The Net Value of Health Care for Patients with Type 2 Diabetes, 1997 to 2005." *Annals of Internal Medicine* 151 (6): 386–93.

Eggleston, Karen, Brian K. Chen, Ying Isabel Chen, Talitha Feenstra, Toshiaki Iizuka, Janet Tinkei Lam, Gabriel M. Leung, Jui-fen Rachel Lu, Joseph P. Newhouse, Jianchao Quan, Beatriz Rodriguez-Sanchez, and Jeroen Struijs. 2019. "Are Quality-Adjusted Medical Prices Declining for Chronic Disease? Evidence from Four Health Systems." Working paper, Stanford Asia Health Policy Program, March.

Quan, Hude, Vijaya Sundararajan, Patricia Halfon, Andrew Fong, Bernard Burnand, Jean-Christophe Luthi, L. Duncan Saunders, Cynthia A. Beck, Thomas E. Feasby, and William A. Ghali. 2005. "Coding Algorithms for Defining Comorbidities in ICD-9-CM and ICD-10 Administrative Data." *Medical Care* 43 (11): 1130–39.

Quan, Jianchao, Deanette Pang, Tom K. Li, Cheung Hei Choi, Shing Chung Siu, Simon Y. Tang, Nelson M. Wat, Jean Woo, Zheng Yi Lau, Kelvin B. Tan, and Gabriel M. Leung. 2019. "Derivation and Validation of Risk Prediction Scores for Mortality, Cerebrovascular Disease, and Ischemic Heart Disease amongst Chinese People with Type 2 Diabetes: HKU-SG Risk Scores." Working paper.

Tanaka, Shiro, Sachiko Tanaka, Satoshi Iimuro, Hidetoshi Yamashita, Shigehiro Katayama, Yasuo Akanuma, Nobuhiro Yamada, Atsushi Araki, Hideki Ito, Hirohito Sone, and Yasuo Ohashi, for the Japan Diabetes Complications Study Group and the Japanese Elderly Diabetes Intervention Trial Group. 2013. "Predicting Macro- and Microvascular Complications in Type 2 Diabetes." *Diabetes Care* 36 (5): 1193–99.

UK Prospective Diabetes Study (UKPDS) Group. 1998. "Intensive Blood-Glucose Control with Sulphonylureas or Insulin Compared with

Conventional Treatment and Risk of Complications in Patients with Type 2 Diabetes (UKPDS 33)." *The Lancet* 352 (9131): 837–53.

Index

The authorized representative in the EU for product safety and compliance is:
Mare Nostrum Group
B.V Doelen 72
4831 GR Breda
The Netherlands

www.ingramcontent.com/pod-product-compliance
Lightning Source LLC
Chambersburg PA
CBHW020338270326
41926CB00007B/227